Hope: An International Human Becoming Perspective

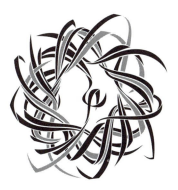

Rosemarie Rizzo Parse, RN, PhD, FAAN

NATIONAL LEAGUE FOR NURSING SERIES

Hope: An International Human Becoming Perspective

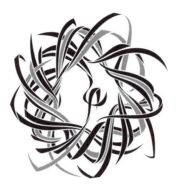

Rosemarie Rizzo Parse, RN, PhD, FAAN
Professor and Niehoff Chair
Marcella Niehoff School of Nursing
Loyola University Chicago
Editor, *Nursing Science Quarterly*
President, Discovery International, Inc.
Pittsburgh, Pennsylvania

JONES AND BARTLETT PUBLISHERS
Sudbury, Massachusetts
BOSTON   TORONTO   LONDON   SINGAPORE

World Headquarters
Jones and Bartlett Publishers
40 Tall Pine Drive
Sudbury, MA 01776
978-443-5000
info@jbpub.com
www.jbpub.com

Jones and Bartlett Publishers Canada
P.O. Box 19020
Toronto, ON M5S 1X1
CANADA

Jones and Bartlett Publishers International
Barb House, Barb Mews
London W6 7PA
UK

PRODUCTION CREDITS
ACQUISITIONS EDITOR   Greg Vis
PRODUCTION EDITOR   Linda S. DeBruyn
MANUFACTURING BUYER   Kristen Guevara
DESIGN   Argosy
EDITORIAL PRODUCTION SERVICE   Argosy
TYPESETTING   Argosy
COVER DESIGN   Stephanie Torta
PRINTING AND BINDING   Braun-Brumfield, Inc.

The Library of Congress has catalogued the hardcover edition of this title as follows:
Hope : an international human becoming perspective /
   Rosemarie Rizzo Parse.
      p.   cm.
   Includes bibliographical references and index.
   ISBN 0-7637-0958-1
      1. Nursing—Philosophy.   2. Hope.   3. Self-actualization
   (Psychology)   I. Parse, Rosemarie Rizzo.
RT84.5.H66   1999
610.73'01—DC21   98-43161
                                                          CIP

ISBN 0-7637-0976-X (pbk)

Printed in the United States of America
03 02 01 00 99   10 9 8 7 6 5 4 3 2 1

Hope is a waking dream.

—*Aristotle (384–322 B.C.)*

Hope is not prognostication . . . and is definitely not the same as optimism. It is not the conviction that something will turn out well, but the certainty that something makes sense, regardless of how it turns out.

—*Vaclav Havel. (1988).* Letters to Olga

Preface

There is growing interest among healthcare professionals in the lived experience of hope as a phenomenon significant to health and quality of life. While hope has been studied from a variety of perspectives and works have been published reflecting various natural science approaches to the phenomenon, little has been published from a human science perspective. This is evident in Chapter 2, where there is an extensive review of literature on hope.

The intent of this work is to report research findings from international qualitative human science studies on hope conducted in nine countries: Australia, Canada, Finland, Italy, Japan, Sweden, Taiwan, the United Kingdom, and the United States. All of these studies were guided by the human becoming theory and were conducted using the Parse research methodology. Each study involved different participant groups: For example, in Taiwan, the study participants were persons living in a leprosarium, in Canada the participants were family members of persons who live in chronic care settings, and in one U.S. study the participants were Native Americans. The findings from these qualitative research studies enhance the knowledge base on the phenomenon of hope, shed new light on its meaning, and expand understanding of human becoming. The findings are rich with information for healthcare professionals, since the participants themselves told stories about their meanings of hope. These stories are included to enhance understanding of hope and health, which is becoming increasingly more important for healthcare professionals as the next century dawns with the focus on technology and cost effectiveness. Phenomena for further research are included, as well as some challenges with conducting translinguistic research studies.

This work is written for undergraduate students, graduate students, and healthcare professionals in nursing and other disciplines who wish to enhance their understanding of the experience of hope as a humanly lived experience of health and quality of life.

Contributors

Steven L. Baumann, RN, PhD, CS, NP
Associate Professor of Nursing
Hunter College of The City University of
    New York
New York, New York

Debra A. Bournes, RN, MSc
Doctoral Student
Loyola University Chicago
Chicago, Illinois

Sandra Schmidt Bunkers, RN, PhD
Associate Professor and Chair of Nursing
Augustana College
Sioux Falls, South Dakota

William K. Cody, RN, PhD
Associate Professor and Chairperson
Family and Community Nursing
University of North Carolina at Charlotte
Charlotte, North Carolina

John Daly, RN, PhD
Associate Professor and Head
School of Nursing
Charles Sturt University, Riverina
Wagga Wagga, NSW, Australia

James E. Filler, RNC, MSN, ACRN
Lecturer
Family and Community Nursing
University of North Carolina at Charlotte
Charlotte, North Carolina

Lois S. Kelley, RN, DEd
Associate Professor of Nursing
School of Nursing and Health Sciences
College of Science and Technology,
    Texas A&M University–Corpus
    Christi
Corpus Christi, Texas
*(Work on this study was completed while the
researcher was Associate Professor at
Augustana College, Sioux Falls, South
Dakota, and was partially funded by an
ARAF research grant.)*

Brian Millar, RN, MN
Lecturer in Nursing Studies
School of Nursing
University of Wales College of Medicine
Cardiff, Wales, UK

Erja Muurinen, RN, MScN
Dean
Lahti Polytechnic
Faculty of Social and Health Care
Lahti, Finland

Rosemarie Rizzo Parse, RN, PhD, FAAN
Professor and Niehoff Chair
Marcella Niehoff School of Nursing
Loyola University Chicago
Chicago, Illinois
Editor, *Nursing Science Quarterly*
President, Discovery International, Inc.
Pittsburgh, Pennsylvania

Lynn Allchin-Petardi, RN, PhD
Assistant Clinical Professor
School of Nursing
University of Connecticut
Storrs, Connecticut

F. Beryl Pilkington, RN, PhD
Nurse Researcher, Sunnybrook Health
  Science Centre
Assistant Professor, Faculty of Nursing,
  University of Toronto
Toronto, Ontario, Canada

Teruko Takahashi, RN, PhD
Associate Professor
School of Nursing
The Jikei University Tokyo
Tokyo, Japan

Tuulikki Toikkanen, RN, MScN
Principal Lecturer
Lahti Polytechnic
Faculty of Social and Health Care
Lahti, Finland

Ching-eng Hsieh Wang, RN, PhD,
  CCRN
Assistant Professor
College of Nursing
Wayne State University
Detroit, Michigan

Ania M. L. Willman, RN, PhD
Senior Lecturer
Department of Nursing
Malmö University
Malmö, Sweden

Renzo Zanotti, RN, AFD, PhD
Professor of Nursing, Padova University,
  Padova, Italy
Assistant Professor, Case Western
  Reserve University, Cleveland, Ohio
Director of ISIRI, International
  Institute of Nursing Research, Italy
Director of ACIENDO, European
  Association for Nursing Diagnoses,
  Interventions and Outcomes,
  London, UK

Contents

Chapter 1

Hope: A Lived Experience of Human Becoming

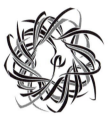

ROSEMARIE RIZZO PARSE

"Hope" is the thing with feathers –
That perches in the soul –
And sings the tune without the words –
And never stops – at all –

And sweetest – in the Gale – is heard –
And sore must be the storm –
That could abash the little Bird
That kept so many warm –

I've heard it in the chillest land –
And on the strangest Sea –
Yet, never, in Extremity,
It asked a crumb – of Me.

Emily Dickinson (c.1891/1960)

Hope–no-hope is a paradoxical lived experience of health and quality of life. It is a humanly lived phenomenon inherent in becoming. According to the stories of the research participants reported in this book, hope is what gets people through their days and nights. It is a rainbow, an inspiration, a oneness, a spark, a moving beyond the moment—it is always present, but it is more noticeable during difficult times. The purposes of this chapter are to describe the ontology of the human becoming school of thought, explain hope from this perspective, and describe the research methodology used in the 13 studies reported in this book.

HUMAN BECOMING

Human becoming is a school of thought encompassing nontraditional beliefs about the human-universe-health process. A school of thought is a theoretical perspective held by a community of scholars (Parse, 1997b). Each school of thought is a knowledge tradition that includes the ontology, epistemology, and congruent methodologies. The ontology includes assumptions and principles. The epistemology is the specification of the knowledge sought in sciencing. The methodologies are approaches to research and practice.

Assumptions of Human Becoming

(Parse, 1998, pp. 19–20)

1. The human is coexisting while coconstituting rhythmical patterns with the universe.
2. The human is an open being, freely choosing meaning in situation, bearing responsibility for decisions.
3. The human is unitary, continuously coconstituting patterns of relating.
4. The human is transcending multidimensionally with the possibles.
5. Becoming is unitary human-living-health.

6. Becoming is a rhythmically coconstituting human-universe process.
7. Becoming is the human's pattern of relating value priorities.
8. Becoming is an intersubjective process of transcending with the possibles.
9. Becoming is unitary human's emerging.

Assumptions About Human Becoming

(Parse, 1998, p. 29)

1. Human becoming is freely choosing personal meaning in situation in the intersubjective process of living value priorities.
2. Human becoming is cocreating rhythmical patterns of relating in mutual process with the universe.
3. Human becoming is cotranscending multidimensionally with the emerging possibles.

Principles of Human Becoming

(Parse, 1981, p. 41)

1. Structuring meaning multidimensionally is cocreating reality through the languaging of valuing and imaging.
2. Cocreating rhythmical patterns of relating is living the paradoxical unity of revealing-concealing and enabling-limiting while connecting-separating.
3. Cotranscending with the possibles is powering unique ways of originating in the process of transforming.

A careful reading of the ontology of human becoming shows the belief that humans are unitary beings who cannot be known by a study of the parts. The notion of *unitary* refers to a wholeness that is recognized through pattern. Unitary is not a combination of entities or pieces that make up a whole. There is always more to the unitary human than can be explicitly known.

The unitary human is free to choose in situation and bears responsibility for all choices, even though emerging outcomes are not fully known when choices are made. The human in a mutual rhythmical ever-changing process with the universe cocreates situations. The rhythmical ever-changing process is lived in the day-to-day paradoxes of human experience. The paradoxes are not opposites, but they are dimensions of the same rhythm lived multidimensionally all-at-once. For example, with hope–no-hope, the hope is only clearly known in light of the ever-present possibility of no-hope, and no-hope only has meaning in light of hope (Parse, 1990).

The term *multidimensional* refers to the explicit-tacit knowings of the was, is, and will-be that humans live all-at-once with the predecessors, contemporaries, and successors at many realms of the universe. To say that the human-universe process is mutual and multidimensional means it is a nonlinear all-at-onceness. The human with the universe cocreates reality, giving rise to emerging seamless meanings that come into being through *imaging*, *valuing*, and *languaging*. The human lives speaking–being-silent and moving–being-still in confirming the cherished beliefs of explicit-tacit knowings. The cocreation of reality is living the meanings of situations through the paradoxical rhythms of *revealing-concealing, enabling-limiting,* and *connecting-separating.* Humans reveal and conceal all-at-once the who that they are becoming. Humans, as emerging mysteries, cannot disclose all there is to know about themselves to themselves or others. They make decisions, all of which are enabling-limiting. There are opportunities and restrictions in all choices as humans connect and separate rhythmically while pushing-resisting in *powering* being with non-being. Humans push-resist in the mutual human-universe process as they live with the known of the now and the unknown potentials of the yet-to-be. Humans create anew in *originating* what is not-yet while conforming–not-conforming in the certainty-uncertainty of day-to-day living as new insights arise in *transforming* the unfamiliar with the familiar in cocreating the seamless symphony of becoming.

Health is the ever-changing process of becoming. It is the human emerging with what is not-yet. Health and quality of life can be described only by the individual, since these are a unique and personal incarnation of that which the individual is becoming. Hope is inextricably woven with health and quality of life as a "thing with feathers . . . the tune without the words . . . and [it] never stops – at all" (Dickinson, c.1891/1960).

HOPE

From the human becoming perspective, hope is a dimension of the paradoxical rhythm, hope–no-hope. It is a chosen way of living in the moment that is the structured meaning of a situation. Hope is anticipating the possibles in imagining the knowings of what might be, as cherished beliefs arise with speaking–being-silent and moving–being-still. It emerges with the connecting-separating of enabling-limiting human-universe engagements. As the human engages with others, ideas, objects, and situations, hope–no-hope is an ever-present rhythm surfacing as expectations of possible achievements. The human reveals and all-at-once conceals personal meanings incarnating hope in choosing the opportunities and restrictions of becoming.

Hope, as a universal lived experience of health, is a way of propelling with envisioned possibilities in everyday living. It springs forth in cocreation with the universe as the desires, wishes, aspirations, and expectations that move humans beyond the moment. When hope is in the foreground of the hope–no-hope paradox, there are always glimpses present of the hopeless, the impossible, and the despondent. The human is powering the being of what is now with the non-being, the unknowns of the not-yet. The hope–no-hope paradoxical rhythm is a lived phenomenon that can be described by people in true presence with a researcher and with a nurse in practice. Epistemologically, it is the lived experience that is the knowledge sought. The methodologies of the human becoming school of thought specify ways to research hope–no-hope and ways to be guided by an understanding of this phenomenon in practice.

THE HUMAN BECOMING METHODOLOGIES

The human becoming school of thought encompasses research and practice methodologies that flow directly from the ontology. The practice methodology will not be discussed here, but can be found in detail in *The Human Becoming School of Thought* (Parse, 1998). There are three research methodologies arising from the ontology of human becoming. The Parse method (Parse, 1987) and the human becoming hermeneutic method (Cody, 1995) are both basic research methods, and the descriptive qualitative preproject-process-postproject method is an applied science method (Parse, 1998). The Parse research method will be described here in detail, since it was the method used by the principal investigator and coinvestigators in the international translinguistic study that created the major content for this book. Details of the other methods are specified in *The Human Becoming School of Thought* (Parse, 1998).

PARSE RESEARCH METHOD

The assumptions (Parse, 1992, p. 41) underlying the method follow:

1. Humans are open beings in mutual process with the universe. The construct *human becoming* refers to the human-universe-health process.
2. Human becoming is uniquely lived by individuals. People make reflective and prereflective choices in connection with others and the universe that incarnate their health.
3. Descriptions of lived experiences enhance knowledge of human becoming. Individuals and families can describe their own experiences in ways that shed light on the meaning of health.
4. Researcher-participant dialogical engagement uncovers the meaning of phenomena as humanly lived. The researcher in true presence with the participant can elicit authentic information about lived experiences.
5. The researcher, through inventing, abiding with logic, and adhering to semantic consistency during the extraction-synthesis and heuristic interpretation processes, creates structures of lived experiences and weaves the structure with the theory in ways that enhance the knowledge base of nursing.

Phenomena and Structure

Phenomena for study in this method are universal human health experiences surfacing in the human-universe process reflecting being-becoming, value priorities, and quality of life. Examples of phenomena for inquiry include joy-sorrow, hope, laughing, courage, grieving, and feeling peaceful (Parse, 1994, 1995, 1996, 1997a).

The *structure* of the phenomenon emerging through this method is the paradoxical living of the remembered, the now-moment, and the not-yet, all-at-once.

Research Question

The research question for all of the studies reported in this book was "What is the structure of the lived experience of hope?"

Processes of the Method

Participant Selection. Participants are selected carefully and according to the interest of the researcher. The phenomena for study with this method must be universal lived experiences, and the participants are persons who are willing to describe through words, movements, symbols, metaphors, poetry, drawings, music, or any other medium the meaning of the experience under study. Based on the ontology, it is assumed that persons who volunteer to participate give an accurate account of the meaning of the experience. An adequate sample for this method is two to ten participants. For this nine-country study on hope with seventeen investigators, participants were selected based on the interest of the investigator in each study. The participants included ten persons from each site on four different continents. The Australian participants were persons with heart disease, and the Canadians were family members of persons confined to a chronic care facility. The Finnish, the Italian, and the Japanese participants were from the general public. The Swedish participants were persons confined to an acute care facility, and those from Taiwan were from a leprosarium. Participants from the United Kingdom were persons who had some injury or terminal illness or were family members of those with injuries or a terminal illness. In the United States, one study had participants from a shelter in North Carolina, and another had participants from transitional housing in New York City. One study from South Dakota had participants from an Indian reservation, and another from South Dakota had participants who worked with homeless persons. In another study, the participants, from various parts of the United States, were women with children.

Participants were recruited in various ways, usually by public bulletin or personal contacts within the community of the coinvestigators. Each coinvestigator or research assistant informed participants about the purpose of the study, their right to withdraw, and the method of protecting anonymity and confidentiality. All participants gave either oral or written consent to be in audio-recorded dialogue with the researcher or research assistant. A university review board for the protection of human subjects approved the study in general. In addition, each coinvestigator received permission from the sites they chose. The rights of all participants were protected, and audio recordings and transcriptions were destroyed at the completion of each of the studies.

Dialogical Engagement. Dialogical engagement is a discussion between the researcher and the participant. The dialogue is not an interview, but rather a true presence during which the researcher is fully attentive as the participant unfolds the meaning of the phenomenon under study. Each dialogue in this study began when the researcher or research assistant said to the participant,

"Tell me about your experience of hope." The researcher only interjected with comments like "go on" or "can you say more about that and hope." The dialogue took place in various settings such as homes, healthcare facilities, and health centers, depending on the desires of the participants. Before entering a dialogue, each researcher or assistant centered and prepared to be truly present with the participant. The dialogues were transcribed from the various languages into English by the coinvestigator. The coinvestigator consulted with at least one other person familiar with English to make sure the translations were clear and accurate.

Extraction-Synthesis. Extraction-synthesis is culling the essences from the dialogue in the language of the participant and conceptualizing these essences in the language of science to form the structure of the experience (Parse, 1995, p. 153). The researcher dwells in quiet contemplation with the transcribed, audiotaped, and videotaped descriptions. The immersion with the descriptions involves five processes. The coinvestigator for each hope study, with assistance from the principal investigator, wrote the participants' stories, extracted-synthesized the essences from the entire dialogue, and wrote the essences in the language of the participant. These essences were synthesized and extracted at a more abstract level of discourse in the researcher's language. A proposition was formulated from the essences for each participant. Core concepts were extracted-synthesized through dwelling with propositions from all of the participants in each study. A structure of the lived experience was synthesized from the extracted core concepts. The structure answered the research question for each study. The structures were somewhat different for each of the thirteen studies, as can be seen in their reports in subsequent chapters in this book.

Heuristic Interpretation. Heuristic interpretation is the process of incrementally moving the structure across levels of discourse to the level of nursing science. Structural transposition is an expression of the structure at a higher level of abstraction, and conceptual integration specifies this structure with the principles of human becoming and beyond to forge new ideas for further research and practice. The principal investigator worked with each coinvestigator in arriving at the heuristic interpretations as written in this work. Subsequent chapters specify the findings from the thirteen studies, and a final chapter illuminates the meaning of hope from a human becoming perspective arising from the 130 participants in this transcultural, translinguistic study on the lived experience of hope.

SUMMARY

The Parse method processes were implemented by the principal and coinvestigators from the nine countries represented here with thirteen studies in which the lived experience of hope was investigated. Coinvestigators engaged in dialogue in the native language of the ten participants of their choice. The transcripts of the tape recordings were then translated into English. The essences were extracted-synthesized in English, and the structure was discovered and moved to the level of theory through heuristic interpretation. The principal investigator worked closely with the coinvestigators throughout the project. The stories of the participants, along with the essences, structures, and heuristic interpretations, are presented in the remaining chapters of this book.

REFERENCES

Cody, W. K. (1995). Of life immense in passion, pulse, and power: Dialoguing with Whitman and Parse, A hermeneutic study. In R. R. Parse (Ed.), *Illuminations: The human becoming theory in practice and research.* New York: National League for Nursing Press.

Dickinson, E. (1960). No. 254. In T. H. Johnson (Ed.), *The complete poems of Emily Dickinson* (p. 116). Boston: Little, Brown and Co. (Original work published c.1891)

Parse, R. R. (1981). *Man-living-health: A theory of nursing.* New York: Wiley.

Parse, R. R. (1987). *Nursing science: Major paradigms, theories, and critiques.* Philadelphia: Saunders.

Parse, R. R. (1990). Parse's research methodology with an illustration of the lived experience of hope. *Nursing Science Quarterly, 3,* 9–17.

Parse, R. R. (1992). Human becoming: Parse's theory of nursing. *Nursing Science Quarterly, 5,* 35–42.

Parse, R. R. (1994). Quality of life: Sciencing and living the art of human becoming. *Nursing Science Quarterly, 7,* 16–21.

Parse, R. R. (Ed.). (1995). *Illuminations: The human becoming theory in practice and research.* New York: National League for Nursing Press.

Parse, R. R. (1996). Building knowledge through qualitative research: The road less traveled. *Nursing Science Quarterly, 9,* 10–16.

Parse, R. R. (1997a). The human becoming theory: The was, is, and will be. *Nursing Science Quarterly, 10,* 32–38.

Parse, R, R. (1997b). The language of nursing knowledge: Saying what we mean. In I. M. King & J. Fawcett (Eds.), *The language of nursing theory and metatheory* (pp. 73–77). Indianapolis, IN: Sigma Theta Tau International.

Parse, R. R. (1998). *The human becoming school of thought.* Thousand Oaks, CA: Sage.

Chapter 2

The Many Facets of Hope

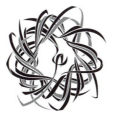

F. BERYL PILKINGTON

Who against hope believed in hope.

> Romans *4:18 (King James Version)*

To hope till Hope creates
From its own wreck the thing it contemplates.

> *Shelley*, Prometheus Unbound. *Act iv, 1. 573*

The subject of hope has been widely discussed in the popular literature and in the literature of philosophy, theology, psychology, the social sciences, and nursing. There are many facets of hope from different theoretical perspectives, and the diverse research approaches and findings show that there are many meanings of this phenomenon.

POPULAR LITERATURE

The importance of hope as a topic of public discourse was evidenced by the devotion of the entire December 1974 issue of *Saturday Review/World* to "An Inventory of Hope." Although this special issue was published two decades ago, the broad themes it addressed are still current. Editor Norman Cousins (1974) stated that the purpose of this issue was to examine and, if possible, to dissipate the apparent gloom of the American people. He wrote:

> In the present mood, it is not likely that any serious problems will be imaginatively approached, much less solved. The main trouble with despair is that it is self-fulfilling. People who fear the worst tend to invite it. Heads that are down can't scan the horizon for new openings. Bursts of energy do not spring from a spirit of defeat. Ultimately, hopelessness leads to helplessness. (p. 4)

Cousins believed that hope could be renewed through the restoration of people's confidence in themselves, their government, and the future. According to him, hope does not depend on facts or logic, nor can it simply be ordered into being, although it can be encouraged. Rather, hope originates in feelings, and its power is "generated by the longing for something better . . . which gives human beings a sense of destination and the energy to get started" (p. 5). Cousins suggested that the possibility of regenerating hope would only become impossible

> . . . when human beings are no longer capable of calling out to one another, when the words in their poetry break up before their eyes, when their faces become frozen toward their young, and when they fail to make pictures out of clouds racing across the sky. (p. 5)

Cousins's call for hope for the future of humankind laid the groundwork for a number of guardedly optimistic articles by important world leaders and visionaries of the day. For instance, former United Nations Secretary-General Maurice Strong (1974) asserted, "I believe that there is a case for hope, that doomsday is not inevitable" (p. 7). He based the case for hope on several conditions:

> [It] must begin with a realistic acknowledgment of the fact that we do indeed face risks to our survival and, perhaps more importantly, to the survival of the qualities and values which endow human life with its higher purposes and meaning. Doomsday is possible—even probable—if we continue on our present course. . . . [Nevertheless] it is possible to opt for a future of unparalleled promise and opportunity for the human species. But this future can come about only if we make a radical change in our present course. (p. 7)

René Dubois (1974), Pulitzer Prize–winning author and microbiologist, based his hope for the future on the capacity of the human species to choose to manifest its humanity, rather than its bestiality. Citing the teachings of an ancient Persian prophet who entreated that the good in human nature should prevail, Dubois observed:

> Instead of being slaves to their genes and hormones, as animals are, human beings have the kind of freedom which comes from possessing free will and moral judgment. . . . Human beings can choose not only between good and evil but also between other traits in their nature. (p. 77)

Dubois asserts that humans are different from animals in their capacity for a unique form of happiness that originates in the "deep awareness that their personal life is the realization of their dreams and their collective life a creative enterprise which gives concrete forms to the dreams of humankind" (p. 80). Convinced that humankind could overcome determinism, his hope was for humanity "to participate in the continuous process of self-creation" (p. 80).

In the same issue of *Saturday Review/World*, Yehudi Menuhin (1974), the world-famous violinist, expounded on art as hope for humanity. For Menuhin, great works of art are both gifts from heaven and high points in the living process; the aesthetics of art provide "the assurances of continuity, of direction, and of design or logic in everyday life" (p. 82). In Menuhin's opinion, politicians are driven by aggressive and dominating instincts, whereas the artist, as "the individual in the unique cultural environment, creates" (p. 83). He believed that if artists held sway over politicians, there could be hope for the future:

> I do not doubt for a moment that humankind will find creative alternatives to rigidity, and I do not doubt that art will play a functional, pragmatic role in our salvation. This is, at any rate, my faith. (p. 83)

In another magazine, *Modern Maturity*, E. Boyd (1994) discussed the importance of hope for surviving. According to Boyd, a survivor clings to a sense of hope, which enables one to remain open to positive alternatives, fresh options, and new prospects for the future. In contrast, negativity, despondency, bitterness, fear of tomorrow, and loss of confidence indicate a person who is having difficulty surviving.

PHILOSOPHY AND THEOLOGY

Hope has been a topic of inquiry for a number of philosophers and theologians, according to whom hope is essential to life (Fromm, 1968; Lynch, 1965; Marcel, 1951; Schrag, 1977; Wu, 1972). For example, Lynch (1965) asserted that "hope comes close to being the very heart and center of a human being" (p. 31). Schrag (1977) described hope as "a concrete, lived-through experience" (p. 270) that is both simple and complex:

> On the one hand, hope is a simple phenomenon, experienced as a unitary and undivided global content, but, on the other hand, this global content only shows itself through a diversity of profiles and perspectives. (p. 270)

Schrag identified three typological regions of hope: praxis, soteriology, and semantics. His region of praxis concerned social formation and transformation, whereby "interacting social selves transform the present in response to an envisioned condition of life in the future" (p. 271). Soteriology referred to the ethico-religious dimension of hope, for example, as discussed by Kierkegaard (1849/1980), Moltmann (1967), and others; and semantics involved deciphering the meaning of hope from the symbolic significations that are prevalent in the discourse on hope. Based on his analysis of the phenomenon of hope, Schrag (1977) identified its ontological elements as "space and time, destiny and freedom, and origin and end" (p. 278).

In correspondence with Schrag's (1977) typological region of praxis, some philosophers have addressed the subject of hope with respect to social formation and transformation. For example, Bloch (1959/1986), a Marxist Jew, has written a three-volume treatise on hope as the fundamental principle of a socialist utopia. Bloch's work focused on hope as a social, rather than individual, objective; thus, he was critical of the hope of religion, which he viewed as being "confined to mere inwardness or to empty promises of the other world" (p. 5). Central to Bloch's (1959/1986) philosophy of hope was the idea of the "Not-Yet-Conscious," which involved the psychological processes of approaching the "Not-Yet-Become." Bloch considered hope to be both subjective and objective: Subjectively, it is an expectant emotion that anticipates the not-yet future, and objectively, it is a cognitive act that requires people to "throw themselves actively into what is becoming, to which they themselves belong" (p. 3).

Fromm (1968), too, considered hope as an essential condition for societal, as well as personal, transformation. His classic work, *The Revolution of Hope*, situated society in the 1960s at a crossroads, one road leading to complete mechanization, and the other to a reawakening of humanism and hope. For Fromm, hope is a movement toward transcendence that is paradoxical in its at-once active-passive nature: "It is neither passive waiting nor is it unrealistic forcing of circumstances that cannot occur" (p. 9); rather, it is a state of being ever ready, consciously and unconsciously, for that which is not yet, character-ized by "an inner readiness, that of intense but not-yet-spent activeness" (p. 12). Fromm connected hope with faith, that is, the knowledge of real pos-sibility, and also with fortitude and fearlessness.

Marcel (1951), in *Homo Viator*, encompasses Schrag's (1977) regions of praxis, soteriology, and semantics in exploring the phenomenology and meta-physics of hope from a Judeo-Christian perspective. Marcel views hope as a mystery that is spiritual in nature and that arises in response to personal trials, which he considers a form of captivity. For Marcel (1951), hope is paradoxical in that it arises in seemingly hopeless situations: "The less life is experienced as a captivity, the less the soul will be able to see the shining of that veiled, myste-rious light, which . . . illumines the very centre of hope's dwelling place" (p. 32). To hope is to recognize the limitations in situations, while believing that opportunities also exist; therefore, hope and despair cannot coexist, since "hope is the act by which this temptation is victoriously overcome" (Marcel, 1951, p. 36). Marcel distinguished hope from despair, optimism, and expect-ing. In contrast to the solitariness of despair, hope entails communion and rec-iprocity; unlike optimism, it is rooted in faith and belief, and unlike expecting, it is characterized by humility and patience.

The intersubjectivity of human relationships is fundamental to Marcel's philosophy of hope (Godfrey, 1987). Given the intersubjective nature of hope and the "indissoluble connection which binds together hope and love" (Mar-cel, 1951, p. 66), Marcel finds it absurd to question hope's objectivity; he believes that if one hopes, then one's hope is real. His phenomenological anal-ysis of hope led to the following definition:

> Hope is essentially the availability of a soul which has entered inti-mately enough into the experience of communion to accomplish in the teeth of will and knowledge the transcendent act—the act estab-lishing the vital regeneration of which this experience affords both the pledge and the first-fruits. (Marcel, 1951, p. 67)

This definition highlights the intersubjective, transcendent, and paradoxical nature of hope, whereby one avails oneself to seize upon a promise that seems presently beyond reach.

Casey (1988), a philosopher of religion, drew upon Marcel's writings while examining the role of hope in a community's experience of evil and suffering. Like Marcel, he approaches the mystery of hope and suffering as an individual who is part of a community. Casey assumes that hope arises out of the same con-ditions that give rise to despair, arguing that hope is founded upon the soul's risk-taking premise that good will triumph over evil in the end. He believes that hope can become a formative influence in ethical moral actions; however, in order to flourish in a community, it must be founded in a symbol system derived from the sufferers' common experience. Casey postulates that the celebration of the Sabbath is a symbolic system that enables a community's experience of suffering to be transformed into hope and solidarity.

Kant's (1781/1952) classic treatise, *The Critique of Pure Reason*, deals with hope as a moral concern, rather than as an intersubjective lived experience. Pondering the ground for hope and its relation to happiness and ultimate good, Kant concludes that:

> . . . [E]very one has ground to hope for happiness in the measure in which he has made himself worthy of it in his conduct, and that therefore the system of morality is inseparably (though only in the idea of pure reason) connected with that of happiness. (p. 237)

Therefore, for Kant, hope for happiness follows logically from worthy conduct, in accordance with moral law.

Godfrey (1987) arrived at a philosophy of hope through a detailed analysis of the works of Bloch, Kant, and Marcel, which he divided into two different ontologies: the will-nature model, represented by Bloch and Kant, and the intersubjective model, represented by Marcel. Godfrey identified two kinds of hope, ultimate hope and fundamental hope, which he viewed as having different conative, cognitional, and affective implications. According to him, ultimate hope is "superordinate to all other hopes" and involves movement toward "what is believed desirable and believed possible although difficult to obtain" (p. 55). Fundamental hope, unlike ultimate hope, is not aimed at an objective, yet has an orientation toward the future that is characterized by "an openness of spirit" (p. 64). Unlike Marcel, Godfrey believed that hope could be sound or unsound, justified or unjustified.

The propensity of the hoping person to seek meaning in adversity has often been linked with imagination (Kierkegaard, 1849/1980; Lynch, 1965; Oliver, 1974; Wu, 1972). For instance, Kierkegaard (1849/1980) saw imagination as the wellspring of hope and transcendence. He wrote:

> In order for a person to become aware of self and of God, imagination must raise one higher than the miasma of probability, it must tear one out of this and teach her/him to hope and to fear—or to fear and to hope—by rendering possible that which surpasses a sufficient amount of any experience. (p. 41)

According to Oliver (1974), "The ideas of hope capture the highest aspirations of the human spirit" (p. 86). Likewise, Wu (1972) posits hope as the basis for "imagineering," a combination of "futuristic imagination and realistic engineering" (p. 144) that could be the key to cosmic survival. He suggests that hope arises out of life's discontentment and suffering, within horizons that present meanings and possibilities. Hope, then, is a creative pull between the now and the future, which persistently believes in the possibility of a thing becoming other than what it is. Wu suggests that hope, like the relativity of modern science and unlike the deterministic science of the past, opens up the probabilities of the future. Furthermore, hope is not only "an undying possibility," but also "our big responsibility which affects the total cosmic future" (Wu, 1972, p. 146). Therefore, Wu urges us to hope that a way can be found to bring humankind into harmony with nature.

In his classic work on hope, Lynch (1965) postulates that it is creative imagination that gives hope the ability to transcend the present situation by moving into the future; thus, while hopelessness remains trapped by difficulty, hope transcends it. Lynch considers reality to be hope's great object; hence, the healing of mental illness necessarily entails realistic imagination. He provides a working definition of hope as "the fundamental knowledge and feeling that there is a way out of difficulty, that things can work out" (p. 32). The act of wishing is central in Lynch's psychology of hope. Unlike the existentialists, he believes that humans are basically afraid, not of being free, but of not being free, and that this prevents one from wishing. He postulates that, ultimately, the inability to wish will result in hopelessness and mental illness. Lynch identifies the following qualities of wishing that connect it with hoping: mutuality, waiting, imagining, and the taking of help. Mutuality is important, because it "creates freedom and unconditionality in human wishing" (p. 159); simply put, if persons depend on one another, they can hope in the other. The waiting that accompanies hope is "positive and creative. It waits because it knows what it wishes and wants" (p. 177). Lynch also considers hope and help as inseparable; as he puts it, "Hope is an interior sense that there is help on the outside of us" (p. 40). The other quality of wishing that connects it with hoping is imagining. According to Lynch, "the ideal and healthy form of wishing" (p. 143) is the absolute wish, which is always imaginative; in contrast, the willful act is without imagination, being based merely in fantasy that mocks and negates reality.

Hope is an important theme in the Judeo-Christian tradition, in which God is believed to be a god of hope (Jer. 17:17; Ps. 42:5; Lam. 3:26; Rom. 15:13). In this tradition, hope and faith are considered to be essential to the ultimate hope of becoming a unique self in relationship to God (Metz, 1992). Faith and hope are intertwined, in that faith gives one the power to hope (Kierkegaard, 1849/1980; Marcel, 1951; Metz, 1966; Moltmann, 1967; Steindl-Rast, 1984; Tillich, 1980; van Kaam, 1976). In the New Testament (I Cor. 13:13), hope, faith, and love are presented as three abiding spiritual gifts. According to Steindl-Rast (1984), a Benedictine monk, faith opens the way for hope to flourish by overcoming fear. He describes hope as an expectant desire, an openness for surprise, and a passion for the possibles. Thus, hope is a creative tension between the not-yet and the already that opens the way for discovery in the human quest for meaning (Steindl-Rast, 1984).

According to Oliver (1974), in the Judeo-Christian perspective, hope is "a way of being in the world by which the meaning of life is affirmed in the face of the apparent meaninglessness of death" (p. 85). It is hope that provides continuity between past and future, thereby giving power to find meaning in the worst adversity (Oliver, 1974). Viewed theologically, hope proceeds from a consciousness of sin and guilt and resides in a new life of freedom *from* "the despair of alienation," and *for* a new life ahead (Schrag, 1977, p. 275). Christian theology specifically centers hope in God's promises as incarnated in Jesus Christ and his resurrection (Metz, 1966; Moltmann, 1967; Oliver, 1974). Moltmann (1967) sees Christian hope as being forward-looking and moving, and thus revolutionizing and transforming. In accord, Metz (1966) argues for a "humanism of creative hope" (p. 283) that entails a responsibility to change the world in the direction promised by Jesus Christ.

PSYCHOLOGY AND THE SOCIAL SCIENCES

Theoretical Perspectives

Jacoby (1993) has divided the psychological literature on hope into two general perspectives: dynamic and cognitive-behavioral. According to Jacoby, dynamic theories, including Erickson's (1964a, 1964b) and Menninger's (1959), focus on the role of hope in psychotherapy and tend toward subjective impressions, whereas cognitive-behavioral theories, including those of Stotland (1969), Gottschalk (1974), and Averill (1991), focus more objectively on hope in terms of expectation. In an attempt to incorporate both of these approaches, Jacoby (1993) has characterized hope as a process involving emotional and cognitive responses to overcome threat, which "enables growth, maturation, and creativity in life's developmental and coping processes" (p. 67).

Developmental and psychodynamic theories have widely influenced the psychology literature on hope. These theories situate hope's origins in early development (Erickson, 1964a, 1964b; Gottschalk, 1974; van Kaam, 1976) and view hope as a fundamental human behavior that activates, shapes, and sustains psychological development (Aardema, 1984). Erickson's (1964a, 1964b) theory of psychosocial growth and development posits hope as one of several basic ego qualities, or virtues, each of which has its time of origin and crisis, and yet persists throughout life. For Erickson (1964b), hope is the earliest and most stable of the basic ego qualities and, indeed, is "the most indispensable virtue inherent in the state of being alive" (p. 115). According to Erickson (1964a), hope is the positive outcome of the early stage of trust versus mistrust, and arises out of the mutuality of infant and caretakers. It is "the enduring belief in the attainability of fervent wishes, in spite of the dark urges and rages which mark the beginning of existence" (Erickson, 1964b, p. 118). Erickson suggests that hope acquires new qualities at different stages of development; for instance, in its mature form, the infant's hope becomes faith.

Van Kaam (1976) considers the early mother-child relationship to be "of essential significance for the wholesome unfolding of one's personal as well as one's spiritual life" (p. 85). Like Lynch (1965) and Erickson (1964a, 1964b), van Kaam believes that hope can flourish only in a relationship of mutuality. He considers faith, hope, and love to be an inseparable triad of God-given potentialities that are inherent in human nature, and that enhance and deepen each other; this triad enables us to abandon ourselves in a transcendent act of self-surrender (van Kaam, 1976).

The cognitive-behavioral perspective of hope is epitomized by Stotland's (1969) classic work. This author defines hope as "an expectation greater than zero of achieving a goal. The degree of hopefulness is the level of this expectation or the person's perceived probability of achieving a goal" (p. 2). Essentially a theory of behavior motivation, Stotland's theory of hope originated in cognitive theories from social psychology (Snyder, 1995). The theory stipulated seven propositions and six directional hypotheses regarding the relationships between the determinants and indicators of motivation. According to Stotland, the determinants of motivation are (a) the importance of the goal and (b) the expectation of achieving it; the indicators are (a) overt and covert action toward the goal and (b) selective attention to instrumental aspects of the environment. Stotland's (1969) theory suggests that hope produces behavior aimed at attaining goals: "With hope, man acts, moves, achieves. Without hope, he is often dull, listless, moribund" (p. 1). In an elaboration on Stotland's theory, Snyder et al. (1991) define hope as "a cognitive set that is based on a reciprocally derived sense of successful (a) agency (goal-directed determination) and (b) pathways (planning of ways to meet goals)" (p. 571). Staats (1987) has shifted the cognitive emphasis to focus on the affective aspect of hope, which she has defined as "the expectation of desirable future events" (p. 357). According to Staats (1991), hope is "intrinsically a positive, affective cognition in the subjective present" (p. 22), which increases one's intentions to act.

In sharp contrast to the cognitive-behaviorist perspective, Frankl (1946/1962) considers hope as fundamentally a process of choosing personal meaning in life. An existentialist psychiatrist, Frankl was imprisoned at the Auschwitz concentration camp during World War II, an experience that led him to rewrite the manuscript of his life's work. An underlying theme of that experience was not giving up hope, which he called the *meaning to live*. Frankl believes that the human's primary motivator in life is the search for meaning. He theorized that many of the Auschwitz prisoners who died from sickness or suicide did so because they had given up hope. According to Frankl, one arrives at meaning in life by rising above seemingly hopeless situations through *the will to meaning*. Based in this premise, his psychoanalytic approach, called *logotherapy*, sought to find concrete meaning in personal existence.

Many authors share Frankl's belief that hope is essential for survival. For instance, several physicians (Cousins, 1979, 1983; Keith, 1991; Tate, 1992) and psychologists (Jevne, 1992, 1994; Linge, 1990) have written personal accounts of the importance of hope to surviving a life-threatening illness or injury. Linge (1990), for example, credited his recovery from a serious head injury to the hope, faith, and love that were nurtured through family relationships. Jevne (1994), a psychologist whose practice focuses on the seriously ill, has recounted the development of hope in her own life. It is her belief that "hope has a unique meaning for each of us. It can't be prescribed. It can't be injected. . . . It's hard to define. It's easier to tell a story about it" (p. 8). Jevne's story of hope centered on her relationships with others and a longing to belong. Echoing certain philosphers (Fromm, 1968; Marcel, 1951; Steindl-Rast, 1984; Wu, 1972), she wrote about hope as a process issuing out of the creative tension between what is and what is believed possible:

> As we move between the dichotomies of life, we feel the pulse of life, the pull homeward. We feel the tension between giving up and going on. A pulsing logic develops between a sense of being apart and being connected. Hope happens in the space between. Between the secular and the sacred. Between trust and skepticism. Between the concrete and the intangible. Between evidence and intuition. Between religion and spirituality. Between doubt and faith. (Jevne, 1994, pp. 134–135)

Jevne (1992) includes hope in a family of concepts, such as coping, courage, faith, resilience, and empowerment, which she considers essential to living with chronic illness. Gottschalk (1985) and Cousins (1979, 1983, 1989) have suggested that hope is one of a group of positive emotions that lessen an organism's susceptibility to serious illness and potentiate healing, through their effects on physiological homeostasis and immune competence. Klenow (1991–1992) developed a typology of hope sources in life-threatening illnesses, which he categorized according to cognitive and behavioral dimensions. For example, according to this typology, the religion-cognitive category of hope sources encompassed prayer, belief, and faith, while the religion-behavioral category included seeking faith healers. The identified sources of hope included religion, medical science, fallibilism, self-discipline and renewal, and deception by others (false hope). Klenow advocated the use of this typology to advance theory about hope in life-threatening illness.

A number of authors consider hope to be an essential element of therapeutic relationships (Aldridge, 1995; Hoffman, 1991; Linge, 1990; Mehler & Argentieri, 1989; Ruvelson, 1990). For instance, music therapy has been suggested as a way to promote hope and spirituality in persons and caregivers in palliative care, thus enhancing their quality of life (Aldridge, 1995). In the belief that faith and hope are psychodynamically related, Carni (1988) has advocated that psychotherapy for cancer patients should aim to restore their faith in life. According to Buechler (1995), the emotional aspect of hope is a motivating force in psychoanalytic treatment. Many writers consider the restoration of hope to be an important goal of psychotherapy, requiring skillful intervention in the psychodynamic processes of hope and hopelessness (Aardema, 1984; Carni, 1988; Hanna, 1991; Mehler & Argentieri, 1989; Ruvelson, 1990). For example, Aardema (1984) developed a model for assessing, generating, and therapeutically using hope to effect client change, based on Erickson's developmental theory. In an inquiry into the development of hope in psychotherapy, Vaughn (1991) analyzed the role of empathy and self-object transference based on Marcel's phenomenology of hope. According to Vaughn, intersubjectivity is the common ground of hope in psychoanalytic and theological perspectives; on these grounds, hope depends on one's loving and being loved in an open community of face-to-face relationships.

Research

Psychology and social science research on hope has generally focused on its objective specification and its relationship to various other psychosocial variables. As Jevne (1992) has observed, psychology and the helping professions lack a common definition and appropriate research methodologies for studying hope; consequently, it is difficult to make comparisons across studies. The predominant conceptualization of hope, originating with Stotland's (1969) hope theory, is one of a positive motivational state and cognitive set that is based upon positive affect (Elliot, Witty, Herrick & Hoffman, 1991; Erickson, Post & Paige, 1975; Gardner, 1985; Harris, 1990; Irving, 1993; Snyder, 1989, 1995; Snyder et al., 1991).

Stotland's theory has provided the basis for several measurement instruments, the earliest being the Gottschalk Hope Scale (GHS) (Gottschalk, 1974), which was designed to assess hope in verbal behavior. A psychiatrist, Gottschalk defined hope as "a measure of optimism that a favorable outcome is likely to occur, not only in one's personal earthly activities but also in cosmic phenomena and even in spiritual or imaginary events" (p. 779). Scoring the GHS involves content analysis of audiotaped speech samples, which are assigned to seven predefined categories. The reliability and validity of the GHS were established through testing with a normative sample of 109 children and 91 adults, as well as 68 outpatients undergoing psychiatric treatment. Construct validation was carried out with measures of depression, anxiety, sleep disturbance, ego weakness, and belonging (Gottschalk, 1974). Several studies utilizing the GHS have found evidence supporting the biological basis of hope (Gottschalk, Fronczek & Buchsbaum, 1993; Udelman, 1986; Udelman & Udelman, 1985). For instance, Gottschalk et al. (1993) studied the relationship between hope and cerebral glucose metabolic rates, using a sample of ten young adult males. Their results indicate that there are distinctly different cerebral locations for hope and hopelessness, both of which involve the functions of cognition, language, perception, vision, audition, and emotions. There is also evidence that hope (measured by the GHS) enhances immunocompetence in response to physical or emotional stress (Udelman, 1986; Udelman & Udelman, 1985).

Erickson's Hope Scale (HS) (Erickson et al., 1975), the Beck Hopelessness Scale (BHS) (Beck, Weissman, Lester & Trexler, 1974), and the Snyder Hope Scale (SHS) (Snyder, 1989, 1995) are also based on Stotland's theory. The HS asks respondents to rate twenty common future-oriented goals and the probability of reaching each goal (Erickson et al., 1975). These goals focus narrowly on the rational aspect of hope, suggesting a Western cultural bias. The limitation of this restrictive operationalization may explain why the HS has largely disappeared from the hope literature in the past ten years (Farran, Herth & Popovich, 1995). The Beck Hopelessness Scale (BHS) is a twenty-item, dichotomous (true-false) scale based on affective, motivational, and cognitive dimensions of hopelessness (Beck et al., 1974). The BHS has been used as an indirect measure of hope (Rabkin, Williams, Neugebauer, Remien & Goetz, 1990) and also for the concurrent validation of various hope measures (Brackney & Westman, 1992; Farran et al., 1995; Harris, 1990).

The SHS is a twelve-item scale containing two factors (agency and pathways), each consisting of four items, plus four distracters. The agency factor represents the will to meet personal goals, while the pathways factor represents the means to meet goals successfully (Snyder, 1989, 1995; Snyder et al., 1991). The reliability and validity of the SHS have been demonstrated in psychometric evaluation with several thousand respondents (Snyder, 1995), including the general adult population, college students (Ahmed & Duhamel, 1994; Babyak, Snyder & Yoshinobu, 1993; Range & Penton, 1994; Snyder, 1995; Snyder et al., 1991), and subjects with traumatically acquired physical disabilities (Elliot et al., 1991). Research findings have lent the following support to construct validity: The level of hope (SHS) was reportedly a significantly better predictor of goal-setting and persistence than the level of optimism (Harris, 1990); SHS scores of college students and psychiatric patients were predictive of coping strategies and goal-related activities (Snyder et al., 1991); and in undergraduate college students, hope (SHS) and hopelessness (BHS) were negatively correlated (Range & Penton, 1994).

The Hope Index (HI) (Staats, 1987, 1989), like the GHS, HS, and SHS, also assumes the dual cognitive-affective nature of hope; however, it places more emphasis on the affective component (Staats, 1987, 1991; Staats & Partlo, 1993; Stassen & Staats, 1988). Developed for use in social indicators research, the HI presents sixteen conditions that respondents individually rate on a six-point Likert scale, according to their wishes (affective component) and expectations (cognitive component) for the condition to ensue. The HI has been tested in several surveys, in which adults' levels of hope (HI) and happiness were positively correlated (Staats, 1987); however, discrepancies have been found between measures of hope, satisfaction, and happiness among American and Canadian college students (Stassen & Staats, 1988). A third study compared American students' and parents' levels of hope in 1988 to those during the 1991 Persian Gulf war and the 1992 recession. Findings revealed that both students' and parents' hope for peace increased during the Gulf war; in addition, hope for national productivity increased during the 1992 recession, but only for parents (Staats & Partlo, 1993).

In other survey research, a positive correlation was found between hope and the following variables: psychosocial development, a sense of personal control (Brackney & Westman, 1992), and self-esteem (Snyder et al., 1991). Brackney and Westman (1992) used two measures of hope in their study with young adults: a single ten-point rating scale and the Miller Hope Scale (Miller

& Powers, 1988). Results showed that with both hope scales, greater hopeful-ness was associated with greater psychosocial maturity, and lesser hopefulnesses with a lack of personal control; however, the hope measures were not signifi-cantly correlated. In explaining this anomaly, the researchers speculated that the scales may assess different aspects of hope, namely, affective and cognitive.

Several intervention studies have been conducted to test the relationship between hope and various psychosocial variables. For instance, Sherwin (1994) tested the hypothesis that persons reminded of their membership in a socially desirable group would manifest higher hope and self-esteem than those who were not so reminded. Results substantiated an association between hope and collective self-esteem and social identity; nevertheless, the interpretation of these findings was confounded by significant correlations between these measures. Irving (1993) investigated the relationships among hope (dispositional and situational) and cancer-related health beliefs, knowledge, and behavior in college women ($N = 156$). Based on assessment as being high, medium, or low in hope, Irving randomly assigned equal numbers of subjects to view a cancer videotape in one of three different conditions: (a) a hopeful videotape, (b) a neutral videotape, or (c) a control videotape about educational programs at the study site. The results sug-gest that greater hope is associated with viewing cancer as less threatening, having greater personal control and greater cancer knowledge, and being more likely to engage in cancer-preventative behavior. Irving concluded that hope is a negoti-ated version of reality, wherein linking oneself with positive events and distancing oneself from negative outcomes is associated with promotion of well-being.

In another intervention study, Staats (1991) used an experimental design to examine the effects of training sessions on hope (HI) and quality of life for persons over 50 years of age. Subjects ($N = 239$) were randomly assigned to three treatment groups and a control group. The treatment consisted of four training sessions to increase happiness and positive activities. Results indicated that the correlation of hope with quality-of-life measures tended to increase over time. Staats concluded that training is effective in increasing older per-sons' hope and expected quality of life.

Some researchers have investigated hope in specific social populations. For example, Peck (1988) examined the relationships among hope, religious convic-tion, and coping in prison inmates ($N = 97$), mostly in their twenties, who were serving life without parole sentences. Peck created case studies from interviews with seven subjects, which supported the hypothesized association between reli-giously inspired hope of release and coping. Another study by Gardner (1985) investigated the effect of hope on constructive actions of young adult Black males classed as productive ($N = 60$) or unproductive ($N = 61$), depending on whether they were employed or in school. Based on Stotland's (1969) theory, Gardner operationalized hope using indicators of motivation. Findings showed no group differences on ratings of the strength and importance of goal expecta-tion, environmental relevance, and goal importance; however, the productive group rated the likelihood of taking action significantly higher. Gardner con-cluded that inability to sustain hope resulted in productivity dysfunction.

Other researchers have focused on hope in children. For example, Hicks and Holden (1994) surveyed hopes and fears for the future in a subsample of children (n unspecified) aged 10 to 18 years, who were among 400 British pupils participating in this study. Findings revealed that more than half of the children thought about their personal futures often or very often. Their hopes were about establishing themselves as adults, getting a good job, having a good life and a good relationship, and doing well at school. Over half the children indicated that they thought about the global future often or very often, and that they thought about it three times more often than they did about the local future. Hopes for the global future included hope for no more war or poverty, no pollution, and better relationships between people and countries. The children expressed greater concern over global futures than personal or local futures; whereas they were generally optimistic about their personal futures, they were generally pessimistic about the global future (Hicks & Holden, 1994).

In other research (O'Keefe, 1993; Scioli, 1991), the Hopelessness Scale for Children (HSC) was used to study hope among school children. O'Keefe (1993) examined the correlation between hopefulness in resilient inner-city children (N = 124) and various aspects of self-esteem, including scholastic and athletic competence, social acceptance, physical appearance, and behavioral conduct. Results showed that hopefulness was strongly predicted by individual aspects of self-esteem; however, there were significant differences between boys and girls. Scioli (1991) investigated the relative importance of structural versus functional variables in determining levels of hope and hopelessness, in a sample of thirty-two children and thirty-two adolescents. Findings indicated that in the areas of problem-solving skills and general information processing, those who scored high on hopelessness performed worse than those who scored low. The researcher concluded that a state of hopelessness may be related to behavioral and cognitive indicators of functioning; however, this relationship appeared to vary greatly with age.

Several studies have examined hope in persons with HIV infection (Jacobson, 1992; Rabkin et al., 1990). Jacobson (1992) conducted semi-structured interviews over a four-month period with five homosexual males living with AIDS, in order to explore specific and global hopes. Emotional states and hopefulness were also tracked by use of an adjective checklist and a hope scale. The findings identified several hope-inspiring factors, including life review and involvement with a caring other (Jacobson, 1992). Rabkin et al. (1990) investigated psychiatric and psychosocial correlates of hope in a community sample (N = 208) of HIV-positive and HIV-negative homosexual men. Hope was measured using the Beck Hopelessness Scale. Findings showed that overall there were high levels of hope and low levels of depressive symptoms. The authors concluded that despite HIV infection, participants were able to preserve faith in their future.

Most of the above research has used quantitative approaches based on theoretically derived operational definitions and measurement instruments; however, some studies have employed more inductive methods to delineate people's hopes. For example, Nekolaichuk (1995) explored the meaning of hope in health and illness in three subsamples: healthy adults (n = 146), persons with chronic and life-threatening illness (n = 159), and nurses (n = 206). A multidimensional structure of hope was delineated through the use of the semantic differential technique and factor analytic procedures. Three identified hope factors were personal spirit, risk, and authentic caring. According to Nekolaichuk, the predominant factor, personal spirit, consisted of a holistic formation of hope elements characterized by the core theme of meaning.

Roberts (1992) interviewed 103 adults aged 19 to 83 years, in order to determine their perceptions of their future selves. Participants were asked to project themselves into the oldest age imaginable, to describe their hopes and fears for that age, and to identify role models for their hopes and fears. Findings showed that the length of future perspective and number of hopes for the future declined with age. As expected, participants could name role models representing both their hopes and fears for aging, but the former were more often identified. In discussing these findings, Roberts suggests that personal hopes and fears for the distant future may serve as motivators for the present.

A number of studies have investigated the nature of hope in persons whose role it is to help or care for others. For example, Cuthbert (1994) interviewed eleven cancer survivor volunteers working with recently diagnosed cancer patients. Five patterns related to having and giving hope were identified: feelings of fear, survivor's guilt, satisfaction, helpfulness, and hopefulness. These patterns were clustered into two themes: self-doubt and self-renewal. In two other studies, researchers (Rumsfeld, 1991; Sutherland, 1993), using unstructured interviews, explored hope from the perspective of psychotherapists (seven in each study). From the findings of his study, Sutherland (1993) concluded that hope is a complex, interpersonal phenomenon that is best understood in the context of adversity and that involves perceived trust, control, and choice. The psychodynamic therapists in Rumsfeld's (1991) study believed it was critical to have and to convey hope to their clients; thus, he concluded that the development of realistic hope is key to the work of psychotherapy.

Other researchers have explored the impact of medical personnel on seriously ill persons' experience of hope. Based on interviews with ten physicians and ten patients, Sardell and Trierweiler (1993) developed fifty-seven statements describing the circumstances of diagnostic disclosures. An additional fifty-six patients rated these statements on a bipolar scale according to hopefulness and favorability. Results suggested broad areas of diagnostic disclosure where physicians might attempt to enhance hope. In another study, Perakyla (1991) used an ethnographic approach rooted in symbolic interaction theory to determine the interactions whereby staff and terminally ill patients shaped their "medical identities." According to Perakyla, medical identities were shaped in terms of the hopefulness of the situation, which was called "hope work." Three types of hope work were identified: curative, palliative, and dismantling hope. Conflicts arose when different parties engaged in different types of hope work. Perakyla (1991) concluded that hope work appeared to be linked to maintaining physicians' legitimacy with regard to the dying process.

Levy (1990) conducted a qualitative inquiry into the role of hope in family members of persons with brain injury, basing the research on the presupposition that denial can serve as an adaptive function for years after the traumatic event. Nine family members were interviewed from five different families whose close relative had sustained a severe head injury in the previous six to eight years. Findings indicated that participants generally believed that their relative would recover completely, despite having a poor prognosis. According to Levy, denial appeared to support the growth of optimism and hope and helped families to adapt; participants gradually replaced the "myth of complete recovery" with more realistic goals, but they still had hope that their relative would progress. Levy concluded that denial and acceptance could coexist.

NURSING LITERATURE

Totality Paradigm Perspective

The burgeoning nursing literature on hope is largely situated within nursing's totality paradigm. In this paradigm, humans are viewed as composites of bio-psycho-social-spiritual parts, and human-environment interrelationships are believed to be linear and causal in nature (Parse, 1987); thus, hope is generally construed as a state or a linear process involving the human's psychosocial and spiritual domains (Brown, 1989; Farran et al., 1995; Forbes, 1994; Haase, Britt, Coward, Leidy & Penn, 1992; Stephenson, 1991). The goals of nursing from this perspective concern health promotion, illness prevention, and the care and healing of the sick (Parse, 1987). In regard to these goals, hope is considered to be essential, particularly for survival (Bushkin, 1993; Douville, 1994; Dubree & Vogelpohl, 1980; Hickey, 1989), healing (Brown, 1993; Holahan, 1995; Wagner, 1993), quality of life (Rustoen, 1995), and dying with dignity (Herth, 1990a; Hickey, 1986; Scanlon, 1989; Yates, 1993). In the totality paradigm, it is generally assumed that hope may be induced through the interventions of expert caregivers; hence, instilling, fostering, or maintaining hope have been advocated as important goals of nursing interventions with patients and families (Brown, 1989; Dubree & Vogelpohl, 1980; Gamlin & Kinghorn, 1995; Gewe, 1994; Hickey, 1986, 1989; Hockley, 1993; Kim, 1989, 1990; Lange, 1978; Limandri & Boyle, 1978; Miller, 1985, 1991; Poncar, 1994; Scanlon, 1989; Vaillot, 1970). To this end, several nurse scholars (Farran, Wilken & Popovich, 1992; Herth, 1992; Nowotny, 1986, 1991) have developed tools to enable clinicians to assess clients' hope.

According to Vaillot (1970), "Hope springs from the depths of one's being" (p. 271). One of the earliest of authors to consider hope as a vital concern of nursing, Vaillot believed that hope was essential for restoring the fullness of being, and that it was possible even when dying. A contemporary of Vaillot, Travelbee (1971) focused on nursing as an interpersonal process. She viewed hope as a mental state that was strongly associated with dependence on others, and that motivated human behavior. Following these pioneering attempts to carve out the concept of hope for nursing, a number of other scholars have endeavored to develop conceptualizations of hope through review and analysis of the multidisciplinary literature (Brown, 1989; Farran et al., 1995; Forbes, 1994; Lange, 1978; McGee, 1984; Rustoen, 1995). Unfortunately, nurse scholars have often blended diverse and incompatible theoretical perspectives in a quest for comprehensiveness, thereby obscuring rather than clarifying the concept of hope.

Fowler (1995) discovered ten definitions of hope in a review of the nursing literature. Common among these definitions were the notions of energy, power, and an action orientation or transcendence. Nurse scholars have variously characterized hope as a mental state (Grimm, 1990; Haase, Britt, Coward, Leidy & Penn, 1992; Herth, 1989; Miller & Powers, 1988; Thompson, 1994; Travelbee, 1971), an attribute (Nowotny, 1989), a process involving feelings, behaviors, and relationships (Brown, 1989; Dufault & Martocchio, 1985; Farran et al., 1995; Stephenson, 1991), and a stimulus for action (McGee, 1984). With regard to the relationship between hope and hopelessness, one view is that they exist on a continuum, the extremes of which represent mutually exclusive, polar opposites (Campbell, 1987; McGee, 1984); another view is that they are in a dialectic relationship and vary proportionately in circumstances ranging from ordinary living to crisis situations and pathological states (Farran et al., 1995).

Several authors (Farran et al., 1995; Forbes, 1994; Haase et al., 1992; Stephenson, 1991) have used formal concept analysis methods to systematically analyze the concept of hope with respect to its antecedents, consequences, and defining and critical attributes. Forbes (1994) and Stephenson (1991) used the method developed by Walker and Avant (1988), while Haase et al. (1992) created a simultaneous method to compare the concepts of hope, spiritual perspective, acceptance, and self-transcendence. Among the identified antecedents of hope were the following: loss, crisis, difficult situations (Stephenson, 1991), life experiences, connectedness, and positive attributes (Haase et al., 1992). The identified consequences of hope included a new perspective (Stephenson, 1991); energy and improved psychological and physiological functioning (Forbes, 1994); personal competency, a winning position, peace, and self-transcendence (Haase et al., 1992). Among the defining attributes of hope were the following: a sense of mutuality and relatedness to others; anticipation of and belief in the future; and spiritual beliefs, confidence in ability to affect outcome, and active involvement (Forbes, 1994). Critical attributes of hope included uncertainty, having a general or particular goal (Haase et al., 1992), or having a personally meaningful object (Brown, 1989; Stephenson, 1991).

Farran et al. (1995) have analyzed hope and hopelessness as clinical constructs, beginning with the following working definition of hope:

> Hope constitutes an essential experience of the human condition. It functions as a way of feeling, a way of thinking, a way of behaving, and a way [of] relating to oneself and one's world. Hope has the ability to

be fluid in its expectations, and in the event that the desired object or outcome does not occur, hope can still be present. (p. 6)

The following processes were identified as "central attributes" of hope: an experiential process (the pain of hope), a spiritual or transendent process (the soul of hope), a rational thought process (the mind of hope), and a relational process (the heart of hope) (p. 6). These authors differentiate hope from wishing and optimism with respect to goals, affect, cognition, behavior, and outcome; nevertheless, they suggest that wishing and optimism may serve as first steps in the hoping process, and might also function simultaneously with hope.

Many authors (Brown, 1989; Farran et al., 1995; Gamlin & Kinghorn, 1995; Herth, 1989, 1990b; Kim, 1989, 1990; McGee, 1984; Rustoen, 1995; Scanlon, 1989) link hope with coping. For example, Farran et al. (1995) deal with hope as an antecedent to coping, a coping strategy, and an outcome of adaptive coping, while Brown (1989) characterizes hope as "a gestalt of coping behaviors" (p. 97). The linkage of hope with coping has bolstered the notion that hope may be unrealistic or unjustified in some situations (Ersek, 1992; Hinds, 1988; Miller, 1989; O'Malley & Menke, 1988; Stoner & Keampfer, 1985), and the belief that hope must be reality-based in order to be actualized (Brown, 1989; Dufault & Martocchio, 1985; Hickey, 1986; McGee, 1984; Skolny & Riehl, 1974). Other authors, however, have contested the idea that nurses can or should judge another person's view of reality (Hall, 1990; Hockley, 1993; Yates, 1993). Hall (1990), for instance, contends that hope has value at all times, inasmuch as it maintains emotional well-being. In Yates's (1993) view, insisting on realistic hope from the nurse's point of view is an imposition upon cancer patients. Rather, she has called for a reconceptualization of hope that "take[s] into account that cancer patients have their own reality, a reality that may be quite different from those around them" (p. 705).

Research. In the totality paradigm perspective, phenomena for research are generally reduced to variables to enable the study of causal or associative relationships (Parse, 1987). Data are usually collected using measurement instruments or observational techniques and are analyzed through the reductive techniques of descriptive or inferential statistics. While quantification is the primary mode and ultimate goal of research, qualitative methods are deemed appropriate in preliminary research aimed at identifying variables for future research. In such research, content analysis is a commonly used reductive technique for analyzing qualitative data. Whether qualitative or quantitative in approach, nursing research on hope has often been conceptualized using theoretical frameworks borrowed from other disciplines, such as Lazarus and Folkman's (1984) stress, appraisal, and coping model (Grimm, 1990; Herth, 1989; Nowotny, 1989; Raleigh, 1992; Yancey, Greger & Coburn, 1994); Erickson's (1964a) model of psychosocial development (Curl, 1992; Mays, 1984); and Stotland's (1969) theory of hope (Artinian, 1984; Farran & McCann, 1989; Herth, 1989; Stoner & Keampfer, 1985).

One qualitative study (Marden & Rice, 1995) examined abused women's use of hope as a coping mechanism in relationships with their abusers, within the framework of social psychology theories on domestic violence, cognitive dissonance, and hope. The researchers conducted four focus group sessions with twenty-four women in abusive relationships. Findings indicated that the women maintained hope in four dimensions: hope for change in their partner's behavior, hope for survival, hope as something to cling to, and hope for control of the situation. Marden and Rice concluded that hope served as a form of coping and as a way of reducing cognitive dissonance, and they recommended that abused women be directed into therapy to reduce cognitive dissonance and enhance coping strategies.

A number of other qualitative studies have been conducted in order to describe the phenomenon of hope and identify its constituent factors, in well and chronically ill adults (Dufault & Martocchio, 1985; Ersek, 1992; Hall, 1990, 1994; Laskiwski & Morse, 1993; Marden & Rice, 1995; Miller, 1989; Morse & Doberneck, 1995; Raleigh, 1992; Ross, 1995; Thompson, 1994) and children (Artinian, 1984; Hinds, 1988). Findings from these studies characterize hope as a multidimensional experience involving interpersonal relations, a future focus, and goal achievement. A classic work frequently cited in the nursing literature is that of Dufault and Martocchio (1985). Using participant observation, these researchers collected data from thirty-five elderly cancer patients over two years, following which they re-analyzed data, also collected during a two-year period, from another forty-seven terminally ill persons aged 14 years or older. On the basis of this analysis, the authors developed a definition of hope as a multidimensional, process-oriented, "dynamic life force characterized by a confident yet uncertain expectation of achieving a future good which, to the hoping person, is realistically possible and personally significant" (p. 380). According to Dufault and Martocchio, confidence and uncertainty reflect different dimensions of hope and, thus, can coexist in the hoping person. Their research findings resulted in the creation of a hope taxonomy consisting of two spheres (generalized and particularized) and six dimensions (affective, cognitive, behavioral, affiliative, temporal, and contextual), which, considered together, "provide a gestalt of hope" (p. 381). The Herth Hope Scale (HHS) (Herth, 1991, 1992) was developed based on this model of hope and has been utilized to measure hope in a number of studies (Harrison, 1993; Herth, 1989, 1990a, 1990b, 1991, 1993a, 1993b; Yancey et al., 1994).

Dufault and Martocchio (1985) delineated six dimensions of hope as follows: In its cognitive dimension, hope is "reality-based from the perspective of the hoping person" (p. 384); that is, persons hope until they can no longer ground their hope in reality. The affiliative dimension concerns the sensations and emotions of the hoping process. The behavioral dimension involves the psychologic, physical, social, and religious actions taken "to directly effect the desired outcome or to achieve a hope" (p. 385). The affiliative dimension refers to "the hoping person's sense of relatedness or involvement beyond self" (p. 386), while the temporal dimension indicates that hope is directed toward the future but is also influenced by past and present experiences. Finally, the contextual dimension pertains to the life situations surrounding one's experience of hope. The researchers concluded that "hope and hopelessness are not the opposite ends of one continuum nor is hopelesssness the absence of hope. . . . Some sphere or dimension of hope is always present" (p. 389). They recommended that these spheres and dimensions be used to guide nursing interventions to help persons achieve or maintain hope.

More recently, Morse and Doberneck (1995) used their own concept development method to delineate the concept of hope. These researchers constructed a prototype of hope consisting of abstract and universal attributes, and then verified this prototype using interview data from four different participant groups: patients undergoing heart transplant, patients with spinal cord injury, breast cancer survivors, and mothers intending to continue breastfeeding while employed. The process resulted in the delineation of seven universal components of hope: "a realistic initial assessment of the predicament or threat, the envisioning of alternatives and the setting of goals, a bracing for negative outcomes, a realistic assessment of personal resources and of external conditions and resources, the solicitation of mutually supportive relationships, the continuous evaluation for signs that reinforce the selected goals, and a determination to endure" (p. 277). The researchers also specified the following unique patterns of hope for the different groups: waiting for a chance (transplant patients); incremental hope (spinal-cord injured patients); hoping against hope (breast cancer survivors); and provisional hope (breastfeeding mothers).

A number of qualitative research studies have focused on identifying the basis of hope among the disabled (Laskiwski & Morse, 1993), seriously ill persons (Cutcliffe, 1995; Ersek, 1992; D. C. Owen, 1989), and well individuals (Hinds, 1988); all of these, except for the study by Laskiwski and Morse (1993), used a grounded theory approach. This methodology was developed by sociologists Glaser and Strauss (1967) for the purpose of building mid-level sociological theories from empirical data (Mitchell & Cody, 1993). For instance, Hinds (1988) purposively sampled three populations (total $N = 117$) of well and ill adolescents, resulting in the following definition of hopefulness: "the degree to which an adolescent possesses a comforting or life-sustaining, reality-based belief that a positive future exists for self or others" (p. 85). In another study, Ersek (1992) explored the process of maintaining hope in twenty adults undergoing bone marrow transplantation for leukemia. The identified basic social process of "maintaining hope" consisted of two core categories: "dealing with it" and "keeping it in its place." Ersek considered these categories to be conflicting; thus, to integrate them, she created an overarching concept, "the dialectic of maintaining hope." Ersek specified this concept as an interactive process of dealing with the threat in order to limit it, a strategy that she suggested was used to maintain hope. However, she cautioned that such hope could be illusory in nature; hence, she recommended further research to identify the adaptive or maladaptive potential of unrealistic hopefulness.

Hope and despair emerged as central themes in an ethnographic study of patients with spinal cord injury residing in a long-term care facility (Laskiwski & Morse, 1993). According to Laskiwski and Morse, when patients realized that the spinal cord injury was permanent, they modified their hope to a "realistic level consistent with their injury" (p. 143). In discussing the apparently contradictory coexistence of hope and despair in the patients' lives, these authors suggested that hope was both a constant background state and an essential affect. In their view, expressions of despair were "a part of the process essential to the modification of hope, and the process of learning to accept a changed life" (p. 152).

Other researchers (Fryback, 1993; Hall, 1994) have identified hope as an important concept in the experience of living with a terminal illness. Fryback (1993), for example, conducted a "naturalistic" inquiry into the meaning of health for ten persons with a terminal diagnosis, using the constant comparison method of data analysis (Glaser & Strauss, 1967). The emergent concept of hope was classified under the domain of mental/emotional health. Fryback (1993) described hope as "a future-orientated attitude" (p. 151) that helped persons to maintain their struggle while they continued to enjoy life. Hall (1994), using interpretive interactionism to guide data analysis, explored the experiences of ten adults living with AIDS. She identified the following four ways of maintaining hope: miracles, religion, involvement in work or vocations, and the support of family and friends.

A number of studies have included the professional's perspective in examining the process of promoting hope for patients and families (Artinian, 1984; Cutcliffe, 1995; Kirkpatrick et al., 1995; D. C. Owen, 1989). For example, Artinian (1984) investigated the hope-fostering process for parents and fifteen patients, aged 10 to 20 years, who were undergoing bone marrow transplant. A research team collected data through interviews with parents, nurses, and children; anecdotal nurses' notes, chart entries, parents' diaries, and letters from parents were also used. The findings focused on the hope-fostering role of support from the perspective of patients, parents, and professionals. Based on these findings, Artinian developed a "probabilistic model" (p. 68) with directional propositions for fostering hope in practice with parents and children.

D. C. Owen (1989) and Cutcliffe (1995), using a grounded theory approach, explored nurses' perspectives of hope in the seriously ill. Through analysis of interview data obtained from six oncology clinical nurse specialists, D. C. Owen (1989) found that "hope is a dynamic process in which patients respond to changing life events" (p. 78), and that during the hoping process, "energy [is] exchanged, transformed, or moved resulting in the preservation or loss of hope" (p. 79). Cutcliffe's (1995) research explored the process whereby psychiatric nurses instill hope in patients terminally ill with HIV. Findings resulted in a theory of hope inspiration consisting of the following core variables: reflection in action, affirmation of worth, creating a partnership, and the totality of the person. Cutcliffe concluded that hope inspiration is essential to nursing practice and to the concept of caring.

Many studies have attempted to specify relationships among hope and other variables using quantitative methods. To this end, a number of nurse researchers have developed instruments to measure hope (Grimm, 1990; Herth, 1991, 1992; Miller & Powers, 1988; Nowotny, 1989; Raleigh & Boehm, 1994; Shang, 1994; Stoner & Keampfer, 1985). Mainly survey and correlational methods have been used to explore the role of hope in promoting health or well-being among healthy adults (Carson, Soeken & Grimm, 1988; Escallier, 1995; Farran & McCann, 1989; Farran & Popovich, 1990; Herth, 1990b; Mays, 1984; Zorn, 1992), and as a way of responding to, or coping with, difficult situations among ill persons or their families (Carson, Soeken, Shanty & Terry, 1990; Grimm, 1990; Harrison, 1993; Herth, 1989, 1990a, 1993a, 1993b; McGill, 1992; Mickley & Soeken, 1993; Mickley, Soeken & Belcher, 1992; O'Malley & Menke, 1988; C. L. Owen, 1990; Popovich, 1991; Raleigh, 1992; Ruth, 1990; Stoner & Keampfer, 1985; Yancey et al., 1994).

Findings from these exploratory studies indicate that hope is related to the following variables: psychosocial maturity (Curl, 1992); coping ability (Herth, 1989, 1990b; Popovich, 1991; Stewart & Hirth, 1994); spiritual well-being and/or religiousness (Carson et al., 1988; Carson et al., 1990; Mickley et al., 1992; Mickley & Soeken, 1993; Ruth, 1990); length of illness and level of fatigue (Herth, 1992); self-esteem and life satisfaction (Mays, 1984); stressful life events and mental health (Farran & Popovich, 1990; O'Malley & Menke, 1988); functional or health status (McGill, 1992; Popovich, 1991; Zorn, 1992); perceived health or disease status (Harrison, 1993; LeClair, 1995; C. L. Owen, 1990); suffering (Holahan, 1995); and support of family and friends (Farran & Popovich, 1990; Khanobdee, 1994; C. L. Owen, 1990; Raleigh, 1992; Yarcheski, Scoloveno & Mahon, 1994; Zorn, 1992). Based on their findings, several researchers have developed models to explain or predict hope and have recommended further research to test these intervention models (Farran & McCann, 1989; Farran & Popovich, 1990; Herth, 1993b).

One intervention study was conducted to determine the effects of positive mental imagery on hope, anxiety, coping, and other variables in persons with chronic obstructive pulmonary disease (COPD) (Aubuchon, 1990). The Nowotny Hope Scale (Nowotny, 1986) and the Beck Hopelessness Inventory (Beck et al., 1974) were used to measure hope. The subjects ($N = 83$), community-living persons with COPD, were randomly assigned to one of two treatment groups or a control group. Treatments consisted of listening to a tape emphasizing positive selves, or relaxation. Findings indicated that hope was altered by the treatments ($F = 5.1$, $p = .027$), while anxiety was not.

Few studies were found that used a nursing conceptual framework. One study (McGill, 1992; McGill & Paul, 1993) used Roy's adaptation model as the framework to explore the relationship between functional status and hope in elders with and without cancer. Hope was viewed as an indicator of adaptation and was measured using the Miller Hope Scale (MHS) (Miller & Powers, 1988). Functional status was linked with Roy's four adaptive modes and was measured using the Philadelphia Geriatric Center's Multi-level Assessment

Instrument. With multiple regression analysis, the only variables significantly related to MHS scores were physical health, income, and education. McGill concluded that while declining physical health and lower socioeconomic status threatened the hope of elders, the diagnosis of cancer did not.

A study conducted by Tollett and Thomas (1995) used a mid-level nursing theory, Miller's model of patient power resources (Miller, 1992), as the conceptual framework. Using a quasi-experimental, pretest–post-test design, the researchers randomly assigned veterans ($N = 40$) admitted to a homeless evaluation unit to either a usual treatment group or an intervention condition designed to instill hope. Dependent variables were hope (measured by the MHS), depression, self-efficacy, and self-esteem. Results showed that at the end of four weeks, the intervention and control groups differed signficantly in levels of hope ($F = 8.93$, $p = .006$). The authors concluded that there was preliminary support for Miller's model and recommended that the research be replicated.

Hope surfaced in the findings of two other studies that explored different health phenomena. One study, conducted by Schorr, Farnham, and Ervin (1991), and using Newman's (1986) model as the theoretical framework, explored the health patterns of aging women as expanding consciousness. The study explored the interrelationships among powerlessness, chronic illness, hopelessness, death anxiety, and future temporal orientation using a correlational design. Hope was measured using the Generalized Expectancies Scale (GES), a measure of hopelessness. Participants were sixty female volunteers aged 65 or older, living in seniors' centers in the western United States. No significant correlation was found between powerlessness and any other study variables. An unexpected finding was that subjects were "hopeful rather than depressed regarding their expectations of life" (p. 59). In discussing this finding, the authors suggested that expressing hope for the future "may reflect an emerging awareness of health as the pattern of the whole, and may be more appropriately investigated using qualitative methods" (p. 61).

Johnson (1995) conducted a phenomenological inquiry into a family's experience with head injury. Rogers's (1970) science of unitary human beings was identified as the theoretical perspective; however, its explication was brief and inaccurate. Unstructured interviews were used to collect data from the participants, including a 16-year-old accident survivor, his parents, and four siblings aged 10 to 15 years. Data were analyzed using Van Manen's (1990) approach. One of three themes identified was *helplessness and the need to hope*. Unfortunately, the findings were not connected with Rogers's theoretical perspective and, hence, do not expand knowledge about hope. Nevertheless, it is noteworthy that hope was identified as important for families in this context.

A number of researchers have combined quantitative and qualitative approaches with the aim of enhancing the validity of findings (Curl, 1992; Herth, 1990a, 1993a, 1993b; Kirkpatrick et al., 1995; Popovich, 1991). Populations sampled in these studies included the elderly (Curl, 1992), terminally ill persons (Herth, 1990a), family caregivers of terminally ill persons (Herth, 1993a), critically ill persons (Miller, 1989), stroke patients (Popovich,

1991), cancer patients (Thompson, 1994), and psychiatric clinicians (Kirkpatrick et al., 1995). The factors shown to promote or diminish hope included supportive relationships (Herth, 1990a, 1993a, 1993b; Jacobson, 1992; Kirkpatrick et al., 1995; Miller, 1989; Thompson, 1994); attainable aims, spiritual beliefs, and cognitive strategies (Herth, 1990a, 1993a, 1993b; Miller, 1989; Thompson, 1994); and a determined mental attitude (Miller, 1989). From the perspective of psychiatric clinicians, factors important for instilling hope in patients include facilitating success, connecting to successful role models, managing the illness, and educating clients (Kirkpatrick et al., 1995).

The body of research on hope that has been conducted from the totality paradigm perspective shares some general limitations. A methodological concern is that the instruments developed by nurse researchers, while frequently used, are still undergoing psychometric evaluation; thus, their reliability and validity are open to question. Moreover, generalizations from the findings are often extrapolated beyond what is warranted, given the usually small sample sizes and uncontrolled research designs. In addition, even though the conclusions drawn from findings are tentative at best, recommendations for hope-instilling interventions are usually made as though the findings were conclusive.

An even more serious criticism concerns the number and variety of borrowed theories that have been used to guide the research. This theoretical eclecticism is problematic for several reasons: first, the resultant findings do not build a cohesive body of knowledge around any given perspective; second, they do not expand the body of *nursing* knowledge; and third, the basis for nursing practice arising from research on these theoretical perspectives is debatable.

Simultaneity Paradigm

A new view of hope is emerging from nursing's *simultaneity paradigm*. This worldview considers humans as unitary beings and the human-universe interrelationship as a mutual process (Parse, 1987). The goal of nursing is quality of life from the person's own perspective (Parse, 1987). Quality of life is shaped through lived experiences of health, which must be understood from the person's viewpoint (Parse, 1994). In this perspective, hope is a lived experience of unitary human beings; it is "a way of propelling self toward envisioned possibilities in everyday encounters with the world" (Parse, 1990, p. 12). Viewed from Parse's (1981, 1992, 1995) human becoming perspective, "hope–no-hope is the paradoxical rhythm from which hope arises. . . . The living of this hope–no-hope is a way of becoming; thus, it is an experience of health" (Parse, 1990, p. 13).

A related concept, *considering tomorrow*, was created by Bunkers (1998) from a synthesis of the literature on hope and imagination, framed in the perspective of Parse's (1981) human becoming theory. According to Bunkers (1998), "Considering tomorrow is contemplating what might be while living moment to moment in the now. It is not a human experience that can be managed, avoided, coped with, or manipulated. It is essential to one's becoming" (p. 57). Thus hope and considering tomorrow are universal lived experiences of human becoming.

Research. The phenomenological approach is congruent with the ontological basis of the simultaneity paradigm, in that it is concerned with understanding phenomena as humanly lived. Three phenomenological studies on hope were found (Brunsman, 1988; Parse, 1990; Stanley, 1978), although only one has been published (Parse, 1990). In Stanley's (1978) dissertation research, van Kaam's method was used with a purposive sample of 100 undergraduate students between 19 and 25 years of age. The students were asked to write a description of a situation in which they experienced hope. Seven common elements were identified in the descriptions, which were combined to form a general structure of hope for healthy young adults. The general structure was this: "The lived experience of hope is a confident expectation of a significant future outcome accompanied by comfortable and uncomfortable feelings, characterized by a quality of transcendence and interpersonal relatedness, and in which action to affect the outcome is initiated" (p. 165).

Brunsman's (1988) master's thesis was a phenomenological study, framed in the perspective of Parse's (1981) theory, on hope in two families with a chronically ill child. The general structural description that emerged from the families' descriptions follows:

> Hope is the process that becomes known as one anticipates a future outcome. It arises from a struggle with the paradoxical nature of day to day experiences. It is in living these paradoxes that choices surface which lead the individual to choose a different view of the situations. That view then becomes the anchor for the individual and fosters movement, which both enables and limits the individual, in creating a new context of the situation. (p. 105)

Linking this finding with the concepts of Parse's theory, Brunsman created the following propositional statement: "Hope is originating the enabling-limiting of imaging" (p. 116).

Parse (1990) studied the lived experience of hope for ten adults on hemodialysis, using her newly created phenomenological-hermeneutic methodology. The structure of the lived experience of hope was this: "Hope is anticipating possibilities through envisioning the not-yet in harmoniously living the comfort-discomfort of everydayness while unfolding a different perspective of an expanding view" (Parse, 1990, p. 15). Conceptually interpreted, the structure of the lived experience was "Hope is imaging the enabling-limiting of transforming" (p. 16). Thus the findings of these phenomenological studies similarly conceptualized hope as anticipating the not-yet, while living the paradoxical patterns of comfort-discomfort amid opportunities and limitations unfolding in creating an expanding view.

The literature on hope is varied and it is certain that hope remains a mystery, but through uncovering structures of hope as described by persons willing to share their stories, a greater understanding of it can be gleaned. It is clear that hope is a phenomenon of great concern to nurses and others, since it is closely connected with health and quality of life.

REFERENCES

Aardema, B. L. (1984). The therapeutic use of hope. *Dissertation Abstracts International, 46*(1), 293–B.

Ahmed, S. M., & Duhamel, P. (1994). Psychometric properties of the scale of individual differences—measure of hope. *Psychological Reports, 74*((3, Pt. 1), 801–802.

Aldridge, D. (1995). Spirituality, hope and music therapy in palliative care. *The Arts in Psychotherapy, 22*(2), 103–109.

Artinian, B. (1984). Fostering hope in the bone marrow transplant child. *Maternal Child Nursing Journal, 13*(1), 57–71.

Aubuchon, B. L. (1990). *The effects of positive mental imagery on hope, coping, anxiety, dyspnea, and pulmonary function in persons with chronic obstructive pulmonary disease: Tests of a nursing intervention and a theoretical model.* Doctoral dissertation. The University of Texas at Austin. (University Microfilms No. 9116811)

Averill, J. R. (1991). Intellectual emotions. In C. D. Spielberger & I. G. Sarason (Eds.), *Stress and emotions* (pp. 3–16). New York: Hemisphere.

Babyak, M. A., Snyder, C. R., & Yoshinobu, L. (1993). Psychometric properties of the Hope Scale: A confirmatory factor analysis. *Journal of Research in Personality, 27* (2), 154–169.

Beck, A. T., Weissman, A., Lester, D., & Trexler, L. (1974). The measurement of pessimism: The Hopelessness Scale. *Journal of Consulting and Clinical Psychology, 42*(6), 861–865.

Bloch, E. (1986). *The principle of hope* (N. Plaice, S. Plaice & P. Knight, Trans.). Oxford: Basil Blackwell. (Original work published 1959)

Boyd, E. (1994). What makes a survivor? *Modern Maturity, 4*–5, 72.

Brackney, B. E., & Westman, A. S. (1992). Relationships among hope, psychosocial development, and locus of control. *Psychological Reports, 70*(3, Pt. 1), 864–866.

Brown, L. (1993). Hope as healing: Patient voices. In D. A. Gaut & A. Boykin (Eds.), *Caring as healing: Renewal through hope* (pp. 167–177). New York: NLN Press.

Brown, P. (1989). The concept of hope: Implications for care of the critically ill. *Critical Care Nurse, 9*(5), 97–105.

Brunsman, C. S. (1988). *A phenomenological study of the lived experience of hope in families with a chronically ill child.* Unpublished master's thesis, Michigan State University.

Buechler, S. (1995). Hope as inspiration in psychoanalysis. *Psychoanalytic Dialogues, 5*(1), 63–74.

Bunkers, S. S. 1998. Considering tomorrow: Parse's theory-guided research. *Nursing Science Quarterly, 11*, 56–63.

Bushkin, E. (1993). Signposts of survivorship. *Oncology Nursing Forum,* 20(6), 869–875.

Campbell, L. (1987). Hopelessness: A concept analysis. *Journal of Psychosocial Nursing and Mental Health Services,* 25(2), 19–22.

Carni, E. (1988). Issues of hope and faith in the cancer patient. *Journal of Religion and Health,* 27(4), 285–290.

Carson, V., Soeken, K. L., & Grimm, P. M. (1988). Hope and its relationship to spiritual well-being. *Journal of Psychology and Theology,* 16(2), 159–167.

Carson, V., Soeken, K. L., Shanty, J., & Terry, L. (1990). Hope and spiritual well-being: Essentials for living with AIDS. *Perspectives in Psychiatric Care,* 26(2), 28–34.

Casey, B. L. (1988). Hope, suffering, and solidarity: The power of the Sabbath experience. *Dissertation Abstracts International,* 50(05), 1336-A. (University Microfilms No. AAG8914925)

Cousins, N. (1974, December 14). Hope and practical realities. *Saturday Review/World. An Inventory of Hope* (Special Issue), 4–5.

Cousins, N. (1979). *Anatomy of an illness as perceived by the patient.* New York: Norton.

Cousins, N. (1983). *The healing heart.* New York: Norton.

Cousins, N. (1989). *Head first: The biology of hope.* New York: E. P. Dutton.

Curl, E. (1992). Hope in the elderly: Exploring the relationship between psychosocial developmental residual and hope. *Dissertation Abstracts International,* 53(4), 1782–B.

Cutcliffe, J. R. (1995). How do nurses inspire and instill hope in terminally ill HIV patients? *Journal of Advanced Nursing,* 22(5), 888–895.

Cuthbert, P. D. (1994). *The importance of both having and giving hope: The cancer survivor volunteer's experience of working with recently diagnosed cancer patients* [CD ROM]. Abstract from: ProQuest File: Dissertation Abstracts Item: 9502054.

Douville, L. M. (1994). The power of hope. *American Journal of Nursing,* 94(12), 34–36.

Dubois, R. (1974, December 14). The humanizing of humans. *Saturday Review/ World. An Inventory of Hope* (Special Issue), 76–80.

Dubree, M., & Vogelpohl, R. (1980). When hope dies, so does the patient. *American Journal of Nursing,* 80, 2046–2049.

Dufault, K., & Martocchio, B. C. (1985). Hope: Its spheres and dimensions. *Nursing Clinics of North America,* 20(2), 379–391.

Elliot, T., Witty, T., Herrick, S., & Hoffman, J. (1991). Negotiating reality after physical loss: Hope, depression, and disability. *Journal of Personality and Social Psychology,* 61(4), 608–613.

Erickson, R., Post, R., & Paige, A. (1975). Hope as a psychiatric variable. *Journal of Clinical Psychology,* 31(2), 324–330.

Erickson, E. H. (1964a). *Childhood and society* (2nd ed.). New York: W. W. Norton.

Erickson, E. H. (1964b). *Insight and responsibility.* New York: W. W. Norton.

Ersek, M. (1992). The process of maintaining hope in adults undergoing bone marrow transplantation for leukemia. *Oncology Nursing Forum, 19*(6), 883–889.

Escallier, L. A. (1995). Prenatal predictors of colic: Maternal-fetal attachment, maternal state anxiety and maternal hope. *Dissertation Abstracts International, 56*(05), 2847–B. (University Microfilms No. AAI9531268)

Farran, C. J., Herth, C. J., & Popovich, J. M. (1995). *Hope and hopelessness: Critical clinical constructs.* Thousand Oaks, CA: Sage.

Farran, C. J., & McCann, J. (1989). Longitudinal analysis of hope in community-based older adults. *Archives of Psychiatric Nursing, 3*(5), 272–276.

Farran, C. J., & Popovich, J. M. (1990). Hope: A relevant concept for geriatric psychiatry. *Archives of Psychiatric Nursing, 4*(2), 124–130.

Farran, C. J., Wilken, C., & Popovich, J. M. (1992). Clinical assessment of hope. *Issues in Mental Health Nursing, 13*(2), 129–138.

Forbes, S. B. (1994). Hope: An essential human need in the elderly. *Journal of Gerontological Nursing, 20*(6), 5–10.

Fowler, S. B. (1995). Hope: Implications for neuroscience nursing. *Journal of Neuroscience Nursing, 27*(3), 298-304.

Frankl, V. E. (1962). *Man's search for meaning* (3rd ed.). New York: Simon & Schuster. (Original work published 1946)

Fromm, E. (1968). *The revolution of hope.* New York: Harper & Row.

Fryback, P. B. (1993). Health for people with a terminal diagnosis. *Nursing Science Quarterly, 6*, 147–159.

Gamlin, R., & Kinghorn, S. (1995). Using hope to cope with loss and grief. *Nursing Standard, 9*(48), 33–35.

Gardner, W. E. (1985). Hope: A factor in actualizing the young adult Black male. Special Issue: The Black male: Critical counseling, developmental, and therapeutic issues: II. *Journal of Multicultural Counseling & Development, 13*(3), 130–136.

Gewe, A. (1994). Hope: Moving from theory to practice. *Journal of Christian Nursing, 11*(4), 18–21, 54–55.

Glaser, B. G., & Strauss, A. L. (1967). *The discovery of grounded theory.* New York: Aldine de Gruyter.

Godfrey, J. J. (1987). *A philosophy of human hope.* Dordrecht, The Netherlands: Martinus Nijhoff.

Gottschalk, L. A. (1974). A hope scale applicable to verbal samples. *Archives of General Psychiatry, 30*, 779–785.

Gottschalk, L. A. (1985). Hope and other deterrents to illness. Annual meeting of the American Psychiatric Association (1984, Los Angeles, CA). *American Journal of Psychotherapy, 39*(4), 515–524.

Gottschalk, L. A., Fronczek, J., & Buchsbaum, M. S. (1993). The cerebral neurobiology of hope. *Psychiatry, 56*, 270–281.

Grimm, P. M. (1990). Hope, affect, psychological status and the cancer experience. *Dissertation Abstracts International, 50*(9), 3918–3919-B.

Haase, J. E., Britt, T., Coward, D. D., Leidy, N. K., & Penn, P. E. (1992). Simultaneous concept analysis of spiritual perspective, hope, acceptance, and self-transcendence. *Image: Journal of Nursing Scholarship, 24*(2), 141–147.

Hall, B. A. (1990). The struggle of the diagnosed terminally ill person to maintain hope. *Nursing Science Quarterly, 3,* 177–184.

Hall, B. A. (1994). Ways of maintaining hope in HIV disease. *Research in Nursing and Health, 17*(4), 283–293.

Hanna, F. J. (1991). Suicide and hope: The common ground. *Journal of Mental Health Counseling, 13*(4), 459–472.

Harris, C. B. (1990). Hope: Construct definition and the development of an individual differences scale. *Dissertation Abstracts International, 51*(5), 1552-A. (University Microfilms No. DA9020074)

Harrison, R. L. (1993). The relationship among hope, perceived health status and health-promoting lifestyle among HIV seropositive men. *Dissertation Abstracts International, 54*(3), 1333-B. (University Microfilms No. DA9317666)

Herth, K. (1989). The relationship between level of hope and level of coping response and other variables in patients with cancer. *Oncology Nursing Forum, 16*(1), 67–72.

Herth, K. (1990a). Fostering hope in terminally-ill people. *Journal of Advanced Nursing, 15,* 1250–1259.

Herth, K. (1990b). Relationship of hope, coping styles, concurrent losses, and setting to grief resolution in the elderly widow(er). *Research in Nursing and Health, 13,* 109–117.

Herth, K. (1991). Development and refinement of an instrument to measure hope. *Scholarly Inquiry for Nursing Practice: An International Journal, 5*(1), 39–51.

Herth, K. (1992). Abbreviated instrument to measure hope: Development and psychometric evaluation. *Journal of Advanced Nursing, 17,* 1251–1259.

Herth, K. (1993a). Hope in the family caregiver of terminally ill people. *Journal of Advanced Nursing, 18,* 538–549.

Herth, K. (1993b). Hope in older adults in community and institutional settings. *Issues in Mental Health Nursing, 14,* 139–156.

Hickey, S. S. (1986). Enabling hope. *Cancer Nursing, 9*(3), 133–137.

Hickey, S. S. (1989). Hope as a key element in cancer survivorship. *Journal of Psychology Oncology, 7*(4), 111–118.

Hicks, D., & Holden, C. (1994). Tomorrow's world: Children's hopes and fears for the future. *Educational and Child Psychology, 11*(4), 63–70.

Hinds, P. S. (1988). Adolescent hopefulness in illness and health. *Advances in Nursing Science, 10*(3), 79–88.

Hockley, J. (1993). The concept of hope and the will to live. *Palliative Medicine, 7,* 181–186.

Hoffman, L. W. (1991). Hope and its expressions in psychotherapy: A psychological/theological analysis. *Dissertation Abstracts International, 51*(11), 5576-B.

Holahan, L. (1995). A study of suffering, hope, healing, and demographic factors in persons receiving hemodialysis. *Dissertation Abstracts International, 56*(07), 3693-B. (University Microfilms No. 9539817)

Irving, L. M. (1993). Hope and cancer-related health beliefs, knowledge, and behavior: The advantage of the "negotiated" reality principle. *Dissertation Abstracts International, 54*(4), 2204-B. (University Microfilms No. 9323020)

Jacobson, A. A. (1992). Hope and AIDS. *Dissertation Abstracts International, 52*(11), 6086-B.

Jacoby, R. (1993). 'The miserable hath no other medicine, but hope': Some conceptual considerations on hope and stress. *Stress Medicine, 9*, 61–69.

Jevne, R. (1992). Enhancing hope in the chronically ill. In The National Institutes of Health, Immunity, & Disease (Ed.), *Clinical approaches to behavioral medicine: The healing methods of a new generation* (pp. 127–132). Mansfield Center, CT: Editor.

Jevne, R. F. (1994). *The voice of hope: Heard across the heart of life.* San Diego: LuraMedia.

Johnson, B. P. (1995). One family's experience with head injury: A phenomenological approach. *Journal of Neuroscience Nursing, 27*(2), 112–118.

Kant, I. (1952). The critique of pure reason. In R.M. Hutchins (Ed.), *Great books of the western world. 42. Kant.* Chicago: Encyclopaedia Britannica Inc. (Original work published 1781)

Keith, S. J. (1991). Surviving survivorship: Creating a balance. *Journal of Psychosocial Oncology, 9*(3), 109–115.

Khanobdee, C. (1994). *Hope and social support of Thai women experiencing a miscarriage* [CD ROM]. Abstract from: ProQuest File: Dissertation Abstracts Item: 9434817

Kierkegaard, S. (1980). *The sickness unto death* (V. Hong & E. H. Hong, Eds. & Trans.). Princeton: Princeton University Press. (Original work published 1849)

Kim, T. (1989). Hope as a mode of coping in amyotrophic lateral sclerosis. *Journal of Neuroscience Nursing, 21*(6), 342–347.

Kim, T. S. (1990). Hoping strategies for the amyotrophic lateral sclerosis patient. *Loss, Grief, & Care, 4*(3–4), 239–249.

Kirkpatrick, H., Landeen, J., Byrne, C., Woodside, H., Pawlick, J., & Bernardo, A. (1995). Hope and schizophrenia. *Journal of Psychosocial Nursing, 33*(6), 15–19.

Klenow, D. J. (1991–1992). Emotion and life threatening illness: A typology of hope sources. *Omega: Journal of Death & Dying, 24*(1), 49–60.

Lange, S. P. (1978). Hope. In C. E. Carlson & B. Blackwell (Eds.), *Behavioral concepts and nursing intervention* (2nd ed.) (pp. 171–190). Philadelphia: J. B. Lippincott.

Laskiwski, S., & Morse, J. M. (1993). The patient with spinal cord injury: The modification of hope and expressions of despair. *Canadian Journal of Rehabilitation, 6*(3), 143–153.

Lazarus, R. S., Folkman, S. (1984). Appraisal, coping, and adaptational outcomes. In R. S. Lazarus & S. Folkman (Eds.), *Stress, appraisal and coping* (pp. 181–225). New York: Springer.

LeClair, S. A. (1995). Disease longevity, long-term complications, short-term complications, and hope level of adults with type I diabetes mellitus. *Dissertation Abstracts International, 56*(06), 3127-B. (University Microfilms No. AAI9533393)

Levy, B. (1990). Denial and hope in family members of the traumatically brain-injured. *Dissertation Abstracts International, 51*(1), 435-B. (University Microfilms No. 9016063)

Limandri, B., & Boyle, D. (1978). Instilling hope. *American Journal of Nursing, 78*, 79–80.

Linge, F. R. (1990). Faith, hope, and love: Nontraditional therapy in recovery from serious head injury, a personal account. *Canadian Journal of Psychology, 44*(2), 116–129.

Lynch, W. F. (1965). *Images of hope: Imagination as healer of the hopeless.* Baltimore: Helicon Press.

Marcel, G. (1951). *Homo viator* (E. Craufurd, Trans.). Chicago: Henry Regnery Co.

Marden, M. O., & Rice, M. J. (1995). The use of hope as a coping mechanism in abused women. *Journal of Holistic Nursing, 13*(1), 70–82.

Mays, M. J. (1984). Hope and its relationship to selected variables in the elderly. *Dissertation Abstracts International, 44*(10), 134-A.

McGee, R. F. (1984). Hope: A factor influencing crisis resolution. *Advances in Nursing Science, 6*(4), 34–43.

McGill, J. S. (1992). Functional status as it relates to hope in elders with and without cancer. *Dissertation Abstracts International, 53*(2), 771-B.

McGill, J. S., & Paul, P. B. (1993). Functional status and hope in elderly people with and without cancer. *Oncology Nursing Forum, 20*(8), 1207–1213.

Mehler, J. A., & Argentieri, S. (1989). Hope and hopelessness: A technical problem? *International Journal of Psycho-Analysis, 70*, (Part 2), 295–303.

Menninger, K. (1959). Hope. *International Journal of Psychiatry, 116*, 481–491.

Menuhin, Y. (1974, December 14). Art as hope for humanity. *Saturday Review/World. An Inventory of Hope* (Special Issue), 82–83.

Metz, J. B. (1966). The responsibility of hope. *Philosophy Today, 10*(4/4), 280–287.

Metz, P. (1992). Despair's demand: An appraisal of Kierkegaard's argument for God. *Philosophy of Religion, 32*, 167–182.

Mickley, J. F., & Soeken, K. (1993). Religiousness and hope in Hispanic- and Anglo-American women with breast cancer. *Oncology Nursing Forum, 20*(8), 1171–1177.

Mickley, J. R., Soeken, K., & Belcher, A. (1992). Spiritual well-being, religiousness and hope among women with breast cancer. *Image: Journal of Nursing Scholarship, 24*(4), 267–272.

Miller, J. F. (1985). Inspiring hope. *American Journal of Nursing, 85*(2), 23–25.

Miller, J. F. (1989). Hope-inspiring strategies of the critically ill. *Applied Nursing Research, 2*(1), 23–29.

Miller, J. F. (1991). Developing and maintaining hope in families of the critically ill. *AACN Clinical Issues in Critical Care Nursing, 2*(2), 307–315.

Miller, J. F. (1992). *Coping with chronic illness: Overcoming powerlessness* (2nd ed.). Philadelphia: F. A. Davis.

Miller, J. F., & Powers, M. J. (1988). Development of an instrument to measure hope. *Nursing Research, 37*(1), 6–10.

Mitchell, G. J., & Cody, W. K. (1993). The role of theory in qualitative research. *Nursing Science Quarterly, 6,* 170–178.

Moltmann, J. (1967). *Theology of hope.* New York: Harper & Row.

Morse, J. M., & Doberneck, B. (1995). Delineating the concept of hope. *Image: Journal of Nursing Scholarship, 27*(4), 277–285.

Nekolaichuk, C. L. (1995). An exploration of the meaning of hope in health and illness. *Dissertation Abstracts International, 56*(11), 6445-B. (University Microfilms No. AAINN01738)

Newman, M. A. (1986). *Health as expanding consciousness.* St. Louis: Mosby.

Nowotny, M. L. (1986). Measurement of hope as exhibited by a general adult population after a stressful event. *Dissertation Abstracts International, 47*(08), 3296-B. (University Microfilms No. 8626494)

Nowotny, M. L. (1989). Assessment of hope in patients with cancer: Development of an instrument. *Oncology Nursing Forum, 16*(1), 57–61.

Nowotny, M. L. (1991). Every tomorrow, a vision of hope. *Journal of Psychological Oncology, 9*(3), 117–126.

O'Keefe, S. M. (1993). Correlates of hopefulness in inner-city children: Resilience in context. *Dissertation Abstracts International, 54*(4), 1244-A. (University Microfilms No. DA9314617)

Oliver, H. H. (1974). Hope and knowledge: The epistemic status of religious language. *Cultural Hermeneutics, 2,* 75–88.

O'Malley, P. A., & Menke, E. (1988). Relationship of hope and stress after myocardial infarction. *Heart and Lung, 17*(2), 184–190.

Owen, C. L. (1990). The relationship of selected variables to the level of hope in women with breast cancer. *Dissertation Abstracts International, 51*(5), 2288-B. (University Microfilms No. 9023878)

Owen, D. C. (1989). Nurses' perspectives on the meaning of hope in patients with cancer: A qualitative study. *Oncology Nursing Forum, 16*(1), 75–79.

Parse, R. R. (1981). *Man-living-health: A theory of nursing.* New York: Wiley.

Parse, R. R. (1987). *Nursing science: Major paradigms, theories, and critiques.* Philadelphia: Saunders.

Parse, R. R. (1990). Parse's research methodology with an illustration of the lived experience of hope. *Nursing Science Quarterly, 3,* 9–17.

Parse, R. R. (1992). Human becoming: Parse's theory of nursing. *Nursing Science Quarterly, 5,* 35–42.

Parse, R. R. (1994). Quality of life: Sciencing and living the art of human becoming. *Nursing Science Quarterly, 7*, 16–21.

Parse, R.R. (1995). *Illuminations. The human becoming theory in practice and research.* New York: National League for Nursing Press.

Peck, D. L. (1988). Religious conviction, coping, and hope: The relation between a functional corrector and a future prospect among life without parole inmates. *Case Analysis, 2*(3), 201–219.

Perakyla, A. (1991). Hope work in the care of seriously ill patients. *Qualitative Health Research, 1*(4), 407–433.

Poncar, P. J. (1994). Inspiring hope in the oncology patient. *Journal of Psychosocial Nursing, 32*(1), 33–38.

Popovich, J. M. (1991). Hope, coping and rehabilitation outcomes in stroke patients. *Dissertation Abstracts International, 52*(2), 750-B (University Microfilms No. DA9120838)

Rabkin, J. G., Williams, J. B., Neugebauer, R., Remien, R. H., & Goetz, R. (1990). Maintenance of hope in HIV-spectrum homosexual men. *American Journal of Psychiatry, 147*, 1322–1326.

Raleigh, E. D. (1992). Sources of hope in chronic illness. *Oncology Nursing Forum, 19*(3), 443–448.

Raleigh, E. D., & Boehm, S. (1994). Development of the Multidimensional Hope Scale. *Journal of Nursing Measurement, 2*(2), 155–167.

Range, L. M., & Penton, S. R. (1994). Hope, hopelessness, and suicidality in college students. *Psychological Reports, 75*(Special Issue 1, Part 2), 456–458.

Roberts, P. (1992). I think of Ronald Reagan: Future selves in the present. *International Journal of Aging & Human Development, 34*(2), 91–107.

Rogers, M. (1970). *An introduction to the theoretical basis of nursing.* Philadelphia: Davis.

Ross, L. (1995). The spiritual dimension: Its importance to patients' health, well-being, and quality of life and its implications for nursing practice. *International Journal of Nursing Studies, 32*(5), 457–468.

Ross, T. L. (1995). *The lived experience of hope in young mothers with human immunodeficiency virus infection: A phenomenological inquiry* [CD ROM]. Abstract from: ProQuest File: Dissertation Abstracts Item: 9533351

Rumsfeld, V. (1991). The dance of hope: An inquiry into the psychological nature and function of hope. *Dissertation Abstracts International, 51*(8), 4035-B.

Rustoen, T. (1995). Hope and quality of life, two central issues for cancer patients: A theoretical analysis. *Cancer Nursing, 18*(5), 355–361.

Ruth, J. (1990). Spiritual well-being, religiousness, and hope: Some relationships in a sample of women with breast cancer. *Dissertation Abstracts International, 51*(5), 2288-B.

Ruvelson, L. (1990). The tense tightrope: How patients and their therapists balance hope and hopelessness. *Clinical Social Work Journal, 18*(2), 145–154.

Sardell, A. N., & Trierweiler, S. J. (1993). Disclosing the cancer diagnosis. Procedures that influence patient hopefulness. *Cancer, 72*(11), 3355–3365.

Scanlon, C. (1989). Creating a vision of hope: The challenge of palliative care. *Oncology Nursing Forum, 16*(4), 491–496.

Schorr, J. A., Farnham, R. C., & Ervin, S. M. (1991). Health patterns in aging women as expanding consciousness. *Advances in Nursing Science, 13*(4), 52–63.

Schrag, C. O. (1977). The typology of hope. *Humanitas, 13*(3), 269–281.

Scioli, A. (1991). The development of hope and hopelessness: Structural and functional aspects. *Dissertation Abstracts International, 52*(1), 544B–545B. (University Microfilms No. DA9108029)

Shang, T. C. (1994). Development and testing an instrument of hope: The hope indicator questionnaire. *Dissertation Abstracts International, 56*(05), 2935-B. (University Microfilms No. AAI9527975)

Sherwin, E. D. (1994). Hope and social identity: An investigation into the relationship between the self and the environment. *Dissertation Abstracts International, 55*(10), 4633-B (University Microfilms No. AAI9507152)

Skolny, M. A., & Riehl, J. (1974). Hope: Solving patient and family problems by using a theoretical framework. In J. P. Riehl & C. Roy (Eds.), *Conceptual models for nursing practice*. New York: Appleton-Century-Crofts.

Snyder, C. R. (1989). Reality negotiation: From excuses to hope and beyond. *Journal of Social and Clinical Psychology, 8*, 130–157.

Snyder, C. R. (1995). Conceptualizing, measuring, and nurturing hope. *Journal of Counseling and Development, 73*, 355–360.

Snyder, C. R., Harris, C., Anderson, J. R., Holleran, S. A., Irving, L. M., Sigmon, S. T., Yoshinobu, L., Gibb, J., Langelle, C., & Harney, P. (1991). The will and the ways: Development and validation of an individual-differences measure of hope. *Journal of Personality & Social Psychology, 60*(4), 570–585.

Staats, S. R. (1987). Hope: Expected positive affect in an adult sample. *Journal of Genetic Psychology, 148*(3), 357–364.

Staats, S. R. (1989). Hope: A comparison of two self-report measures for adults. *Journal of Personality Assessment, 53*, 366–375.

Staats, S. R. (1991). Quality of life and affect in older persons: Hope, time frames, and training effects. *Current Psychology: Research & Reviews, 10*(1&2), 21–30.

Staats, S., & Partlo, C. (1993). A brief report on hope in peace and war, and in good times and bad. *Social Indicators Research, 29*(2), 229–243.

Stanley, A. T. (1978). The lived experience of hope: The isolation of discreet descriptive elements common to the experience of hope in healthy young adults. *Dissertation Abstracts International, 39*(03), 1212-B. (University Microfilms No. AAG7816899)

Stassen, M. A., & Staats, S. R. (1988). Hope and happinesss: A comparison of some discrepancies. *Social Indicators Research, 20,* 45–58.

Steindl-Rast, D. (1984). *Gratefulness, the heart of prayer.* New York: Paulist Press.

Stephenson, C. (1991). The concept of hope revisited for nursing. *Journal of Advanced Nursing, 16,* 1456–1461.

Stewart, M. J., & Hirth, A. M. (1994). Hope and social support as coping resources for adults waiting for cardiac transplantation. *Canadian Journal of Nursing Research, 26*(3), 31–48.

Stoner, M. H., & Keampfer, S. H. (1985). Recalled life expectancy information, phase of illness and hope in cancer patients. *Research in Nursing and Health, 8,* 269–274.

Stotland, E. (1969). *The psychology of hope.* San Francisco: Jossey-Bass.

Strong, M. (1974, December 14). The case for optimism. *Saturday Review/World. An Inventory of Hope* (Special Issue), 7–11.

Sutherland, P. M. (1993). *The lived experience of hope: A qualitative study of psychologists* [CD ROM]. Abstract from: ProQuest File: Dissertation Abstracts Item: NN82123.

Tate, D. A. (1992). Health, hope, and healing: A survivor's perspective. In The National Institutes of Health, Immunity, & Disease (Ed.), *Clinical approaches to behavioral medicine: The healing methods of a new generation* (pp. 304–321). Mansfield Center, CT: Editor.

Thompson, M. (1994). Nurturing hope: A vital ingredient in nursing. *Journal of Christian Nursing, 11*(4), 10–17.

Tillich, P. (1980). *The courage to be.* New Haven: Yale University Press.

Tollett, J. H., & Thomas, S. P. (1995). A theory-based nursing intervention to instill hope in homeless veterans. *Advances in Nursing Science, 18*(20), 76–90.

Travelbee, J. (1971). *Interpersonal aspects of nursing.* Philadelphia: F.A. Davis.

Udelman, D. L. (1986). Hope and the immune system. *Stress Medicine, 2,* 7–12.

Udelman, H. D., & Udelman, D. L. (1985). Hope as a factor in remission of illness. *Stress Medicine, 1,* 291–294.

Vaillot, M. C. (1970). Living and dying: Part I. Hope, the restoration of being. *American Journal of Nursing, 70*(2), 268–272.

van Kaam, A. (1976). *The dynamics of spiritual self direction.* Denville, NJ: Dimension Books.

Van Manen, M. (1990). *Researching lived experience.* New York: State University of New York Press.

Vaughn, S. B. (1991). Intersubjectivity as the ground of hope: Psychoanalytic and theological perspectives. *Dissertation Abstracts International, 52*(3), 970-A.

Wagner, A. L. (1993). A journey with breast cancer: Telling my story. In D. A. Gaut & A. Boykin (Eds.), *Caring as healing: Renewal through hope* (pp. 178–182). New York: NLN Press.

Walker, L. O., & Avant, K. C. (1988). *Strategies for theory construction in nursing.* Norwalk, CT: Appleton & Lange.

Wu, K.-W. (1972). Hope and world survival. *Philosophy Forum, 12,* 131–148.

Yancey, D., Greger, H. A., & Coburn, P. (1994). Effects of an adult cancer camp of hope, perceived social support, coping, and mood states. *Oncology Nursing Forum, 21*(4), 727–733.

Yarcheski, A., Scoloveno, M. A., & Mahon, N. E. (1994). Social support and well-being in adolescents: The mediating role of hopefulness. *Nursing Research, 43*(5), 288–292.

Yates, P. (1993). Towards a reconceptualization of hope for patients with a diagnosis of cancer. *Journal of Advanced Nursing, 18,* 701–706.

Zorn, C. (1992). Factors contributing to hope among noninstitutionalized elderly. *Dissertation Abstracts International, 53*(4), 1792-B.

Chapter 3

The Lived Experience of Hope for Australian Families Living with Coronary Disease

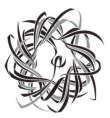

SANDRA SCHMIDT BUNKERS
JOHN DALY

The profession of nursing was called into being for the purpose of contributing to the betterment of humankind. Nursing, from the human becoming perspective, engages in the betterment of humankind by "being with" others as they cocreate meanings of their lived experiences of health (Parse, 1981, 1992, 1994, 1995a, 1995b). Hope is one universal experience of health. The depiction of hope in the presenting research illustrates the lived experiences of persons who cocreate with close others new meaning when faced with the challenges of changing patterns of health. In the following study, families living with coronary disease described hope as an energetic endeavor to find new meaning and purpose with intimate others as challenges to their health and quality of life prevailed. The lived experience of hope emerged in this study as *anticipating possibilities amid anguish, while enduring with vitality in intimate affiliations.*

PARTICIPANTS

Participants in this study included ten persons (three women and seven men) ranging from 34 to 79 years of age. All participants were Australian and were able to understand, read, and speak English and to focus on and describe the lived experience of hope. The discussions were audiotaped and ranged from 30 to 70 minutes, depending on how long the participant wished to discuss hope. All participants were recruited from South Western Sydney (SWS), Sydney, Australia. This is a rapidly expanding/developing area of Sydney. The major portion of the population of Sydney live in the Greater West. SWS is multicultural, with ethnic groups of Vietnamese, Arabs, Aboriginals, Chinese, Lebanese, Cambodian, and European-born Australians. The area is socio-economically disadvantaged with a high birthrate and young population.

DIALOGICAL ENGAGEMENT

The dialogical engagements took place either in the participant's home or at an agreed-upon location. The discussion began with the researcher's statement, "Tell me about the experience of hope in your life."

EXTRACTION-SYNTHESIS

Alan's Story

Alan, a 75-year-old man suffering from coronary disease, states quietly, "Hope is the will to live. If anything happened to me, the Mrs. would have no one to look after her. See, you must have something to keep you going, a goal. And to meet that goal you have to keep fit. It's too easy to die, far too easy. I could just say, 'That's it' and fold up, but I've got to fight this illness. Hope is the determination not to succumb to the illness." Alan goes on to tell of experiencing two heart attacks in a short period of time and struggling with medication-related side effects. "As I was wondering if it was worth carrying on or just letting myself succumb to the heart attack, my granddaughter was killed in a car accident," Alan continues with sadness in his voice.

> She was riding a motorcycle and got run over by a car. Ironically, the first car that run her over just broke her wrist, but the second car run over her and killed her. Looking at things, I said to myself, "Well that's it! She died so I could live." So I was determined from then on to live. All thoughts of anything else was put aside and that was it. I started with five minutes of exercise a day and gradually increased my walking. I'm glad to say now that I am okay. The Mrs. and I have been together now for 52 years, so it is important that we stay together. Hope for me is to be here, to look after the Mrs., and carry on our lives together.

Essences: Participant's Language

1. Hope is a determination to keep fit and carry on while wondering whether to succumb to an illness.
2. Hope involves a goal to look after and be with the Mrs.; for the participant it is knowing that a granddaughter died so he could live.

Essences: Researcher's Language

1. Vitality amid despair surfaces with a tenacious resolve to press onward.
2. Contemplating mortality emerges while engaging with intimate affiliations.

Proposition. The lived experience of hope is contemplating mortality while engaging with intimate affiliations, as vitality amid despair surfaces with a tenacious resolve to press onward.

Alice's Story

Alice, a 68-year-old woman, began her description of hope by talking about her family.

> My hope was always to have a good life for my kids and for ourselves. We decided to come out here from Germany to a new country and start all over again. So that we did. We came without any money, no language speaking . . . nothing. And we have been very lucky so far. The little bit we have makes us happy. We have had a bit of sadness, too. My granddaughter was killed about six months ago. That's something that can't be helped . . . something you hope never to have happen, but it is just one of those things.
>   My experience of hope has included cheating death. Honestly, I'd say about three times. Once when I was 3 years old I fell in a gutter where there was grime. They told me they just got me out at the last minute. Then when I was 10 years old I nearly drowned. When I woke up they had pumped all the water out of me. After that I thought,

"Oh my God, thank God I'm alive." The third time was during a bombing in Germany when the war was on. I was standing outside when we heard a big splinter which landed on my hands, not on my head. I cried again, "Thank God." The splinters cut all my hands open. If they would have hit my head, I would have been gone. That's all the hope I have in my life. I really have a good life and I'm hoping for more of that kind of good life.

Essences: Participant's Language

1. Hope is cheating death three times with the help of God; for the participant it is having a good life with family.
2. Hope is deciding to start over in a new country, considering new projects, and being happy even with the sadness of a granddaughter being killed.

Essences: Researcher's Language

1. Enduring adversity surfaces with intimate alliances.
2. Contemplating innovative endeavors emerges with joy amid anguish.

Proposition. The lived experience of hope is contemplating innovative endeavors emerging with joy amid anguish, as enduring adversity surfaces with intimate alliances.

Thomas's Story

Thomas, a 70-year-old man whose wife had suffered a heart attack, talks openly about hope. He states, "When Emma had her heart attack, naturally, my hope was that she would get better, and I'm still hoping that there will never be another one. That is the biggest thing I have ever hoped for." Thomas goes on, however, and relates other experiences of hope. "When we left Germany, we had no hope at all over there, but we had great hopes about coming to Australia. This country promised anyone that wanted to work anything in the world. That's why we are here and have never gone back. Hope for me is having a good life and something to look forward to. See, today I am getting old, but we still have a really good life." Suddenly Thomas shakes his head and states sadly:

> I come from a big family. My father died when I was 2, so I never had a father. I saw other kids getting brought to school by their father, but I never had that. In those days I was hoping to have a father. I had uncles and all of that, but that's not a father. I don't think it ever occurred to my mother to get married again. It's hard to explain or put in words, but there was no father in my life, and now all these things are coming back to me. My father-in-law wanted me to call him Dad, but I couldn't do that because I never had one. So, when Emma and I got married, we had our own family. My kids at least got a father

and I tried to be a good father. I was pretty strict, but my kids appreciated it. I put them all on the right track and they got their apprenticeships. They still call me today and ask, "Dad, what do you think?" See, that is a good understanding between us, but they always stand on their own feet.

Thomas looks up and says, "I'm too old now for anything, but, anyway, that was always my hope, to have a father. . . . I almost got everything I hoped for."

Essences: Participant's Language

1. Hope is working and having a good life after having no hope; it is something to look forward to.
2. Hope is being a good father even though the participant had none and hoping his wife will get better and not have another heart attack.

Essences: Researcher's Language

1. Anticipating possibilities emerges with contentment amid despair.
2. Achieving a longed-for worthiness surfaces with preserving intimate alliances.

Proposition. The lived experience of hope is anticipating possibilities emerging with contentment amid despair, as achieving a longed-for worthiness surfaces with preserving intimate alliances.

Douglas's Story

"My first experience in relation to hope was when I had melanoma cancer twelve years ago. I had the mole removed and then, several months later, I had a secondary growth which proved to be worse. That is when I started to realize that life could be shorter for me than what I expected. Then, with the heart attack, having gone through the whole cancer thing, the heart attack didn't seem so critical." Douglas, aged 48, relates his experiences of having a melanoma and a heart attack as deeply connected to his understanding of hope. "I just hoped I could survive and I have to this day. I had the heart attack in the hospital, which was a good thing for me. I was close by to everyone who could help me. I hadn't lost all my faculties during the heart attack, so I saw what people were doing for me. That boosted my confidence and gave me a lot of hope. So, hope for me is surviving, overcoming all the odds. For me now, I'm hoping things will be all right for me." Douglas settles comfortably in his chair and continues:

> I started to realize with the melanoma that I had to hope I could beat this thing. I enrolled in a meditation course where with other people we formed a body where we all hoped together that we'd get over the affliction. Also, during that time I was a guinea pig for immunotherapy for melanoma. The hope was to get as much information as possible

about immunotherapy, still in its infancy stage. Also, I believe that religion comes into this in more ways than one. I think belief in a superior being assists me in getting through my affliction. One of the biggest hopes I have is to survive because I'm the breadwinner of the family, and what would happen if I did go? I find a definition of hope difficult, but it is the willingness to live . . . the hope to keep going.

Essences: Participant's Language

1. Hope is meditating with other people to beat melanoma after realizing life could be shorter than expected; it is going through immunotherapy to get over the affliction.
2. Hope is the belief in a superior being and people doing things for the participant during a heart attack; it is surviving to be the breadwinner in the family with a willingness to live and keep going.

Essences: Researcher's Language

1. Communal anticipation of treasured possibilities emerges with the awareness of impermanence.
2. Hope is vital endurance amid peril with the ministry of solemn alliances.

Proposition. The lived experience of hope is communal anticipation of treasured possibilities emerging with the awareness of impermanence, while vital endurance amid peril surfaces with the ministry of solemn alliances.

Donna's Story

Donna, 34 years old, began the description of hope in her life by telling about what she calls, "a really bad experience."

> I had an accident and fell on my head and developed a concussion and bruising of the brain. I started seeing doctors, and six months later I started developing anxiety attacks. It just felt like I was dying . . . there was no hope. I was always in bed; I could not get dressed or drive anywhere. After two years with anxiety attacks I was depressed, I'd lost weight, had suicidal feelings, and I could not look after my four kids any more. That is when I met a spiritual healer.

Donna smiles briefly as she begins to describe her experience with the spiritual healer.

> He taught me so much about positive thinking, meditation, and looking at life differently. I've become so strong. I love life, as a matter of fact. I wake up and thank God for each day.
> Hope is a spiritual healer who worked through God with me and I became stronger and feeling really good. The specialists thought I

had a pituitary tumor. My spiritual healer started sending out the "Light," that's meditation with a sending out of the "Light," into my pituitary gland, trying to break the tumor. After a few weeks I went for another blood test and then they were going to put me in the hospital. The specialist said the pituitary tumor had disappeared. So hope for me is a miracle. It is also looking at my four children and appreciating their help to go on. I will say it again: hope is letting God enter your heart. That is your best hope in life. But that happens through someone who puts you on the right track. For me it was my spiritual healer; otherwise, I would not have known hope.

Essences: Participant's Language

1. Hope involves four children and a spiritual healer who worked through God with the participant; it encompasses a miracle, meditation, positive thinking, and looking at life differently.
2. Hope is living every day feeling stronger after experiencing suicidal feelings, anxiety attacks, fear, and no hope.

Essences: Researcher's Language

1. Communing with nurturing affiliations arises with the mystery of envisioning anew.
2. Endurance surfaces with vitality amid trepidation.

Proposition. Hope is communing with nurturing affiliations as mystery arises with envisioning anew, while endurance surfaces with vitality amid trepidation.

Carolyn's Story

"I will start with what I hoped would change in my life." Carolyn, aged 50 and facing cardiac surgery, begins describing hope in her life by talking about some of her most traumatic times.

> One of the times I felt I needed hope was when my father died. I was 12 years old. My mother didn't really worry too much about us children. I felt I had to be the adult. Ten days after my father died I went to bed, and when I woke up the next morning my hair was white. The doctor said that happened because of stress. Then, at 15 I was thrown out of my mother's house and had to live on my own. So I grew up fast. That's when I met my first husband. My real hope came when I met him. I grew to love him and we had a good life.

Carolyn shakes her head slightly and continues.

> I lost a baby when I was six months pregnant. The baby was growing three times the rate it should and it burst the sac. I felt like I wanted to

die . . . like it was the end of my life. My daughter, who was in school, and my six-month-old baby pulled me through that time. I said to myself, "C., you've got to get a hold of yourself. These are your two children; they are alive. They need you." That's when my hope began.

Carolyn shifts the conversation to the present.

My first husband died, and that was a bad time. But I've met my second husband now and we have a great relationship. Everything has gone fine until my heart attack. It feels to be the worst thing that's happened to me because it's so recent. After my heart attack, I changed my lifestyle. I'm eating better. I'm doing everything to make myself have a healthy heart. I was picking up on exercise until I had the angiogram. Now, I've got to survive this operation and go on. I have every reason to live. I have two lovely children, five grandchildren, and a good husband. These things are my hope.

Essences: Participant's Language

1. Hope is her two children and a love relationship with a husband.
2. Hope is wanting to survive after wanting to die; it involves changing a lifestyle and having reasons to go on.

Essences: Researcher's Language

1. Promise arises in engaging with nurturing others.
2. Overriding desire to prevail surfaces with envisioned possibilities amid despair.

Proposition. The lived experience of hope is promise arising in engaging with nurturing others, as an overriding desire to prevail surfaces with envisioned possibilities amid despair.

Regina's Story

"I pray quite a lot to God. If you need hope, you just pray and you get it. God's there to help." Regina, a 77-year-old who experienced a heart attack several months ago, talks about her relationship with God and her family as avenues of hope. "God is here to help, but if it doesn't work out, well then, I just think maybe it is better up there. But I don't want to go yet. I want to stay with my daughters and grandkids. I love them. I think they give me hope because they love me." Regina then discusses her heart attack.

I had quite a shock. I'd never been sick before. My kids called me the "gadabout gran" because I used to put on concerts and things like that. I just prayed and prayed that it wasn't the end for me. I did start to give up until my children came in to see me, my three daughters.

They were pretty upset. My youngest daughter had to be taken out of the room because she was so upset. I thought, "I have got to be all right." So, when she came next time I was cheerful and I think that was giving me hope . . . seeing them smile again and saying "you're going to be okay." They gave me a push and I stopped feeling sorry for myself. What has given me a lot of hope is knowing that I'm doing well. I try not to overwork. I hope to continue for a few more years feeling as good as I do. I am about watching concerts now instead of being in them. I go out in town and things like that. I go to the chiropractor to keep fit. Hope, you see, for me is something you want. If you want something enough then you don't give up. It means wanting something and saying "I'm going to get better" and kind of push like that and not give way. I told myself I was going to get well and I did.

Essences: Participant's Language

1. Hope involves prayer for God's help and love of children and grandchildren.
2. Hope is a push to not give up; it involves keeping fit, continuing on, and wanting something.

Essences: Researcher's Language

1. Engaging with intimate alliances surfaces with envisioning possibilities.
2. Pressing beyond with the desired emerges with vitality amid anguish.

Proposition. The lived experience of hope is envisioning possibilities while engaging with intimate alliances, as pressing beyond with the desired emerges with vitality amid anguish.

Tommy's Story

"To talk about hope, you have got to look at tragedy rather than anything else." Thus began this 79-year-old man's description of hope in his life. "My first wife was at the theater and she had a cerebral thrombosis. She did not survive more than a few hours. I had two boys, one of them 9 and the other age 11. I had to explain to them that Mommy wasn't coming home. That experience left me in a hopeless position. But the thing that gave me strength was the drive to carry on because of the two boys. They gave me the courage to carry on." Tommy smiles briefly and continues:

I remarried, a woman who had one boy. We had many happy years together. So, when you have tragedy, you have to remember there is also a sunny side that can come back to you. I never forgot my first love, but I loved another. Unfortunately, cancer was another killer and I found myself alone again. This time, however, the boys were married and so I found it a lot more difficult because I was older and I had no one dependent on me. That is when my religion gave me great strength. Religion is the thing that got me out of that tragedy. I have remarried again. So, I say, "Don't give up hope; there is a sunny day ahead." Now, I've had a heart attack. When you have a heart attack, it flaws you. I ask, "What's going to happen? Does this mean I am going to die?" I do feel like I'm getting better. It is worthwhile to carry on because I have so much to live for. I have a home, a wife, and I live near the water. I have a boat and a car. Life is good. It is too good to throw away. I need to keep going and make use of every day because every day is something I will treasure for the rest of my life. Hope is looking forward and living a life according to the law of man and the laws of God. A person must always fight on and look forward with hope.

Essences: Participant's Language

1. Hope involves having two boys, the love of a wife, and religion giving strength and courage to fight on in the face of tragedy and hopelessness.
2. Hope is looking forward to sunny days ahead and making use of every day while living a good life according to God's laws.

Essences: Researcher's Language

1. Intimate affiliations surface with enduring amid anguish.
2. Anticipating possibilities emerges while propelling onward with cherished endeavors.

Proposition. The lived experience of hope is anticipating possibilities in propelling onward with cherished endeavors, as intimate affiliations surface with enduring amid anguish.

Patrick's Story

Patrick, a 70-year-old man who has struggled through a heart attack and surgery from cancer, describes hope as "a great family affair." Patrick states:

> When I lost my wife many, many years ago, that was the biggest downfall I have ever had. That was 1974. I had to raise four kids and give them a good home life. And that is exactly what happened. We pulled together and the family life has been great. We had our ups and downs. I hoped that everything would go well and it has. It was a matter of keeping going and doing what had to be done. I carried on. Now, of course, some of the kids have moved away, but we still keep in contact.
>
> Then, the next event was the cancer followed by my heart attack in '96. I have overcome these things. I have to go in for examinations

like a review of my heart. That doesn't matter. I'm going to do it, and, hopefully, there's going to be no change. The hope that I have is to keep the quality of life I have now until the day I die. I don't look on the dark side of life or the dark side of past experiences. That is all gone . . . water under the bridge. I love life, I love doing the things a normal retiree does. Hope for me is to expect more life, to expect a beautiful living world, to expect more of what I'm going through right now. I have the support of my kids and my friends. I want to keep on living, playing golf, doing my walking, going to the theater, and making more friends. Tomorrow is going to be a beautiful day and if you live through the day, then the bonus comes over night time and is that we are still here. It is like going to work and coming home. The bonus of coming home is your family. I have right now a continuing beautiful lifestyle. I hope to live to an old age.

Essences: Participant's Language

1. Hope is pulling together as a family after losing his wife; it is the support of children and friends.
2. Hope is expecting a beautiful life and a beautiful living world involving quality of life with keeping on living, playing golf, walking, going to the theater, and overcoming a heart attack and cancer.

Essences: Researcher's Language

1. Intimate alliances surface in withstanding adversity.
2. Envisioning possibilities emerges with pressing on with prized endeavors.

Proposition. The lived experience of hope is envisioning possibilities in pressing on with prized endeavors, as intimate alliances surface in withstanding adversity.

Vincent's Story

I think I found hope after my son died. He committed suicide. He had been sexually assaulted when he was young and was tormented by that. When my wife and I found him that night hanging, we said, "He's at peace now." I knew I'd done everything I could for him. I'd taken him to counseling for over fifteen years. I found hope because I never neglected the boy. I suppose the hope is that when others realize it happened to our son, people who it has happened to come forward and speak openly about being sexually assaulted. I think it gives people hope to be able to openly discuss and talk about these things. So we have been able to support our family and his close friends and that's what got us through this.

Vincent, 54 years old, discusses hope in light of the hardships in his life.

I'm a person who has had heaps of problems throughout my life. I had a hard bringing up with an alcoholic father. My mother died when I was about 20 and I took care of my sister who was only 9. It gave me hope to keep going, realizing that I had to look after my sister and bring her up. I've always looked after the underprivileged and it was people who were worse off then me that gave me the strength to keep going. I've had a back injury, back surgery, infection in my leg, and then I had a heart attack, which was a terrifying thing. When in the hospital, the specialist told my wife to bring the children. Once I'd seen my kids and grandkids there, that gave me the determination to keep going. I pulled through. A person has to go to their limits. Thinking positive has a lot to do with hope. Hope to me is positive thinking. Hope is being able to talk with people.

Vincent smiles briefly and concludes, "I would be very distressed if I couldn't go out and do something for somebody. That is what my whole life has revolved around."

Essences: Participant's Language

1. Hope is thinking positive, having the support of family and friends, and doing something for family and the underprivileged.
2. Hope involves having the determination to keep going in spite of multiple problems such as surgery, a leg infection, and a heart attack.

Essences: Researcher's Language

1. Anticipating possibilities emerges with benevolent alliances.
2. The tenacity to prevail surfaces with pressing onward amid adversity.

Proposition. The lived experience of hope is anticipating possibilities emerging with benevolent alliances, as the tenacity to prevail surfaces while pressing onward amid adversity.

FINDINGS AND RELATED HUMAN BECOMING LITERATURE

Propositions from all ten participants revealed three core concepts: *anticipating possibilities amid anguish, enduring with vitality,* and *intimate affiliations.* Through heuristic interpretation, the core concepts were taken up levels of abstraction to the theoretical level where the lived experience of hope is understood to be *imaging powering in connecting-separating.* Table 1 displays the core concepts and their progression across levels of abstraction.

The central finding of this study is *the lived experience of hope is anticipating possibilities amid anguish, while enduring with vitality in intimate affiliations.* Propositions of all ten participants describe the various unique ways the meaning of hope was articulated.

TABLE 1.
Progressive Abstraction of Core Concepts with Heuristic Interpretation

Core Concepts	Structural Transposition	Conceptual Integration
Anticipating possibilities amid anguish	Picturing possibles amid tribulation	Imaging
Enduring with vitality	Persevering steadfastness	Powering
Intimate affiliations	Togetherness-aloneness	Connecting-separating

Structure

The lived experience of hope is anticipating possibilities amid anguish, while enduring with vitality in intimate affiliations.

Structural Transposition

The lived experience of hope is picturing possibles amid tribulation, while persevering steadfastness surfaces in togetherness-aloneness.

Conceptual Integration

The lived experience of hope is imaging powering in connecting-separating.

Heuristic Interpretation

Structural transposition begins the process of connecting the findings of the research with the theory of human becoming. The meaning of hope at the structural transposition level of abstraction is *picturing possibles amid tribulation, while persevering steadfastness surfaces in togetherness-aloneness.* At the conceptual integration level, hope is *imaging powering in connecting-separating.*

The first core concept, anticipating possibilities amid anguish, is picturing what can be while struggling with adversity in the moment. The participants described engaging with meaning moments of pain and despair while foreseeing a promise for a new tomorrow. All participants, in experiencing changes in patterns of living health, discovered new insights concerning life's purpose in moving onward. Typical comments of participants follow: "I look at life differently now; I love life, as a matter of fact"; "I have every reason to go on"; "I just told myself that this is just a little relapse. I am going to get well, and I did." The concept of anticipating possibilities amid anguish was derived from essences from the propositions. (See Table 2.)

Related literature supporting the notion of anticipating possibilities amid anguish includes Parse's (1997) study on joy-sorrow, where the concept of "pleasure amid adversity" describes the way people live "the commingling of

TABLE 2.
Essences of the Concept Anticipating Possibilities Amid Anguish

Concept:	**Anticipating possibilities amid anguish**
Structural Transposition:	**Picturing possibilities amid tribulation**
Conceptual Integration:	**Imaging**

1. contemplating mortality . . . amid despair
2. contemplating innovative endeavors . . . amid anguish
3. anticipating possibilities . . . amid despair
4. communal anticipation of treasured possibilities . . . amid peril
5. envisioning anew . . . amid trepidation
6. promise . . . envisioned possibilities amid despair
7. envisioning possibilities . . . amid despair
8. anticipating possibilities . . . amid anguish
9. envisioning possibilities . . . withstanding adversity
10. anticipating possibilities . . . amid adversity

pleasure with the arduous moments of adversity" (p. 84), and Parse's (1990) study of hope in which the concept of "persistent picturing of possibles" involves "the explicit-tacit knowing that their situations would be better" (p. 15). Similarly, Bunkers (1998), in a study on considering tomorrow, discovered the notion of "contemplating desired endeavors" and linked it to "pondering the possibles" (p. 60).

Anticipating possibilities amid anguish is picturing possibles amid tribulation in imaging tomorrow and is connected with the first principle of human becoming. Imaging is "languaging imaged values through speaking - being silent and moving - being still" (Parse, 1995a, p. 7). The participants languaged new meanings of their changing health patterns as they coconstructed with others hope for a better day.

Enduring with vitality, the second core concept, reflects the resolve to prevail in the face of peril. All participants described pushing onward while resisting succumbing to experiences they described as "bad experiences," "traumatic times," and "tragedy." Statements depicting this pushing-resisting process included the following: "The doctor said I'd never walk again without a limp and that made me more determined than ever that I wouldn't do that"; "I was getting better . . . life was so good, too good to throw away . . . I had to keep going"; "Hope is overcoming all the odds." The concept of enduring with vitality was derived from the essences from the propositions. (See Table 3.)

TABLE 3.
Essences of the Concept Enduring with Vitality

Concept:	Enduring with vitality
Structural Transposition:	Persevering steadfastness
Conceptual Integration:	Powering

1. tenacious resolve to press onward
2. enduring adversity . . . with joy
3. achieving a longed-for worthiness . . . with contentment
4. vital endurance
5. endurance surfaces with vitality
6. overriding desire to prevail
7. pressing beyond with the desired emerges with vitality
8. propelling onward with cherished endeavors . . . enduring
9. pressing on with prized endeavors
10. the tenacity to prevail surfaces with pressing onward

Literature consistent with the notion of enduring with vitality includes Smith's (1990) discovery of "sculpting new lifeways in turbulent change through affirming self" for persons struggling through a difficult time. Likewise, Rendon, Sales, Leal, and Pique (1995), in studying the lived experience of aging, found that "forceful enlivening" "reflects a sustaining resolve, a determined curiosity to move forward as possibles emerge" (p. 156). Enduring with vitality is an energizing process of pressing onward in tragedy with tenacious commitment to life dreams. Enduring with vitality reflects an intentional sculpting of new patterns of living health and is lived in the persevering steadfastness of powering. Powering, from a human becoming perspective, is "the force of human existence and underpins the courage to be" (Parse, 1981, p. 57). Hope was lived by the participants in a relentless pressing onward with forbearance for what was yet-to-be.

The third core concept, intimate affiliations, refers to the importance of being with close others in special ways. All participants, in describing experiences of hope, spoke about significant relationships. Participants said: "My hope is the will to live, to look after the Mrs. and carry on our lives together"; "I saw what people were doing for me and that boosted my confidence"; "Hope for me is that I can keep helping people . . . to keep talking to people"; "Hope is looking at my four children. . . . Hope is God because I know through God I've come so far"; "I had to carry on because of the two boys, and that was the thing that kept me going"; "I want to stay with my kids, and I've got grandkids. I love them, too. I think they all give me hope because they love me and couldn't believe I was sick." The concept of intimate affiliations was derived from the essences from the propositions. (See Table 4.)

Human becoming literature consistent with the concept of intimate affiliations as integral in living hope includes Parse's (1997) study on joy-sorrow, where "benevolent engagements" were described by participants as "shifting intimate patterns of relating [in] extending their efforts and time to assist strangers in various ways" (p. 85). Also, Parse's (1996) study on quality of life for persons living with Alzheimer's disease uncovered the theme of "close to–apart from" as "desiring cherished intimacies yields with inevitable distancing in the vicissitudes of life" (p. 129). Bunkers (1998), in her research on considering tomorrow, identified "intimate alliances with isolating distance," (p. 60) which depicted being close to those loved and yet feeling isolated from the community.

Intimate affiliations describes the togetherness with close others cherished by the participants while feeling alone in their struggles with changing patterns of health. This togetherness with aloneness is the process of connecting-separating with persons, ideas, and events as participants live their hope. Connecting-separating is linked to the second principle of the human becoming theory and involves two or more people coming together "in an intersubjective relationship; that is, they are truly present to each other, simultaneously unifying and separating as their togetherness evolves. While these individuals

TABLE 4.
Essences of the Concept Intimate Affiliations

Concept:	Intimate affiliations
Structural Transposition:	Togetherness-aloneness
Conceptual Integration:	Connecting-separating

1. engaging with intimate affiliations
2. intimate alliances
3. preserving intimate alliances
4. the ministry of solemn alliances
5. communing with nurturing affiliations
6. engaging with nurturing others
7. engaging with intimate alliances
8. intimate affiliations
9. intimate alliances
10. benevolent alliances

are participating with each other, they all at once are separating from others" (Parse, 1981, p. 54). Hope, for these participants, was lived by connecting with important others while at the same time being alone in the struggle to find meaning in challenging life experiences.

Implications for research and practice derived from the findings of this study are described in the final chapter of this book with findings from the other studies.

REFERENCES

Bunkers, S. S. (1998). Considering tomorrow: Parse's theory-guided research. *Nursing Science Quarterly, 11,* 56–63.

Parse, R. R. (1981). *Man-living-health: A theory of nursing.* New York: Wiley.

Parse, R. R. (1987). *Nursing science: Major paradigms, theories, and critiques.* Philadelphia: W. B. Saunders.

Parse, R. R. (1990). Parse's research methodology with an illustration of the lived experience of hope. *Nursing Science Quarterly, 3,* 9–17.

Parse, R. R. (1992). Human becoming: Parse's theory of nursing. *Nursing Science Quarterly, 3,* 9–17.

Parse, R. R. (1994). Quality of life: Sciencing and living the art of human becoming. *Nursing Science Quarterly, 7,* 16–21.

Parse, R. R. (1995a). The human becoming theory. In R. R. Parse (Ed.), *Illuminations: The human becoming theory in practice and research* (pp. 5–8). New York: National League for Nursing Press.

Parse, R. R. (1995b). Research with the human becoming theory. In R. R. Parse (Ed.), *Illuminations: The human becoming theory in practice and research* (pp. 151–157). New York: National League for Nursing Press.

Parse, R. R. (1996). Quality of life for persons living with Alzheimer's disease: The human becoming perspective. *Nursing Science Quarterly, 9,* 126–133.

Parse, R. R. (1997). Joy-sorrow: A study using the Parse research method. *Nursing Science Quarterly, 10,* 80–87.

Rendon, D. , Sales, R. , Leal, J. , & Pique, J. (1995). The lived experience of aging in community-dwelling elders in Valencia, Spain: A phenomenological study. *Nursing Science Quarterly, 8,* 152–157.

Smith, M. (1990). Struggling through a difficult time for unemployed persons. *Nursing Science Quarterly, 3,* 18–27.

Chapter 4

The Lived Experience of Hope
for Family Members of Persons Living
in a Canadian Chronic Care Facility

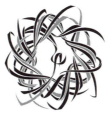

ROSEMARIE RIZZO PARSE

"Hope is sky blue and maybe the top of a mountain early in the morning when the sun is shining on it." "What you are hoping for is a better quality of life for the one you love." "Hope springs eternal." "Hope is beautiful." "Hope keeps us alive." "I never give up hoping." These expressions of hope surfaced during dialogical engagements with ten family members of persons who live in a chronic care setting in Canada.

PARTICIPANTS

Participants in this study were from varied ethnic backgrounds, including Greek, Portuguese, English, Polish, and French Canadian. Hope was described as important to these family members as an intentional way to move beyond day-to-day joys and sorrows. Family members were inspired by one another and by even the little changes in their loved ones, which kept their flame of hope burning as they pictured dreams for tomorrow. The lived experience of hope arose in this study as *persistently anticipating possibilities amid adversity, as intimate engagements emerge with expanding horizons.*

DIALOGICAL ENGAGEMENT

The dialogical engagements with ten family members of persons who live in a chronic care setting in Canada took place in a quiet environment in an institutional facility.

EXTRACTION-SYNTHESIS

Helen's Story

Helen is an 81-year-old woman whose husband had an accident from which he "will not recover." He remains in a chronic care facility. Helen says she has no hope now for her husband's recovery and that it is a challenge to improve his quality of life—"the little things in daily living." She wants to live longer than her husband because she wants to make sure he gets the best attention that can be provided. She and her husband had a wonderful life together before his accident. Helen has been inspired by other patients' family members' stories about their loved ones with brain injuries and has admired how others in similar situations keep on going. She says she has acquired new friends through this experience upon whom she can rely, and this is hopeful. She has faith in God and is grateful to people who helped her to have hope during difficult times.

Essences: Participant's Language

1. Hope is what keeps the participant going; it is a challenge to keep trying to improve her husband's quality of life while facing the reality that there may be no hope. She has great hope for whatever time is left for her and her husband.

2. Hope is being inspired to see things differently by others who have been in situations like hers for many years, and this keeps the participant's perspective in line. She has children, grandchildren, great faith in God, and now some close friends of a different nationality that she would not have had if her husband were not confined to a chronic care facility.

Essences: Researcher's Language

1. Anticipation of persevering amid despair arises with contentment in the moment.
2. Enlivening engagements emerge with clarity of view, expanding horizons.

Proposition. The lived experience of hope is anticipation of persevering amid despair arising with contentment in the moment, as enlivening engagements emerge with clarity of view, expanding horizons.

Sophie's Story

Sophie is a Polish Canadian who says she was born with hope; it is in every minute of her life. She believes people can have hope if they are optimistic. She never gives up hope, even though she had a "hard life" raising her daughter alone for six years after her husband left Poland for Canada. Even after her husband brought her and her daughter to Canada, Sophie had a hard time. She did not speak English or French and her husband left her. She worked two jobs, learned English, made new friends, and remarried, with many struggles for survival. She says that she survived because of hope; she makes things happen. Even though her husband is now ill and in need of therapy, Sophie says she keeps looking forward with hope, for she never says "I can't." She says many people visit her and talk to her about their problems and leave her feeling "lighter." She believes this is giving hope to others. Hope is "something beautiful" and "we don't know what is going to happen. . . . If something goes wrong, I cancel the wrong so fast because my hope is stronger than the 'bad things.'"

Essences: Participant's Language

1. Hope is an optimism you are born with, and it grows with the mutual support of family and friends, but the participant herself makes things happen. She never says she can't; she tries—that is hope.
2. Hope is looking forward to what life could be; it is something very high and it is unclear what will happen, but the participant planned for survival through many disappointments by learning English and typing.

Essences: Researcher's Language

1. An inherent anticipation of possibilities with resolute perseverance arises with nurturing engagements.
2. Persistent uplifting envisioning amid the unsureness of disillusionment surfaces with a deliberate expanding of horizons.

Proposition. The lived experience of hope is an inherent anticipation of possibilities with resolute perseverance arising with nurturing engagements, while a persistent uplifting envisioning amid the unsureness of disillusionment surfaces with a deliberate expanding of horizons.

Georgia's Story

Georgia is a Greek Canadian who says hope is waiting for, expecting, and believing something; it is working hard to make things better. She believes everyone lives with hope because "if there is no hope, there is no life." She says there is always hope for a better tomorrow since hope is beautiful and dreams are hopes. Georgia's daughter has multiple sclerosis, and, even though her daughter continues to worsen, Georgia continues to have hope that doctors will find something to help her daughter. She has great hope for her other daughter, who has many dreams also, and she prays a lot. She believes everyone must have hope.

Essences: Participant's Language

1. Hope is waiting for, expecting, and believing something, since if there is no hope, there is no life. With hope you work hard and try for a better tomorrow.
2. Hope is a dream, hoping for a daughter to finish school, for a cure for multiple sclerosis, for business to go well, just to be free of problems, and have your dreams come true.

Essences: Researcher's Language

1. Prevailing anticipation of possibilities amid potential despair emerges with resolute perseverance.
2. Persistent envisioning of cherished affiliations arises with the unburdening of an expanding view.

Proposition. The lived experience of hope is a prevailing anticipation of possibilities amid potential despair emerging with resolute perseverance, as persistent envisioning of cherished affiliations arises with the unburdening of an expanding view.

Teresa's Story

Teresa is a Portuguese Canadian who believes hope is something that a person wishes for in life, like health, a better day, a happy family, or accomplishing something. Hope is a dream for a good life, even though there are many struggles. Teresa said she hoped she could take her mother home from the chronic care facility because her own life would be better if she could, but she is unable to stay at home to give her mother care. Continuing to hope makes life easier; even if "bad things happen," one can hope for a better day ahead. "Hope is a good thing."

Essences: Participant's Language

1. Hope is a wish for or a dream of something or someone in life, like health, a better day, a happy family, or accomplishing something for the next day or next month.
2. Hope is a positive feeling, without negative thoughts, yet not all that is hoped comes true. But living on hope makes life easier even if "bad things happen."

Essences: Researcher's Language

1. Envisioning possibilities with cherished engagements arises with contemplating expanding horizons.
2. Affirming musings amid potential adversity surfaces with an unburdening.

Proposition. The lived experience of hope is envisioning possibilities with cherished engagements in contemplating expanding horizons, as affirming musings amid potential adversity surfaces with an unburdening.

Margarita's Story

Margarita, a Colombian Canadian, believes hope is beautiful, keeps one alive, and is what makes a person carry on in life. Hope is something to look forward to when planning for a better day, no matter what the obstacles are along the way. Margarita says she lives on hope for a better tomorrow and this helps to accomplish dreams for the future. Hope "helps you go ahead, go forward" and it makes things easier when life is hard.

Essences: Participant's Language

1. Hope is beautiful; it keeps you alive, and when life is hard, it makes it easier and helps you go forward no matter what obstacles are along the way.
2. Hope is looking forward to something, like a better day, or wishing that something will come true and dreams will be accomplished.

Essences: Researcher's Language

1. An uplifting enlivenment in moving beyond emerges with an unburdening amid the adverse.
2. Anticipating new horizons arises with resolutely envisioning possibilities of cherished fulfillment.

Proposition. The lived experience of hope is an uplifting enlivenment in moving beyond that emerges with an unburdening amid the adverse, as anticipating new horizons arises with resolutely envisioning the possibilities of cherished fulfillment.

Maryanne's Story

Maryanne, whose sister has been in chronic care facility since an accident several years earlier, believes hope is a "blue sky and maybe the top of a mountain early in the morning when the sun is shining on it." Maryanne says hope is more than a pleasant expectation, it's an "aspiration—you have optimism, trust, and faith." She believes hope is part of the present and the future and is always there; it is the opposite of despair. She said that at first, after her sister's accident, people gave her materials to read about head injury and often talked about denial without offering to help or understanding the situation. Maryanne believes that hope is "out of the realm of science" and that hope is nourished by nurses and other families in similar situations. She hopes her sister will have less pain, more joy, and a better quality of life, and she believes that deep down her sister hasn't changed.

Essences: Participant's Language

1. Hope is a blue sky and maybe the top of a mountain early in the morning when the sun is shining on it. It is visualizing less pain, more joy, and a better quality of life for her sister, who the participant firmly believes did not really change deep down since her accident.
2. Hope is future-oriented, yet the seeds are in the present, and it is an aspiration, an optimism inspired by others, an unrealized expectation, the opposite of despair, the other side of fear, often disturbingly mistaken for denial.

Essences: Researcher's Language

1. Envisioning a bright uplifting moment with intimate engagements arises with contemplating an affirming shift with a persistent stance.
2. Anticipating the will-be in the now emerges with new possibilities amid disillusionment.

Proposition. The lived experience of hope is envisioning a bright uplifting moment with intimate engagements that arises with contemplating an affirming shift with a persistent stance, while anticipating the will-be in the now emerges with new possibilities amid disillusionment.

Alice's Story

Alice, 81 years old, believes that where there is life, there is hope. She says, "Hope springs eternal," and she wishes for something better for everyone. Alice says, "Hope is everything; without hope you have nothing." She recalled a difficult time when she was 12 years old; her mother told her she was going to die and Alice remembers saying, "Mommy, where there is life, there is hope." She hopes now for a nice place for her husband to live. She says she is forever hoping that there is a happy outcome; without this she would be unhappy.

Essences: Participant's Language

1. Hope springs eternal and is a wish for something better for close others.
2. Hope is everything; without it one has nothing. Where there is life, there is hope, even during difficult times.

Essences: Researcher's Language

1. Infinite anticipation of possibilities emerges with nurturing affiliations.
2. A prevailing expanding view amid potential adversity arises with obscuring a vacuum.

Proposition. The lived experience of hope is the infinite anticipation of possibilities emerging with nurturing affiliations, as a prevailing expanding view amid potential adversity arises with obscuring a vacuum.

Simone and Jacque's Story

Simone and Jacque are French Canadians who believe hope is never giving up, even in the struggles of life and especially in relation to their daughter's situation after a severe accident. Hope is appreciating small progress in the recovery of their daughter who had the accident many years ago. Sharing problems with others in similar situations helped to keep hope alive. Simone believes hope is always there, and when "things get low, hope is inside me and that is where I go to get it." Simone and Jacque pray a lot and stay closely connected to their family members and friends. They believe that hope is not superficial but a part of daily life, and their belief in God keeps them going.

Essences: Participant's Language

1. Hope is never giving up the struggle, even with only a little bit of progress in the recovery of a loved one; it is having a belief in God with expectations, praying, and keeping going.
2. Hope is always there inside when things get low; it is not superficial or despairing but living life.

Essences: Researcher's Language

1. Resolute anticipation emerges with intimate solemn engagements.
2. Persistent envisioning amid disillusionment arises with an expanding view.

Proposition. The lived experience of hope is resolute anticipation of possibilities emerging with intimate solemn engagements, while persistent envisioning amid disillusionment arises with an expanding view.

Anne's Story

Anne, who grew up among close family and helpful friends, is 75 years old. She brought her brother to the long-term care facility and says hope is "having a feeling of confidence in your own day-to-day encounters, whether they are pleasant or unpleasant." She believes that successes are built on hope and struggles, and "nothing is hopeless, everything can be overcome." Even though she lived during the Great Depression and had lots of discouraging, difficult times, she was always hopeful and confident. Anne says hope is "an attitude of mine." She believes it helps to solve large and small problems and gives one confidence to accept the goodwill of others who share similar situations. Hope, she says, is a "thread of life."

Essences: Participant's Language

1. Hope is a confidence-builder in day-to-day encounters, pleasant or unpleasant; everything can be overcome, nothing is hopeless, and one can plan for the future.
2. Successes are built on hope and struggles, and things are often done to overcome lack of hope. It is the greatest thread of life in helping to solve problems.

Essences: Researcher's Language

1. A resolute sureness with diverse engagements emerges with decisiveness for expanding the view.
2. Fulfillment arises with the weaving of a persistent envisioning of unburdening possibilities, despite disheartenments.

Proposition. The lived experience of hope is a resolute sureness with diverse engagements emerging with decisiveness for expanding the view, as fulfillment arises with the weaving of a persistent envisioning of unburdening possibilities, despite disheartenments.

Elizabeth's Story

Elizabeth says "hope is the basis for everything." She hopes for health, peace in the family, and that things will get better for her daughter, who has been ill for over ten years. She believes that she has a lot of hope "because I have faith in God." Elizabeth thinks she could not survive without hope. She says hope is alive and it is always there, even when her expectations are not met. "I am never giving up." Elizabeth and other family members include her daughter in all traditional family celebrations at home. She wants to take her daughter home permanently, but this would require more help and this is difficult for her. She continues to hope that things will get better for herself and for others who she knows are in similar situations.

Essences: Participant's Language

1. Hope is the basis of everything; it is wishing to stay healthy and at peace with family, and that things will get better for an ill loved one and others. It is like faith in God, and one couldn't survive without it.
2. Hope is alive in successes, even though wished-for expectations are not always met.

Essences: Researcher's Language

1. Persistent envisioning of contentment with intimate solemn engagements emerges with an unwavering stance for expanding the view.

2. Anticipating fulfilling possibilities arises amid disheartenments.

Proposition. The lived experience of hope is a persistent envisioning of contentment with intimate solemn engagements emerging with an unwavering stance for expanding the view, as anticipating fulfilling possibilities arises amid disheartenments.

DISCUSSION OF FINDINGS AND RELATED LITERATURE

The central finding of this study is the structure: *the lived experience of hope is persistently anticipating possibilities amid adversity, as intimate engagements emerge with expanding horizons.* Propositions synthesized from each participant's description indicate that the core concepts were expressed in unique ways. (See Tables 1–4.) At the structural transposition level, *hope is an undaunting pursuit of the not-yet amid the wretched, as affable involvements arise with transfiguring.* At the conceptual integration level, *hope is powering imaging in the connecting-separating of transforming.*

TABLE 1.
First Core Concept as Evident in Propositions

Core Concept:	Persistently anticipating possibilities amid adversity
Structural Transposition:	Undaunting pursuit of the not-yet
Conceptual Integration:	Powering imaging

1. anticipation of persevering amid despair
2. anticipation of possibilities amid disillusionment . . . resolute perseverance
3. prevailing anticipation of possibilities amid potential despair
4. possibilities . . . affirming musings amid despair
5. anticipating . . . possibilities amid the adverse . . . resolute
6. anticipating . . . possibilities amid disillusionment . . . persistent stance
7. infinite anticipation of possibilities amid potential adversity
8. resolute anticipation of possibilities amid disillusionment
9. persistent envisioning . . . possibilities amid disheartenments
10. persistent . . . anticipating fulfilling possibilities amid disheartenment

TABLE 2.
Second Core Concept as Evident in Propositions

Core Concept:	Intimate engagements
Structural Transposition:	Affable involvements
Conceptual Integration:	Connecting-separating

1. enlivening engagements
2. nurturing engagements
3. cherished affiliations
4. cherished engagements
5. cherished fulfillments
6. intimate engagements
7. nurturing affiliations
8. intimate solemn engagements
9. diverse engagements
10. intimate engagements

TABLE 3.
Third Core Concept as Evident in Propositions

Core Concept:	Expanding horizons
Structural Transposition:	Transfiguring
Conceptual Integration:	Transforming

1. view . . . expanding horizons
2. deliberate expanding of horizons
3. expanding view
4. contemplating expanding horizons
5. uplifting enlivenment in moving beyond . . . new horizons
6. uplifting moments . . . the will-be . . . new
7. expansion of view
8. expanding the view
9. expanding the view
10. expanding the view

TABLE 4.
Progressive Abstraction of the Core Concepts of the Lived Experience of Hope with Heuristic Interpretation

Core Concepts	Structural Transposition	Conceptual Integration
Persistently anticipating possibilities amid adversity	Undaunting pursuit of the not-yet amid the wretched	Powering imaging
Intimate engagements	Affable involvements	Connecting-separating
Expanding horizons	Transfiguring	Transforming

Structure

Hope is persistently anticipating possibilities amid adversity, as intimate engagements emerge with expanding horizons.

HEURISTIC INTERPRETATION

Structural Transposition

Hope is an undaunting pursuit of the not-yet amid the wretched, as affable involvements arise with transfiguring.

Conceptual Integration

Hope is powering imaging in the connecting-separating of transforming.

Persistently Anticipating Possibilities Amid Adversity

The first core concept, *persistently anticipating possibilities amid adversity*, is described by participants as considering other options even while in adverse situations. Participants believe that hope is constantly present, and they are adamant that it is what moves them through difficult times of despair and disillusionment. Participants' stories show the determination with which they resolutely anticipate what will be beyond the moment.

Persistently anticipating possibilities amid adversity was transposed to the higher level of abstraction as *an undaunting pursuit of the not-yet* and conceptually integrated as *powering imaging*. Powering is the pushing-resisting of being with non-being in the human-universe mutual process, and imaging is envisioning or picturing the explicit-tacit knowing in cocreating reality (Parse, 1981, 1995, 1997). The powering of being with non-being underpins the courage to be, incarnating intentions and possibles all-at-once as reflective-prereflective imaging is shaping personal knowledge (Dilthey, 1961; Parse, 1981; Polanyi, 1959; Tillich, 1954). Powering imaging, then, is the pushing-resisting of being with non-being in the explicit-tacit knowing of what is and will be. The pushing-resisting of being with non-being is expressed when participants insist that while potential despair or adversity is always present, there is an inherent hopefulness that pushes and pulls as the unknown not-yet looms heavy with possibilities in their prereflective-reflective knowings. Hope as a cocreated reality structured by the participants moves them beyond the moment as they transcend with what they each uniquely view as possibilities.

Powering arises from the principle "cotranscending with the possibles is powering unique ways of originating in the process of transforming" (Parse, 1981, p. 55). In persistently anticipating possibilities amid adversity there is certainty-uncertainty in the conformity-nonconformity arising with creating anew with the familiar-unfamiliar. Imaging arises from the principle "structuring meaning multidimensionally is cocreating reality through the languaging of valuing and imaging" (Parse, 1981, p. 42). In persistently anticipating possibilities amid adversity, beliefs are confirmed–not-confirmed as what is imaged is shown through speaking–being-silent and moving–being-still (Parse, 1998). While originating, transforming, valuing, and languaging are all inherently present with the core concept of persistently anticipating possibilities amid adversity, powering imaging is clearly the predominant construct articulating the notion at the theoretical level of discourse.

The concept of persistently anticipating possibilities amid adversity is primarily consistent with a core concept found in an earlier study on hope by Parse (1990), where the concept was stated as "anticipating possibilities through envisioning the not-yet" (p. 15). In that study, this core concept was conceptualized at the theory level as imaging. Also in Thornburg's (1993) work on hope, powering and imaging were concepts named at the theoretical level of discourse. Though not about hope, Gouty's (1996) study on the lived experience of feeling alone while with others showed that imaging powering best described the meaning her participants gave to considering other ways to be in situations, and Kruse's (1996) study on the lived experience of serenity showed that the theoretical concepts powering and imaging best articulated the participants' descriptions of feeling calm, peaceful, and quiet. The notion of hope with imaging and powering is explicated also in the works of several other authors (Bloch, 1959/1986; Bunkers, 1998; Frankl, 1946/1962; Fromm, 1968; Kierkegaard, 1849/1980; Lynch, 1965; Marcel, 1962).

Bloch (1959/1986), a preeminent Marxist Jew, wrote a treatise on hope. While his beliefs about hope are somewhat different from the findings of this study, he does say that hope anticipates the not-yet, which is a notion quite consistent with the concept, persistently anticipating possibilities amid adversity. Also consistent are Fromm's (1968) conceptualization of hope as an always present untapped ready possibility and Marcel's (1962) view that sheds light on hope as a paradoxical mystery arising with adversity. Marcel believes that when individuals experience restrictions, they move to overcome despair with optimism and keen expectancy, a powering of being with non-being in imaging; these ideas are consistent with the first core concept, persistently anticipating possibilities amid adversity. Lynch (1965) links hope with imagining and also with powering. He focuses on the art of wishing, which is willful imagining and future-oriented, moving humans beyond or over difficulties. Lynch's views coincide with Kierkegaard's (1849/1980), in that Kierkegaard believes that hope arises from imagination and thus humans can move beyond fear and restrictions, imaging possibles while powering being with non-being. Bunkers (1998) synthesized notions about hope and imagination, in conceptualizing the phenomenon of considering tomorrow. Her research on this phenomenon led to a structure that included the idea of pondering possibles with considering tomorrow, which corresponds to anticipating possibilities with hope. Frankl (1946/1962) purports that hope is necessary in choosing personal meaning in life; in fact, he writes about it as an essential for survival. Participants of this study also describe relationships as essential to hope.

Intimate Engagements

The second core concept, *intimate engagements*, is described by participants as connections with family members, friends, God, nature, and ideas. Participants wish for "good things" for close others and themselves. Their stories tell about various unique expressions of intimate or cherished engagements. At the structural transposition level, intimate engagements is *affable involvements*, and it is conceptualized with the theory as *connecting-separating*. Connecting-separating is described by Parse (1981, 1992, 1995, 1997) as being with and away from others, ideas, objects, and situations in the was, is, and will-be all-at-once. In engaging with a phenomenon, one connects and all-at-once separates from that phenomenon, just as in distancing from a phenomenon, one separates and connects in a different way with the same phenomenon. Patterns of relating arise with the ebb and flow of the connecting-separating of intimate engagements. Connecting-separating arises from the principle "cocreating rhythmical patterns of relating is living the paradoxical unity of revealing-concealing and enabling-limiting while connecting-separating" (Parse, 1981, p. 50). The concepts revealing-concealing and enabling-limiting are also related to the core concept intimate engagements in that in all engagements one discloses and hides the who that one is, and all engagements emerge with opportunities and restrictions. Connecting-separating, however, most clearly articulates the notion of intimate engagements at the theoretical level of discourse.

Parse is in agreement with van Kaam (1976), who proposes that hope is nurtured in mutual relationships, and Marcel (1962), who refers to the intimate engagements of hope as a communion with others in situations. This is consistent with participants' descriptions of hope in which they specify the importance of various affiliations in expanding their views.

Expanding Horizons

The third core concept, *expanding horizons*, is transposed to a higher level as *transfiguring* and integrated with the theory as *transforming*. Participants' uplifting enlightenments, expanding views, and buoyant moments arise with their deliberate dreaming about and planning for shifting their views of the familiar-unfamiliar. The expanding view obscures the vacuum of despair. Hope is in the participants' expectations of changing the change that is ongoing with loved ones and themselves. The expanding view is that which changes the moment, shedding a different light on the familiar and unfamiliar.

Parse (1981, 1992, 1995, 1997) posits transforming, from the principle "cotranscending with the possibles is powering unique ways of originating in the process of transforming" (Parse, 1981, p. 55), as the changing of change, shifting the unfamiliar to the familiar and the familiar to the unfamiliar all-at-once. Expanding horizons surface with transcendent movement beyond the now. This movement is all-at-once struggling and leaping beyond, cocreating diverse patterns with new meaning. The new meaning stretches the possibilities of the moment. Participants described these moments as ones in which they shifted their views of the familiar and were uplifted to see their situations differently. While powering and originating are also present with this core concept, in that expanding views are powered with creating new ways of becoming, transforming articulates most clearly this notion at the theoretical level of discourse.

Parse's view of transforming and expanding views agrees with van Kaam (1976), when he refers to the experience of hope as a transcendent movement toward potentialities, and Frankl (1946/1962), when he writes about humans as finding meaning when they transcend or rise above an apparent hopelessness. The rising above is a way of expanding views.

SUMMARY

For the participants in this study, hope is the anticipation of possibilities despite the potential despairing moments of day-to-day living, as engagements with others and situations open new vistas. There are many implications for further research and practice related to the findings of this study. These are discussed in the final chapter of this book, along with the findings from the other studies reported in this work.

REFERENCES

Bloch, E. (1986). *The principle of hope* (N. Plaice & P. Knight, Trans.). Oxford: Basil Blackwell. (Original work published 1959)

Bunkers, S. S. (1998). Considering tomorrow: Parse's theory-guided research. *Nursing Science Quarterly, 11*, 56–63.

Dilthey, W. (1961). *Pattern and meaning in history.* New York: Harper & Row.

Frankl, V. E. (1962). *Man's search for meaning* (3rd ed.). New York: Simon & Schuster. (Original work published 1946)

Fromm, E. (1968). *The revolution of hope.* New York: Harper & Row.

Gouty, C. A. (1996). *Feeling alone while with others.* Unpublished doctoral dissertation, Loyola University, Chicago.

Kierkegaard, S. (1980). *The sickness unto death* (V. Hong & E. H. Hong, Eds. & Trans.). Princeton, NJ: Princeton University Press. (Original work published 1849)

Kruse, B. (1996). *The lived experience of serenity: Using Parse's research method.* Unpublished doctoral dissertation, University of South Carolina, Columbia, SC.

Lynch, W. (1965). *Images of hope: Imagination as healer of the hopeless.* Baltimore: Helicon Press.

Marcel, G. (1962). *Homo viator: Introduction to a metaphysics of hope* (E. Craufurd, Trans.). New York: Harper & Row.

Parse, R. R. (1981). *Man-living-health: A theory of nursing.* New York: Wiley.

Parse, R. R. (1990). Parse's research methodology with an illustration of the lived experience of hope. *Nursing Science Quarterly, 3,* 9–17.

Parse, R. R. (1992). Human becoming: Parse's theory of nursing. *Nursing Science Quarterly, 5,* 35–42.

Parse, R. R. (Ed.). (1995). *Illuminations: The human becoming theory in practice and research.* New York: National League for Nursing Press.

Parse, R. R. (1997). The human becoming theory: The was, is, and will be. *Nursing Science Quarterly, 10,* 32–38.

Polanyi, M. (1959). *The study of man.* Chicago: University of Chicago Press.

Thornburg, P. D. (1993). *The meaning of hope in parents whose infants died from sudden infant death syndrome.* Doctoral dissertation, University of Cincinnati, OH. (University Microfilms International No. 9329939)

Tillich, P. (1954). *Love, power, and justice.* New York: Oxford University Press.

van Kaam, A. (1976). *The dynamics of spiritual self-direction.* Denville, NJ: Dimension Books.

Chapter 5

Toivo: Hope for Persons in Finland

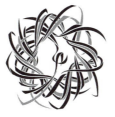

TUULIKKI TOIKKANEN
ERJA MUURINEN

FINLAND AND THE PARTICIPANTS

The purpose of this study, guided by Parse's (1981, 1992) human becoming theory, was to describe the meaning of the lived experience of hope for Finnish people, using Parse's research methodology. Ten people were invited to participate in this study, eight women and two men. The youngest participant was an 18-year-old boy and the oldest was an 83-year-old woman.

Finland, the northernmost country in the world, is situated in northern Europe between Sweden and Russia. The first people reached Finland shortly after the end of the last Ice Age, when the glaciers had retreated and the land risen above the sea. Genetic research has shown that Finnish genes are 65 to 75 percent of European origin and 25 to 35 percent of Asian origin. On the basis of language, Finns are assumed to have belonged to the Fenno-Ugrian family. Finland has stayed independent for eighty years, after having been governed for centuries by the foreign powers of Sweden and Russia. Finland's eighty years of independence have been earned through its people's stubbornness in the face of a difficult geopolitical situation on the one hand and some supremely successful international diplomacy on the other (Eskola, 1995).

Finland is a land of forests and a thousand lakes. In Finland, there are some very specific phenomena, such as the midnight sun, the long polar night, and the northern lights. It is impossible to appreciate the midnight sun fully unless you have actually lived through an entire Finnish winter. During June and July, day and night are separated only by a brief period of twilight in the south, and the sun never sets in the far north. The summertime has a special atmosphere. During December and January, the sun remains below the horizon in the far north and the moon and stars reflect on the snow to create a twilight of their own. The northern lights are caused by the interaction of positively charged particles from outside the atmosphere with atoms of the Earth's upper atmosphere. The ions emit radiation at various wavelengths, thus creating the characteristic colors of the aurora (red and greenish blue). It is a stunning spectacle to observe.

The geopolitical situation, influences from western and eastern cultures, and the natural resources of Finland have created the possibilities for Finnish culture to develop its unique features. The roots of Finnish culture lie deep in prehistory, in the customs and beliefs of the ancient Finns. These are most graphically portrayed in the national epic, the *Kalevala*, compiled by Elias Lönnrot from oral memories of rune singers in the early nineteenth century. Finnish cultural development has also been affected by its long association with Sweden and the Roman Catholic church, ancient trading links with Germany and the Baltic states, and the eastern influence, seen most clearly in the role of the Orthodox church. The absorption of these influences over the centuries can be recognized in the multiple nuances of modern Finnish culture (Eskola, 1995).

The Finnish people are often thought to be shy; some of them truly are, but once you get to know them, they are not. It has also been said that Finns have a tendency toward melancholia. Many of them are depressed and feel hopeless. But maybe the most typical characteristic of the Finns is perseverance, which is the way of living through the dark winter days and hopeless and gray times. This research study has also shown this to be true.

DIALOGICAL ENGAGEMENT

The dialogical engagements took place in quiet, comfortable places selected by the participants.

EXTRACTION-SYNTHESIS

Marja's Story

Marja, a 42-year-old homemaker, lives with her husband and four children in the countryside. Marja believes that experiencing hope is a characteristic and that some people never seem to feel hopeless. She thinks that hope is a main factor in all people's lives, reflecting new life and healing. Marja had a personal problem in her life when she experienced "terrible hopelessness" and she did not seem to have a way out. There was a moment when she felt that she did not have anybody with whom to discuss her situation. However, she kept a diary, which gave her some distance from her own problems. She reported that in the middle of the night she had driven to a dark graveyard, lit by candles. She was afraid at first but the environment made her feel relaxed. When she returned back to her car, she heard a song on her radio and the words "Everyone is worth a song, every life is important." This gave her the feeling that as long as there is life, there is hope. Her grandmother, one of the most important people in her life, was buried at the graveyard and Marja was thinking aloud by her grandmother's grave. She thought that things were well, since she had had children, was healthy, could appreciate nature, could write and draw, and had an optimistic character. Marja says that everyone feels hopeless from time to time, but in the countryside one easily gets near to nature. She lives in the country, and whether she feels good or bad, her feet tend to take her automatically to a certain hill nearby. There she can hear the birds singing, the silence and soughing of the forest wind, and she realizes that nature helps her better than a psychologist or friend. She sees hope as a basis of life from the cradle to the grave.

Essences: Participant's Language

1. Hope is in all people's lives from the cradle to the grave; where there is life, there is hope.
2. Hope is being optimistic and realizing all the good things of life, such as children, health, writing, drawing, and nature.
3. The participant feels hopeful in times of hopelessness when she gets away to her usual places, speaks to a deceased loved one, and takes walks in the forest where she hears the singing birds.

Essences: Researcher's Language

1. Enduring inspiration emerges with the waxing-waning of horizons.

2. Affirming cherished connections arises with expectant contemplation.
3. Promise surfaces amid despair in the repose of familiar patterns.

Proposition. The lived experience of hope is an enduring inspiration emerging with the waxing-waning of horizons, as affirming cherished connections arises with the expectant contemplation of promise amid despair in the repose of familiar patterns.

Kyllikki's Story

Kyllikki is a 48-year-old woman living in a small town in the south of Finland working as a teacher. Kyllikki says that she has not had very many experiences of hope in her life. Life has been "even and gray and hopeless . . . a bottomless swamp at times . . . but how does one get out of the hopelessness?" She says, "It is quite a big process, but the issues of being are found in literature and philosophy . . . so that is one experience of hope." Kyllikki has been interested in psychology and studied it because she thought that through this knowledge she could manipulate other people. At first it had felt "great" but after having read more of it, it had lost its significance. Kyllikki speaks of a dream she had during surgery. She considers that dream a turning point of her life. "I kind of rose in the air and then there were all kinds of teaching points; one—maybe the most significant of them—was where I was told that I have to remember that I have a life to live . . . and I wondered." Kyllikki says that the dream is connected with her experience of hope, so that after it her life turned from hopeless, problem-based, to future, life-oriented. Kyllikki says that for her "hope and life are quite close to each other." She says, "Hope and joy are connected as well as hope and life. I cannot exactly limit what hope is and what joy is and what is life. Hope is that I know something about possibilities for life and joy." Kyllikki has defined health as joy and she sees that hope is connected with health. Other people's similar experiences give hope. Hope and yearning exist in order to be able to share life and joy. Kyllikki says, "If I hide my joy, it does not get a chance to help other people. I tend to give life a chance. That way hope helps meeting other people and experiencing joy. The more one dares to uncover self, the more there are changes."

Essences: Participant's Language

1. Hope is realizing that there is a life to live; through a dream during surgery, the participant's hopelessness and bottomless swamp of problems turned to a future that is life-oriented.
2. Hope is connected with the joy of life and health, and it means that in making progress little by little, there are possibilities.
3. Hope is enhanced in sharing similar experiences and understandings with other people; it is uncovering of self.

Essences: Researcher's Language

1. Vitality with expectation amid despair emerges with enlightenment.

2. Envisioned delightful contentment surfaces with gradual advancement.
3. Inspiration arises with clarifying insights of mutual disclosure.

Proposition. Hope is vitality with expectation amid despair emerging with enlightenment, as envisioned delightful contentment surfaces with gradual advancement, while inspiration arises with clarifying insights of mutual disclosure.

Anja's Story

Anja, a 55-year-old teacher, lives with her husband in a middle-sized town. They have a daughter, who is married. Anja finds many things in her life that are connected with hope. The most significant thing that has affected her life happened thirty years ago when her only child was suddenly taken ill with diabetes when she was eighteen months old. At that time, young children's diabetes was a disaster, almost like a death penalty. It was almost Christmas and that made the situation even worse. Suddenly everything lost significance and the ground of life was gone. She thought only about how the child would have to suffer. Everything was black. After visiting the pediatrician, Anja remembered his words, "This is not the end of life." The person who talked with Anja was wonderful and professional. She spoke to the mother as a mother and to the child as a child. In the discussions Anja found out that treatments had been developed and the results of them had been good. She received written material about diabetes and found that one does not necessarily die of this disease. That was important. The child was treated as her own person, and her attitude was good. Therefore, the parents felt that the situation was not hopeless. Also the child's recovering helped and brought hope. Hope came more and more into the picture, and Anja noticed that she thought more of the child and less of the diabetes. Gradually, grayness started to disappear and the participant started seeing the spring coming: "The sun started shining, trees got their leaves, the birds started singing, and flowers flourished. . . . Hope entered life." Soon Anja started noticing that the child developed and the disease only brought some limitations to the child's life. One did not have to let the health problem interfere with life. From this experience she learned to see that hope is present all the time. "There is not such an impossible situation that there is not hope. This has been a situation of growth—one learns to accept what is coming and given."

Essences: Participant's Language

1. Many things in life are connected with hope; when the participant's daughter was diagnosed with diabetes, everything lost significance and the ground of life was gone and everything was black.
2. Hope entered and the grayness disappeared. Birds sang, flowers flourished, and the sun shone when the participant understood the disease better and saw her child getting better, and she felt the situation was not hopeless.
3. Hope is present all the time; in every situation there is hope with opportunities to grow, while accepting what is given.

Essences: Researcher's Language

1. Inspiration emerges amid despair.
2. Radiant aspiration surfaces with the contentment of enhanced awareness.
3. Persistent anticipation arises with the potential of reconciliation.

Proposition. The lived experience of hope is inspiration emerging amid despair, as radiant aspiration surfaces with the contentment of enhanced awareness, while persistent anticipation arises with the potential of reconciliation.

Venla's Story

Venla is a 63-year-old woman who lives alone in her apartment in a small town. She has two sisters, one living not far from her. The greatest wish Venla ever had was to have a home where her father would not use alcohol. Her father drank almost all his life and was quarrelsome. After decades of waiting, her father quit drinking. Venla's lifelong wish had come true and she was very happy. Venla's father had caused her a lot of worry, disappointment, exhaustion, pain, and fear. Other people's temperate lifestyles had made her jealous and bitter. Having responsibility for her parents and forgetting herself is the way Venla pictures her life. She feels she lost something by abandoning her own life for other people. On the other hand, she feels that it has given her something . . . at least perseverance. She does not regret taking care of her parents until their death. Venla feels that she has not hoped for anything for herself, only for other people. For her father she had hoped for an alcohol-free life and in that way for a fearless and carefree life for the rest of the family. She had also hoped that her sister's son would grow up to be "a good person." A wish came true: Her father quit drinking and stayed sober for the last three and a half years of his life. The best part of her day was when she would come home from work and not have to worry, wait, fear, or start looking for him. Now Venla is deeply grateful for all this. She has an apartment of her own. She feels that she could not hope for more. Her only wish is to be healthy herself, to have peace in the world, and that the youth are blessed.

Essences: Participant's Language

1. Hope is having a long-lasting wish come true; when the participant's father stopped drinking, she was truly happy and was no longer fearful or worried.
2. Hope is wishing good things for other people; the participant feels she has abandoned her own life for others, yet she feels this has given her perseverance.
3. Hope is being deeply grateful for all that the participant has, and she does not wish for anything more, yet she wishes to be healthy, to have peace in the world, and that all the youth are blessed.

Essences: Researcher's Language

1. Persistent envisioning amid the arduous arises with joyful fulfillment.

2. Benevolent desires for affiliations emerge with enduring sacrifice.
3. Inspired gratitude surfaces with the contentment of altruistic aspirations.

Proposition. The lived experience of hope is a persistent envisioning amid the arduous arising with joyful fulfillment, as benevolent desires for affiliations emerge with enduring sacrifice, while inspired gratitude surfaces with the contentment of altruistic aspirations.

Liisa's Story

Liisa is a 52-year-old unemployed, divorced nurse who lives in a small Finnish town. Liisa has had many situations in her life that are related to hope. The most significant one is with her youngest son's developmental process, which took some twenty-six years. The son is disabled. After slowly mastering abilities at the various developmental stages, her son entered kindergarten and enjoyed being there. He was shy and liked to be alone. The social worker did not believe in him but the psychologist kept encouraging him. Later, Liisa, who had been deeply disappointed in his development, started believing in his progress. After kindergarten, the son entered a school for retarded children, which was a good solution. Cooperation between home and school went well. There were difficult tests at school, but the boy managed them somehow because Liisa read all his homework to him. Every time he learned something it gave hope to Liisa to move toward the next step. Liisa says she is happy that her son could continue school to the upper level, despite the fact that some of the teachers disagreed. What was even better, there were teachers who promised to teach her son. The child became more and more independent, and he started helping the caretaker in all his tasks. He entered a vocational school in another town and managed the journeys there by himself. Liisa started believing that he would really be socially normal. At the moment, he lives alone and has a part-time job. Liisa hopes that he will find a girlfriend. Liisa has had to give up her own career, but still she is happy that her son has become independent and that he has found his place in society. Hope is faith in the future; seeing the child progressing and having other people's support maintain hope.

Essences: Participant's Language

1. Hope is witnessing the true miracle of a disabled child's continuous development over twenty-six years in light of the participant's initial, deep disappointment. Hope stayed alive as teachers and a psychologist who believed in the participant's child offered encouragement and support.
2. The participant continues to hope for her son's future and is happy that he is independent and has found a place in society.

Essences: Researcher's Language

1. Expectation amid the arduous surfaces with enduring wonder of the devoted confidence of nurturing affiliations.

2. Persistent anticipation of what will be arises with contented satisfaction.

Proposition. The lived experience of hope is expectation amid the arduous, arising with the enduring wonder of the devoted confidence of nurturing affiliations, while persistent anticipation of what will be arises with contented satisfaction.

Elina's Story

Elina, a 22-year-old woman, is studying nursing and living in a small town in the south of Finland. Elina speaks of hope in light of her latest experience. A tumor had been found in her breast and it might have been a malignant one. However, it proved to be benign. During the weeks when Elina did not know what kind of tumor it was, she was afraid of death. Her worst fear had been that she could not have children if she had to have radiotherapy or cytostatic therapy. Childlessness had worried her most. After learning the results, Elina felt like "she had got the moon or the stars in the sky." That information had relieved her worry and fear. She experienced joy. Everyday things and adversities were nothing. The information brought a lot of hope that life would go on and she could possibly have children. Elina calls that a concrete experience of hope. During these last weeks she said that she had especially experienced hope. The hope had been different from before. She experienced hope more deeply. While Elina waited for the biopsy results she says that friends' concern and presence had helped her see that life is not as black and white as it seemed to her. "Friends kept reminding me of the existence of hope even though I did not see it myself." Elina also says that even though she is not a religious person, during the last few weeks she had prayed and tried to get hope from God. Elina says that she had experienced hope for concrete things before. Now she says that she understands hope more deeply than before. She calls it "hope in life." Now that she does not have cancer, she says that it has given her hope in life. She says that it is something different from what she used to call hope. "This hope follows you all the time; it is present, whatever you do. I think that this hope is life. I experience it more deeply."

Essences: Participant's Language

1. Hope is knowing life will go on after fear of dying and not being able to have children were relieved, in that the participant's tumor was not malignant.
2. Hope is found in friends and in God.
3. The participant used to hope for concrete things; now hope is understood more deeply and she has "hope in life"; it follows you all the time and is present in whatever you do.

Essences: Researcher's Language

1. Anticipatory certitude amid potential despair arises with contented vitality.
2. Promise surfaces with intimate affiliations.

3. Profound comprehension of the expectant emerges as an enduring presence.

Proposition. The lived experience of hope is an anticipatory certitude amid potential despair, arising with contented vitality, while promise surfaces with intimate affiliations, as profound comprehension of the expectant emerges as an enduring presence.

Mikko's Story

Mikko is an 18-year-old young man, the only child in his family. Mikko will graduate from upper-secondary high school in a year. He lives in a medium-sized Finnish town. Mikko's life is peaceful and carefree, and he says that he lives for the here and now—in the moment. Plans for the future are mostly about the next day. There have been situations when Mikko sensed the existence of hope, as when he was getting his driver's license and when he was taking difficult examinations at school. In order to pass the exams, the participant had to attend many boring lectures. He also had to "suffer" (study) by the books at home and prepare himself mentally. Mikko thinks that hope brings some sort of interest to life. Related to hope, Mikko says that if you have hurt someone, you have to explain it later and hope for the relationship to be good again.

Essences: Participant's Language

1. Hope is sensed during difficult and important examinations and it brings interest to life.
2. Hope is related to times when you hurt someone and hope that the relationship will be good again.

Essences: Researcher's Language

1. Inspiration arises with the arduous amid intriguing appeal.
2. Anticipation of conciliatory affiliations emerges with provoked affronts.

Proposition. The lived experience of hope is inspiration arising with the arduous amid an intriguing appeal, as anticipation of conciliatory affiliations emerges with provoked affronts.

Sinikka's Story

Sinikka, aged 51, is a teacher living in a small town with her husband. Sinikka thinks that hope exists at different levels. She says that hope is an important, life-maintaining thing, and that is real hope. Then there are lots of little wishes: "I wish this and I wish that." It is not that important whether these hopes come true or not. Fundamental hope is something else. It has to do with maintaining and continuing life, and it makes a big difference, but that kind of hope must be future-oriented. Sinikka has not had such illness that her life would have been threatened. However, she describes a life-threatening event. It happened long ago and she does not remember it very well. Sinikka had been in

Europe with her husband and another married couple. They had traveled in a small airplane. When they had just taken off at Warsaw, they noticed that there was something wrong with the engine. Sinikka says, "It was so exciting. . . . I kept hoping and hoping that the engine would run . . . just a little bit more! I kept looking at the field and thought that we could make an emergency landing there . . . if the engine turns off . . . what if we all die here. . . . I was glad that I had sent a postcard to my father before leaving. . . . He would know that we had had a very good vacation." Sinikka also tells how she tried to encourage her friend sitting next to her. She did not dare to speak to the men in the cockpit so that they could concentrate on the piloting. They landed back at Warsaw airport and discovered that the defective engine could not have functioned much longer. Sinikka also remembers that she had thought it was wrong to keep up unrealistic hope. She had always thought that it was ethically wrong to give a person hope when it was unrealistic. With age this has changed. Sinikka says, "It is difficult to know what is realistic and what is unrealistic. Now I am careful with my words if they could take away someone's hope." However, Sinikka says that she is careful not to have unrealistic hopes for herself. "I do not dare to hope unrealistic things. It means that I myself act the way that the hope would come true. I can make it come true myself a bit, but there are always things I cannot affect myself; otherwise it would only be planning." Sinikka describes how life and other people bring uncertainty and surprises even to realistic hope. At the moment, Sinikka hopes to be able to work and to be of help to others. "I hope to be able to feel useful in the future. . . . It is related to other people . . . so that I could feel that I am not a burden." She hopes to be able to maintain a hold on her life and to affect it by planning it.

Essences: Participant's Language

1. Hope is an important, life-maintaining thing and lots of little wishes, too; it has to do with continuation of health and living with fears in dangerous situations like the time a plane she was in had a defective engine.
2. Hope is planning for the future to help others by acting in a useful way and not being a burden.
3. Hope that is realistic also brings uncertainty and surprises that life and other people bring to situations.

Essences: Researcher's Language

1. Persistent anticipation amid the arduous arises with an enduring contentment.
2. Envisioning the will-be emerges with benevolent affiliations.
3. Genuine expectancy surfaces with enlivening ambiguity.

Proposition. The lived experience of hope is persistent anticipation amid the arduous, arising with an enduring contentment, as envisioning the will-be emerges with benevolent affiliations, while a genuine expectancy surfaces with enlivening ambiguity.

Ilmari's Story

Ilmari is a 35-year-old man who is studying nursing and living with his family in a small town in the south of Finland. Ilmari has previously had a metal enterprise of his own. He says that hope is present automatically in all situations of life even though it is not always noticed. Hope is in big and small things. He finds hope "when planning something. . . . There is always hope. . . . Now that I started thinking more of hope, when you think of your life you notice that there has always been hope. . . . No matter how difficult situations are, there is always hope." Ilmari says that in difficult situations one starts thinking of ways to survive and "hope is there in the end of the pipeline." Ilmari goes on to say, "For example, when you have a different situation in your life or when something tragic happens, one always thinks of surviving. . . . That is hope. . . . It does not have to be a very difficult thing. . . . It can be related, for example, to purchasing a house. One hopes to get a house of his own sometime and there is this hope present . . . a kind of warm feeling." Ilmari tells that imagining success beforehand is related to hope and it gives him a good feeling. He also tells how hope can bring a slight moment of relief in the difficult situations of life. "When having hard times in life, one falls into self-pity and when the prospects do not look so bright . . . but when you start hoping for better times you find a moment of relief, which is a very short moment but enough. It gives you strength to seek the hoped." Ilmari says that hope is the absolute prerequisite of life. If there were not hope "one could easily think of ending his/her life in different situations."

Essences: Participant's Language

1. Hope is in everything automatically. It is an absolute, always there in big and small things, in planning to succeed in something, to get over something, and in thinking about how things could be better.
2. Hope is a warm, good feeling, and it can bring a slight moment of relief and strength in difficult situations.

Essences: Researcher's Language

1. An inherent expectancy emerges in contemplating the new with cherished connections.
2. Envisioning with contentment arises with the fleeting unburdening of fortification amid adversity.

Proposition. The lived experience of hope is an inherent expectancy emerging in contemplating the new with cherished connections, as envisioning with contentment arises with the fleeting unburdening of fortification amid adversity.

Tellervo's Story

Tellervo is an 83-year-old woman who is living with her husband in a nice apartment in a small town in the south of Finland. They have four children and nine grandchildren, all living in other parts of Finland. Tellervo talks about a situation more than forty years ago when she was extremely hopeless. Their second child, a baby girl, was handicapped. At that time (the 1950s), people did not know very much about handicapped people and they tried to cover it up. Tellervo says that this second child was very different from the first, a healthy boy, but she did not have any feeling that the child was handicapped until the midwife asked her whether she had healthy children. Tellervo says:

> I told her that we had one son; she did not have to ask me a lot more when I started suspecting . . . because this girl was totally different . . . yellow and sleepy . . . different from healthy children in all ways. I asked the midwife directly, "Is this child sick?," and she answered honestly that she was and would be all her life. At first I felt that I fell in a deep well. . . . The situation was very hopeless. . . . My husband and I thought it over. I did not talk about her with anyone and no one asked me anything at the hospital. The room in the ward was big and old-fashioned. We tried to meet a doctor before leaving the hospital, but we did not meet him at all during the time we spent there. At home we started looking for information about her disability. We needed to get information somewhere but it was extremely difficult.

Also professionals left the family alone. Then they started to talk with parents of other handicapped people and found a support group for handicapped people's families. Tellervo has been president of the society for many years. Tellervo says:

> Even when I found out that our child was disabled and had the feeling of falling in a deep well, I started hearing a hymn in my head, "Thank the Good Lord," and somehow I experienced miraculous hope. I cannot explain where it came from. Somehow we went on with our life. . . . Maybe it has helped us to talk with other people in the same kind of situation.
>
> We believe in God and read the Bible. . . . There is the hope. . . . It awakens through the Word of God. . . . If anywhere, hope can be found there. . . . There are so many words of hope. My husband and I have been religious since we were young, and when we got married we had the idea that we are not alone and . . . that we have a resource in God and there is the hope. Most of our friends have thought the same way. It is said in Hebrews: hope is quite like an anchor which is thrown to the other side of the curtain and it has been fastened. I believe that God knows whatever happens in my life. Most things are mysteries that cannot be solved, but very many questions are unnecessary, like, "Why me?" Even with our disabled child, we didn't ask questions. If God wants us to know things, He will let us know. This belief in a loving God . . . is the best hope. . . . There is a lot of pain and worry in

our lives, but still I like to pray that the last moments of life will be good . . . that it would leave good memories for the children.

Essences: Participant's Language

1. Hope is experiencing the miraculous, like the time the participant found out her child was disabled and she felt as though she were falling into a deep well while at the same time she heard a hymn in her head.
2. Hope is being able to go on with life knowing there are others in the same situation; life would be difficult without hope.
3. Hope is an anchor awakened through believing one is not alone but has a resource in a comforting, loving God.

Essences: Researcher's Language

1. Inspiration emerges with sacred wonder amid despair.
2. Propelling with nurturing affiliations arises with easing the arduous.
3. The strong moorings of expectancy surface with a contented communion in the Divine.

Proposition. The lived experience of hope is inspiration emerging with sacred wonder amid despair, as propelling with nurturing affiliations arises with easing the arduous, while the strong moorings of expectancy surface with a contented communion in the Divine.

FINDINGS AND RELATED LITERATURE

For the ten Finnish participants in this study, the structure of hope is *persistent anticipation of contentment arising with the promise of nurturing affiliations, while inspiration emerges amid easing the arduous.* The structure illuminates that hope is a humanly lived phenomenon that can be described. Raised one level of abstraction in the process of structural transposition, the lived experience of hope is *steadfast foresightfulness with the attentive involvements of uplifting vivifications.* Linked conceptually with Parse's theory in the process of conceptual integration, the structure of hope is *imaging the connecting-separating of transforming* (see Table 1).

The first extracted core concept, *persistent anticipation of contentment,* illuminates what the ten participants hope (see Table 2). The participants described examples in their lives when they had experienced hope. They hope and wait for something very important for them. Hope is realizing that there is hope all the time. In this study, one participant told how she kept hoping that her father would not use alcohol. For that participant, hope was having a long-lasting wish come true; when the participant's father stopped drinking she was truly happy and was no longer fearful or worried. Another participant described the experience of her child's being suddenly taken ill with diabetes and how little by little she realized that the child's disease was "not the end of life"; she has learned to see that hope is present all the time.

TABLE 1.
*The Structure and Heuristic Interpretation
of the Lived Experience of Hope*

Core Concepts	Structural Transposition	Conceptual Integration
Persistent anticipation of contentment	Steadfast foresightfulness	Imaging
Promise of nurturing affiliations	Attentive involvements	Connecting-separating
Inspiration amid easing the arduous	Uplifting vivifications	Transforming

Structure

Hope is persistent anticipation of contentment arising with the promise of nurturing affiliations, while inspiration emerges amid easing the arduous.

Structural Transposition

Hope is steadfast foresightfulness surfacing with the attentive involvements of uplifting vivifications.

Conceptual Integration

Hope is imaging the connecting-separating of transforming.

TABLE 2.
Essences of the Concept Persistent Anticipation of Contentment

1. expectant contemplation . . . repose of familiar patterns
2. expectation . . . envisioned delightful contentment
3. persistent anticipation . . . contentment
4. persistent envisioning . . . joyful fulfillment . . . contentment of altruistic aspirations
5. expectation . . . persistent anticipation . . . contented satisfaction
6. anticipatory certitude . . . expectant . . . contented vitality
7. anticipation . . . intriguing appeal
8. expectancy . . . enduring contentment . . . envisioning the will-be . . . persistent anticipation
9. expectancy . . . envisioning . . . contentment
10. strong moorings of expectancy . . . contented communion in the Divine

At the level of structural transposition, persistent anticipation of contentment was conceptualized as *steadfast foresightfulness,* and it relates clearly to Parse's (1981, 1995) concept, *imaging.* Parse (1990) has studied the lived experience of hope and identified imaging as a concept in the theoretical structure of the lived experience of hope; all participants in her study spoke about their experience of hope in relation to possibles, such as living without the machine and picturing themselves in other ways. Persons construct reality through their reflective-prereflective imaging. Parse proposes that imaging is an aspect of questioning as people search for answers. In these research findings, people were actively seeking contentment. Imaging is a "process of assimilating new ideas . . . as one structures meanings compatible with one's world view" (Parse, 1981, pp. 43–44). One participant said, "When having hard times in life, one falls into self-pity and when the prospects do not look so bright. . . . But when you start hoping for better times you find a moment of relief, which is a very short moment but enough. It gives you strength to seek the hoped." Languaging imaged values is structuring meaning and cocreating reality. Parse's first principle relates, "Structuring meaning multidimensionally is cocreating reality through the languaging of valuing and imaging" (Parse, 1995, p. 6). The first core concept, persistent anticipation of contentment, says much about imaging but also reflects valuing and languaging. In the findings of this research, there are also valuing and languaging; these are illuminated through personal value priorities that bring contentment to the participants and arise through choosing, acting, and living personal value priorities.

The second core concept, *promise of nurturing affiliations,* was structurally transposed with the theory of human becoming (Parse, 1992) to *attentive involvements.* At the level of conceptual integration this is expressed as *connecting-separating,* a concept from the second principle of Parse's theory. All ten participants told of how they experienced hope with different kinds of connections. The stories show how rhythmical these connections are and they also show the paradox, hope–not-hope. Examples of essences from participants' stories are cherished connections, nurturing affiliations, and benevolent affiliations (see Table 3).

In this study, involvements with close relations, friends, nature, God, and things were related to hope. One participant spoke of how her friends kept reminding her of the existence of hope even though she did not see it herself and how she had prayed and tried to get hope from God during the weeks when she had waited for biopsy results. Another participant spoke of how she and her husband had talked with other people in the same kind of situation when they found out their child was disabled. Hope is being able to go on with life knowing there are others in the same kinds of situations. This research finding confirms the understanding that hope is found in connections and relations. In many previous studies, it has been discovered that significant relationships with other people, nature, and God maintain hope (Herth, 1993; Raleigh, 1992; Stephenson, 1991).

The second core concept, promise of nurturing affiliations, says much about connecting-separating but also about the other concepts of Parse's

TABLE 3.
Essences of the Concept Promise of Nurturing Affiliations

1. cherished connections . . . promise
2. clarifying insights of mutual disclosure
3. potential of reconciliation
4. benevolent desires for affiliations
5. nurturing affiliations
6. intimate affiliations
7. anticipation of conciliatory affiliations
8. benevolent affiliations
9. cherished connections
10. nurturing affiliations

second theoretical principle, revealing-concealing and enabling-limiting. In the connecting-separating of hope, one is enabled and limited as one reveals-conceals the who one is becoming.

The third extracted core concept, *inspiration amid easing the arduous,* expresses the idea that participants started to see hope amid their difficult life situations. Inspiration amid easing the arduous was structurally transposed with the theory of human becoming (Parse, 1992) as *uplifting vivifications.* Some of the essences of participants' stories are enduring inspiration, radiant inspiration amid despair, and enlivening ambiguity (see Table 4).

Participants realized that there is always hope even in difficult times. For example, one participant told how she realized that in spite of her hopelessness and "bottomless swamp" of problems, there are possibilities for life and joy. Hope arises overtly when one is experiencing problems, like a child's sickness and disability or fears and life-threatening situations. Participants were inspired, and they found in living hopefully that they saw life differently. For example, one participant who experienced "terrible hopelessness" and did not seem to have a way out realized that things were well, since she had her children and was healthy. She appreciated nature and could write and draw. She had an optimistic character. Another participant talked of her hopeless and bottomless experiences and how she found the meaning of hope.

Inspiration amid easing the arduous relates clearly to Parse's (1981, 1992, 1995) concept of *transforming,* or seeing the familiar in a new light. Parse (1981) proposes that "transforming is the changing of change, coconstituting anew in a deliberate way. In the human-universe process, change is ongoing" (p. 62). The human "coparticipates with the universe in mutual emergence" (Parse, 1998, p. 51). Parse's (1981) third principle states "contranscending with the possibles is powering unique ways of originating in the process of

TABLE 4.
Essences of the Concept Inspiration Amid Easing the Arduous

---

1. enduring inspiration . . . despair

2. vitality . . . enlightenment . . . gradual advancement . . . inspiration . . . despair

3. radiant aspiration amid despair . . . enhanced awareness

4. arduous . . . inspired gratitude

5. the arduous surfaces with enduring wonder

6. profound comprehension . . . potential despair

7. inspiration . . . arduous

8. enlivening ambiguity . . . arduous

9. contemplating the new . . . amid adversity

10. inspiration . . . sacred wonder . . . easing the arduous . . . despair

---

transforming" (p. 69). Hoping is one special way of discovering anew and simultaneously viewing the familiar in a new light. Hope is also a mutual process of powering and originating with transforming, relating with the world through the pushing-resisting rhythm, starting anew, and seeing the familiar in a new light. That can be seen, for example, in the essence of one participant: Hope is experiencing the miraculous, like the time the participant found out her child was disabled and she felt as though she were falling into a deep well while at the same time she heard a hymn in her head.

The findings of this study have shed light on the meaning of hope using Parse's (1987, 1995, 1997) research methodology. Each person's hope is personal and unique, just as each person's life is personal and unique. This study has shown the experience of hope as a unitary phenomenon involving the whole person.

Implications for further research and practice based on these findings are discussed in the final chapter of this book, along with findings from other studies.

REFERENCES

Eskola, M. (Ed.). (1995). *Facts about Finland* (M. Wynne-Ellis, Trans.). Helsinki: Otava.

Herth, K. (1993). Hope in the family caregiver of terminally ill people. *Journal of Advanced Nursing, 18,* 538–548.

Parse, R. R. (1981). *Man-living-health: A theory of nursing.* New York: Wiley.

Parse, R. R. (1987). *Nursing science: Major paradigms, theories, and critiques.* Philadelphia: Saunders.

Parse, R. R. (1990). Parse's research methodology with an illustration of the lived experience of hope. *Nursing Science Quarterly, 3,* 9–17.

Parse, R. R. (1992). Human becoming: Parse's theory of nursing. *Nursing Science Quarterly*, 5, 35–42.

Parse, R. R. (Ed.). (1995). *Illuminations: The human becoming theory in practice and research*. New York: National League for Nursing Press.

Parse, R. R. (Ed.). (1997). *Elämyksiä. Ihmisenä kehittymisen teoria käytännössä ja tutkimuksa* (S. Ala-Antti, H. Hausen, K. Ranta-aho, P. Reinikka, & L. Ritanen, Trans.). Helsinki: Kirjayhtymä Oy.

Parse, R. R. (1998). *The human becoming school of thought*. Thousand Oaks, CA: Sage.

Raleigh, E. D. (1992). Sources of hope in chronic illness. *Oncology Nursing Forum*, 19(3), 443–448.

Stephenson, C. (1991). The concept of hope revisited for nursing. *Journal of Advanced Nursing*, 16, 1456–1461.

Chapter 6

Speranza: A Study
of the Lived Experience of Hope
with Persons from Italy

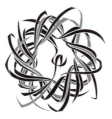

RENZO ZANOTTI
DEBRA A. BOURNES

PARTICIPANTS

The participants in this study range in age from 21 to 60 and live in a northeastern region of Italy called Veneto. According to Julio Cesar, the region was named after the Veneti—the people who inhabited the area in pre-Roman times. People in Veneto have strong beliefs in traditional values like family, religion, and individual freedom, and are well known as entrepreneurs. It is estimated that one of every nine people in Veneto runs his or her own company. Their businesses are predominantly focused on high-technology and fashion manufacturing. Seventy-five percent of what they produce is exported to other countries. The people in Veneto have the highest average annual income in all of Italy. The region also has the country's lowest unemployment. Social policies in the region are traditionally influenced by Catholicism, as in all of Italy.

Treviso, the town where many participants in this study live, is located 30 miles northwest of Venice, the capital of the region. The remainder of the participants live nearby, in either Venice or Padova. In Veneto, people speak a dialect that is a mixture of Italian and Latin with Gaelic influences. The Italian word for hope is "speranza."

The participants from Italy viewed hope as an ever-present optimism noticeable particularly during gray and sad times. They talked about it as an enthused happiness that changed their views of the future. The structure *the lived experience of hope is expectancy amid the arduous, as quiescent vitality arises with expanding horizons* emerged from this study.

DIALOGICAL ENGAGEMENT

The dialogical engagements took place in quiet environments chosen by the participants.

EXTRACTION-SYNTHESIS

Tony's Story

Tony, 60 years old, is a retired teacher, and lives with his wife in a quiet village several miles from the nearest town. Tony spends most of his time gardening and caring for his dogs. For him, hope is the basis of his "experience of life." It is "an anchor of salvation [on] to which man holds." Tony believes the meaning and importance of hope varies with the "passing of years" amid the "vicissitudes" of life. When he was young, Tony's hope focused on the future. He dreamed about doing well in his studies, finding a good job, having his own family, and living happily. As he grew older his hope grew "weaker" and more "concrete." He began to think about the problems in his life more "rationally" and to realize "maturity brings with it the obligations, the duties, [and] the expectations" that demand "a visible result that leaves really little space for flights of fantasy." Tony also believes that as people grow older hope "assumes a new importance." It again becomes "that anchor to which we hold on." He says hoping for the "saving [of] one's soul," "life beyond," or "reincarnation" helps calm the "uncertainty" associated with living at the end of one's life.

Essences: Participant's Language

1. Hope is above all the basis of the participant's experience of life; it is an anchor of salvation in light of uncertainties.
2. Hope varies with age—when one is young there is a lot of hope for the future, but with the passing of years hope is substituted with concreteness until more years pass and hope assumes a renewed, calming importance at the end of life.

Essences: Researcher's Language

1. Persistent expectancy arises with the strong moorings of sustainment amid unsureness.
2. Aspiration emerges with the quiescent vitality of expanding horizons.

Proposition. The lived experience of hope is a persistent expectancy arising with the strong moorings of sustainment amid unsureness, while aspiration emerges with the quiescent vitality of expanding horizons.

Gina's Story

Gina is a 21-year-old student who is specializing in informatics. She spends most of her spare time at home with her parents. Gina believes that "hope is very wide and can assume multiple meanings. It has a thousand facets . . . like a ray of light that strikes a crystal and gets reflected in all different colors and shades." There is a unique ray of light for everyone that reflects personal and "evolving goals or desires." Gina feels there is "a little hope in everything and everyone." She hopes for "a better world" and "divine justice," as well as to finish her university studies, find a satisfying job, and "build a family." She also speaks about young people who "hope for their tomorrow," "poor people who hope to find a piece of bread to satisfy their hunger," "elderly people who hope not to die in solitude," "parents who hope for the best for their children," and "executives who hope their firm will always be on the crest of the wave." She says hope is both a positive and a negative force. In some circumstances it is like "the daily bread," or a "type of spring that pushes us to look ahead." Hope can also make you "a slave to [your] own expectations . . . of [your] own dreams." This happens when you set goals that are beyond your capabilities and then "hope and hope, but in the end your trust in hope has not served for anything. . . . On the contrary, it has left a profound sense of frustration and powerlessness."

Essences: Participant's Language

1. Hope is very wide and can have multiple meanings. It is the daily bread, a positive force, a spring that pushes you to continue to look ahead for satisfactions and calmness. It can also make one a slave to one's own expectations.
2. There is a little hope in everything and everyone since hope has a thousand facets. It is like the ray of light that strikes a sphere of crystal reflecting colors and shades, and each person chooses a different way according to their evolving goals.

Essences: Researcher's Language

1. Diversity with an enlivening propulsion arises with quiescence amid potential languid confinement.
2. Persistent envisioning emerges with expanding unique configurations of radiant distinction.

Proposition. The lived experience of hope is persistent envisioning emerging with expanding unique configurations of radiant distinction, as diversity with an enlivening propulsion arises with quiescence amid potential languid confinement.

Teresa's Story

Teresa is a 35-year-old nurse. She is involved in several health-related projects in Africa and also works on the local "health emergency helicopter squad." Teresa says hope is the "possibility of being able to create an illusion, of being able to believe there is something more, something beyond the daily reality of things that are tangible." Hope is "something hidden. . . . You cannot verify what it is [but] you must trust it." She says hoping for "things that cannot be" creates an "illusion." It helps her feel "pleasant, serene, and calm." Hope is also "associated with the possibility of change." Teresa says she is the "optimistic" type. She is able to see difficult events in positive ways and from there her "hope grows." She looks at hope as "an abstract concept [that] disappears in the moment in which it is fulfilled. . . . [It is] connected to faith, to religion . . . [and] to things that do not have any concrete answers." Sometimes, though, hope is "not able to be fulfilled. . . . Many episodes you hope will go in a positive way then evolve in a negative way."

Essences: Participant's Language

1. Hope is being able to create an illusion beyond reality; it is pleasant, serene, and calm; it is something that cannot be fulfilled and yet it disappears in the moment in which it is fulfilled. Hope is something hidden, not tangible, and something you must trust; it is connected with that which is not concrete, such as faith and religion.
2. Hope is the optimistic possibility of changing things that appear negative into something positive.

Essences: Researcher's Language

1. Fleeting apparitions of the obscure surface with the quiescence of indiscernible theistic assurances.
2. Heartening visions amid the arduous arise with an enlivened potential metamorphosis.

Proposition. The lived experience of hope is the fleeting apparitions of the obscure surfacing with quiescence amid indiscernible theistic assurances, as heartening visions amid the arduous arise with an enlivened potential metamorphosis.

Franco's Story

Franco is a 32-year-old man who has a degree in civil engineering and owns a consulting company. Franco says hope has "two distinct faces," and it is "influenced by the various experiences [one] lives." First, hope "can represent something positive if it in some way helps a person to believe in what he is doing, to look at life differently, or to find a way [to live] with a . . . difficult situation." Franco believes hope "offers a light in the darkness" when something happens that does not "make you happy," or that "undermines your tranquillity." Hope "grants you the opportunity to . . . believe something can change in your favor." Hope is really "extra arms to combat daily battles." For instance, Franco believes hope is a source of "strength" and "conviction" for "all the people who get seriously sick from one of those sicknesses for which science has not yet found a remedy." Hope, however, is not a "totally positive" concept. Franco thinks "there is a reverse side of the medal, an aspect that can . . . be damaging for whom[ever] discovers it." He says he "trusted in [his] hope" that he would be able to solve a complex situation on his own, but felt "powerless" when he realized he did not have the "capacity or the resources" to handle the situation. Hope opens you to the "risk of [being] disappointed."

Essences: Participant's Language

1. Hope is something positive when it helps a person to believe in what he is doing and to look at life optimistically during a difficult situation; it offers light in the darkness.
2. Hope is strength to combat daily battles, especially for those who are sick. On the other side, some may trust in hope without the resources available to solve a situation.

Essences: Researcher's Language

1. Heartening aspiration for expanding possibilities emerges with a vital radiance amid the arduous.
2. Fortification for contention arises with the frailty of naive certitude.

Proposition. The lived experience of hope is a heartening aspiration for expanding possibilities emerging with vital radiance amid the arduous, while fortification for contention arises with the frailty of naive certitude.

Maria's Story

Maria, an assistant manager in a private business, is 28 years old. Maria believes hope "pertains to a field of expectations." It is always "connected with something positive." She says her hope relates to "something that does not exist," but that she wishes for herself or for others, especially for the people she loves. Maria thinks her hope has changed as she has matured. She used to "hope for things without knowing if those things were okay [to hope for]. . . . For example, [she] hoped to pass an exam . . . [but] evidently was not ready to live that situation." Now Maria hopes for "objectives that . . . are reachable . . . not illusions." Her hope is more concrete and she hopes this change "has not limited [her] thoughts." Maria feels another aspect of hope is that being able to reach her objectives depends on her "attitude" and her "spirit." It also depends on "external circumstances." Hope "can be disappointing because it has some characteristics that do not depend on [her] as the only actor in the situation." For Maria, hope also has a "religious aspect." Above all, "to hope is to believe in eternal life."

Essences: Participant's Language

1. Hope pertains to a field of positive expectations. It is concrete and reachable, yet it has some aspects that can be disappointing. When the participant was younger, she hoped for things that did not exist yet, without knowing if these were right.
2. Hope has a religious aspect; to hope is to believe in eternal life.

Essences: Researcher's Language

1. Discernible-indiscernible disheartenment arises amid unwavering anticipation of expanding horizons.
2. Solemn aspiration surfaces with the certitude of immortality.

Proposition. The lived experience of hope is discernible-indiscernible disheartenment arising amid unwavering anticipation of expanding horizons, while solemn aspiration surfaces with the certitude of immortality.

Paolo's Story

Paolo is 41 years old and works as an assistant professor of mathematics at a local university. For Paolo, "Hope is fundamental to the life of a person. . . . [Without] it life would be gray and sad." It is "a very personal concept . . . connected to one's "daily experiences" and to the "culture," "religion," and "society" to which one belongs. Paolo says hope is about "expectations." "It is connected to life, and it is intimately related to one's existence, and to the goals one sets for [oneself]." Hope "is without a doubt a positive thing. It gives an optimistic edge to all things." It is especially helpful to those who are suffering, because they "are naturally induced to hope . . . their state evolves positively." Hope relates to "what one does. . . . It helps one to live better, to be committed, to confront life with enthusiasm . . . and to fulfill . . . dreams." Paolo believes hope can also be negative. If one "hopes for too much" one can be "disillusioned." Hope, therefore, must be used "a little at a time," in the "right measure," and "with a little bit of pessimism."

Essences: Participant's Language

1. Hope is connected to life and to the goals one sets and, when in the right measure, a little at a time. It gives an optimistic edge to all things, even for those who are suffering; without it life would be gray and sad.

2. Hope is quietly personal and plays a part in daily life, which helps one to fulfill dreams and confront life with enthusiasm.

Essences: Researcher's Language

1. Cautious attention with heartening vitality emerges with expectancy amid the inimical.
2. Aspiring uniquely surfaces with the silent familiar of spirited possibles.

Proposition. The lived experience of hope is aspiring uniquely with the silent familiar of spirited possibles, as cautious attention with heartening vitality emerges with expectancy amid the inimical.

Francesca's Story

Francesca is a 26-year-old student. She works as a waitress to make enough money to pay her tuition. She is also very involved in parochial activities. Francesca says hope is "trusting . . . in God." It represents the "vigor of present reality" and "certainty in the future." It is "believing" negative situations have "positive" answers. Hope offers a "gleam" of "possible solutions." It is a "type of human feeling" that is "indispensable. . . . Life would not make sense without it." Francesca cannot imagine a "world or an individual without this feeling." She says it is inevitable that individuals will find themselves in "difficult" situations; "life is like that." Francesca remembers hoping one of her dear friends would recover from cancer. She says she prayed and hoped God would restore his health, yet her feelings about hope did not "change at all" when her friend died. Having hope "does not automatically mean God grants you what you want." Francesca also believes hope is not just for "dramatic" situations. She says she lives hope "in very small things" that might seem "insignificant" to some people. Hope is "having the courage" to face any difficult situation.

Essences: Participant's Language

1. Hope is trust in God that something positive will happen; it is certainty in the future with vigor in the present.
2. Hope is indispensable and one cannot make sense of life without it; it gives one the courage to face difficulty.
3. Hope is a type of human feeling; it is in very small things and sometimes offers a gleam for a possible solution to a situation.

Essences: Researcher's Language

1. Confident sacred aspiration arises with the certitude of the will-be amid the vitality of the now.
2. Requisite expectancy surfaces with fortifying clarity amid the arduous.
3. Inherent anticipation of the familiar emerges with an expanding horizon.

Proposition. The lived experience of hope is the confident sacred aspiration arising with the certitude of the will-be amid the vitality of the now, while requisite expectancy surfaces with fortifying clarity amid the arduous, as inherent anticipation of the familiar emerges with an expanding horizon.

Antonio's Story

Antonio is 57 years old and has a degree in business. He is an entrepreneur in finance consulting and enjoys photography. Antonio believes that to be able to describe hope, "one must have felt the difficulties in life." Hope "is something that derives from certain ways of living and being, from being human, and from cultural togetherness." Antonio describes hope as "trust in Divine Providence," "trust in the joy of living," and "trust in oneself." He says it is possible to hope for "a better future, for a God, for a Father, or for a Son," but this is a "postponing of tomorrow" that "puts you in a situation of passivity, [while] waiting for the future."

Essences: Participant's Language

1. Hope is experienced with difficulties in life; it derives from an enthused way of living; it is part of being human.
2. Hope is calm waiting for a better future with trust in Divine Providence; it is thinking about and postponing tomorrow.

Essences: Researcher's Language

1. Heartening vital visions amid the arduous arise with the indigenous.
2. Quiescent expectancy with a sacred promise surfaces with prolonged contemplation of possibles.

Proposition. The lived experience of hope is heartening vital visions amid the arduous arising with the indigenous, as quiescent expectancy with a sacred promise surfaces with prolonged contemplation of possibles.

Carla's Story

Carla, aged 56, lives with her husband and three sons in a small village. She has a degree in teaching and currently does volunteer work for a local nonprofit organization. Carla believes "humans cannot live without hope." Hope is a "universal concept . . . without which life would be devoid of sense." She says life is full of "uncertainty" about "what will happen tomorrow," or even about what might happen "in an hour, or in a second." It is hope that makes it possible for one "to go on, to continue [with the uncertainty] toward the road one would like to travel." Carla believes people "resort to hope" when they find themselves without the "strength" to resolve difficult situations. She says "faith is hope" regardless of the religion one believes in because "human beings do not have absolute certainty about the existence of a superior entity." Individuals decide to have "faith" in, or to hope for, what is "nonmaterial, intangible, invisible, or unsure." When she was young, Carla feels her hopes "were for futile things like becoming a great doctor and freeing the world from illness." She now cares for persons who are "oppressed by pain" and finds she hopes their "situations will get better." Carla also says she sometimes comes across "problems" in which she feels "powerless to do anything." In these situations, hope helps her "to believe" something can be done, "to wait" for the stoplight to turn green, and "to think" bad moments will soon pass and the road will be free of impediments.

Essences: Participant's Language

1. Hope makes sense of life and allows one to go on quietly, since without it one would die and not have a future.
2. Hope is present in difficult, uncertain situations; it is having faith in the intangible.

Essences: Researcher's Language

1. Heartening emerges with the clarity of the silent fortification of vitality in expanding horizons.
2. Persistent expectancy amid obscure adversity arises with the discernible-indiscernible.

Proposition. The lived experience of hope is heartening, emerging with the clarity of the silent fortification of vitality in expanding horizons, while persistent expectancy amid obscure adversity arises with the discernible-indiscernible.

Rosa's Story

Rosa is 28 years old and works as a statistician. Rosa believes hope is "a necessary thing . . . like an element of energy for being able to reach [something] you want." It gives "thickness" and "positive direction" to your life. Rosa feels hope is not "innate." It is "cultivated, learned, and enriched" through experiences and relationships with others. Rosa describes her parents as individuals "very rich in hope." She says they lived and had success despite "many difficulties." Knowing this helps her to "believe in the goodness of hope." Rosa remembers a "period of darkness" in her adolescent life during which she had difficulty "managing her relationships with people." She says it was during that time of "isolation" that she first understood the necessity of hope. She believes "hope is the ability to [avoid] feeling isolated." Rosa describes her hopes as "intimate and personal." They are for "realizable and concrete things." Hope helps her "live well," "give the right dimension to negative things," and "maintain [herself] in a storm in the sea." For Rosa, hope is "happy, serene, and tranquil." She says the feeling of "tranquility" arises when she "reaches a goal" she had "never imagined" would happen. Rosa hopes "to know how to live adverse [situations] in a positive manner." In her experience, "people who have lived through tragedies have a certain strength around them." She describes this strength as "an umbrella of hope."

Essences: Participant's Language

1. Hope is a necessary thing; it is an element of energy for being able to reach that which you want to reach; it gives thickness to your life in the sense that it directs your way in a positive manner.
2. Hope is happiness and a sense of serenity and tranquillity; it is formed and cultivated through personal experiences and relationships.
3. Hope is a course that helps you maintain yourself in a storm, and it is an umbrella over a person living a tragedy; it is the ability to not feel isolated in difficult situations.

Essences: Researcher's Language

1. Vital expectancy emerges with propelling auspicious possibles.
2. Quiescence surfaces with the blossoming of unique convergences.
3. Unwavering envisioning arises with turbulent anguish amid the shield of easing seclusion.

Proposition. The lived experience of hope is vital expectancy emerging with propelling auspicious possibles, as quiescence surfaces with the blossoming of unique convergences, while unwavering envisioning arises with turbulent anguish amid the shield of easing seclusion.

FINDINGS AND RELATED LITERATURE

The structure of the lived experience of hope that emerged from this study with Italian participants is *the lived experience of hope is expectancy amid the arduous, as quiescent vitality arises with expanding horizons.* This structure arose from dwelling with propositions from each participant's dialogue. It synthesizes the three core concepts discovered in all ten participants' propositions: *expectancy amid the arduous, quiescent vitality,* and *expanding horizons.* The structure of the lived experience of hope was structurally transposed as *prospectivity amid the laborious as a lulled potency arises with the shifting familiar-unfamiliar.* It was conceptually integrated as *imaging enabling-limiting in the powering of transforming* (see Table 1). In this section, each core concept is further explicated in light of the human becoming theory and relevant theoretical and research literature for the purpose of enhancing understanding of the meaning of the lived experience of hope.

Expectancy Amid the Arduous

The first core concept, *expectancy amid the arduous,* was raised through structural transposition to *prospectivity amid the laborious.* Through conceptual integration it was then linked to the theoretical construct *imaging enabling-limiting* (see Table 2). Imaging is one of three concepts related to the first principle of the human becoming theory: "Structuring meaning multidimensionally is cocreating reality through the languaging of valuing and imaging" (Parse, 1998, p. 35). The theme of this principle is meaning. It relates to the

TABLE 1.
*Progressive Abstraction of the Core Concepts
of the Lived Experience of Hope*

Core Concepts	Structural Transposition	Conceptual Integration
Expectancy amid the arduous	Prospectivity amid the laborious	Imaging enabling-limiting
Quiescent vitality	Lulled potency	Powering
Expanding horizons	Shifting familiar-unfamiliar	Transforming

Structure

The lived experience of hope is expectancy amid the arduous, as quiescent vitality arises with expanding horizons.

Structural Transposition

The lived experience of hope is prospectivity amid the laborious as a lulled potency arises with the shifting familiar-unfamiliar.

Conceptual Integration

The lived experience of hope is imaging enabling-limiting in the powering of transforming.

way human beings continuously structure the meaning of multidimensional experiences that are lived all-at-once (Parse, 1981, 1998). In this principle, imaging is linked with the speaking–being-silent of languaging and the confirming–not-confirming of valuing.

Imaging refers to knowing at both explicit and tacit realms all-at-once (Parse, 1981, 1992, 1998). It is inherent in constructing reality, searching for answers, and coming to understand the world through the integration of new ideas (Mitchell, 1992; Parse, 1981). Imaging can include creative imagining, which Parse (1990a) described as "the picturing of what a situation might be like if lived in a particular way" (p. 138). Creative imagining immerses the person with what is pictured. It "is a way of experiencing a change and learning about what might be while evolving with the imaged possibles" (Parse, 1998, p. 74).

Enabling-limiting refers to the simultaneous existence of infinite opportunities and restrictions in all choices. Individuals choose ways to be with situations, and, in choosing, they enable themselves to move in one direction while simultaneously restricting their movement in another direction. Individuals are enabled and limited by all choices (Parse, 1981). Enabling-limiting evolves from the second principle of the human becoming theory: "Cocreating rhythmical

TABLE 2.
First Core Concept as Evident in Propositions

Core Concept:	Expectancy amid the arduous
Structural Transposition:	Prospectivity amid the laborious
Conceptual Integration:	Imaging enabling-limiting

1. expectancy . . . amid unsureness
2. envisioning . . . amid potential languid confinement
3. heartening visions amid the arduous
4. heartening aspiration . . . amid the arduous
5. aspiration amid disillusionment
6. expectancy amid the inimical . . . aspiring
7. requisite expectancy . . . amid the arduous
8. visions amid the arduous arise with expectancy
9. expectancy amid obscure adversity
10. envisioning arises with turbulent anguish

patterns of relating is living the paradoxical unity of revealing-concealing and enabling-limiting while connecting-separating" (Parse, 1998, p. 42). The theme of this principle is rhythmicity. Humans live rhythmical patterns of relating, which are paradoxical in nature and cocreated with the human-universe process (Parse, 1992). In this principle, enabling-limiting is associated with the simultaneous disclosing and hiding inherent in the paradoxical rhythm revealing-concealing. Parse's second principle also links enabling-limiting with the rhythmical process of moving together and moving apart intrinsic to humans' connecting and simultaneously separating with people, places, and events that are important to them.

Imaging enabling-limiting, as a construct, best describes the participants' meaning at the theoretical level. For participants in this study, imaging enabling-limiting is envisioning opportunities-restrictions. Imaging enabling-limiting refers to the ways participants speak about their desires and expectations for the future amid the arduousness of "uncertainties," "hardships," "frustrations," and "disappointments," which are the all-at-once opportunities and restrictions. It also relates to the participants' awareness that, in choosing to have expectations and desires, there is risk. For instance, one participant says, "Hope opens you to the risk of being disappointed." Another says, "Hope can make you a slave to your own expectations. This happens when you set goals . . . and then hope and hope, but in the end your trust in hope has not served for anything. . . . On the contrary, it has left a profound sense of frustration and powerlessness." Excerpts from participants' dialogues are illustrative of their choices to trust in their desires and expectations of future possibilities despite recognition of both opportunities and restrictions inherent in those choices. For example, one person envisioned a close friend recovering from cancer; yet, when he died, she says her feelings about hope "did not change at all." Another person pictures a world where "poor people find [something] to satisfy their hunger," and "elderly people do not have to die alone," yet acknowledges the opportunities and restrictions with this kind of hope, since it can be disappointing "when you set goals that are beyond your capabilities."

Several authors have written about hope in ways consistent with the ideas captured by the core concept, expectancy amid the arduous. Their works support the notion that hope is an expectant desire enabling and limiting possible surprises and opportunities for the future (Bloch, 1959/1986; Boyd, 1994; Godfrey, 1987; Staats, 1987; Steindl-Rast, 1984) that arises with life's discontentments and sufferings, amid horizons of new meanings and possibilities (Wu, 1972). Hope is about recognizing restrictions, while risking believing that situations can become other than they are (Casey, 1988; Marcel, 1951). In particular, the words of one person in this current study illuminate this point. He says, "Hope grants you the opportunity to believe that something can change in your favor." Other excerpts from the dialogical engagements linked with the first core concept, expectancy amid the arduous, demonstrate that participants in this study recognize constraints yet envision what they want and believe possible for the future. For instance, one person hopes to be able to reach her goals but cautions that "hope can be disappointing." Another participant, who says "hope is about expectations," believes that restrictions surface, since "if one hopes for too much, one can be disillusioned. Hope must be used a little at a time, in the right measure, and with a little pessimism."

In three other phenomenological studies, one of which used Parse's (1990b) research method, the lived experience of hope was also described, in various ways, as an expectation of a desirable outcome in the future that arose with the opportunities-restrictions of envisioning new possibles while living with day-to-day struggles (Brunsman, 1988; Parse, 1990b; Stanley, 1978). Thornburg (1993) and Wang (1997) reported similar findings from their Parse method investigations of the lived experience of hope; however, the notion of opportunities-restrictions, as connected with the theoretical concept enabling-limiting, was not reported as a major finding of their studies.

In this current study, participants' illustrations of expectancy amid the arduous were given in concert with explications of the calming, fortifying, and sustaining nature of hope. This reflects quiescent vitality, the second core concept in the structure of the lived experience of hope.

Quiescent Vitality

Quiescent vitality, the second core concept, was structurally transposed as *lulled potency* and conceptually integrated as *powering* (see Table 3). Powering

TABLE 3.
Second Core Concept as Evident in Propositions

Core Concept:	Quiescent vitality
Structural Transposition:	Lulled potency
Conceptual Integration:	Powering

1. quiescent vitality
2. enlivening propulsion . . . quiescence
3. quiescence . . . enlivened
4. vital radiance . . . fortification
5. unwavering . . . solemn certitude of immortality
6. vitality . . . with the silent familiar
7. vitality . . . confident sacred . . . fortifying clarity
8. quiescent . . . sacred promise . . . vital
9. silent fortification . . . vitality
10. propelling . . . quiescence . . . blossoming

is one of the three concepts in the third principle of the human becoming theory: "Cotranscending with the possibles is powering unique ways of originating in the process of transforming" (Parse, 1998, p. 46). The theme of the third principle is transcendence. It is about the ways in which humans change and unfold in life as they reach beyond what was and is with what is not yet (Parse, 1981). Powering is the energizing force, the pushing-resisting rhythm, that propels humans beyond the moment with cherished plans, hopes, and dreams (Parse, 1981). To be is to power. Powering is "the continuous affirming of self in light of the possibility of non-being" (Parse, 1981, p. 57). It happens in light of threats that may not only lead to non-being, or death, but also in light of threats of "being rejected . . . or not recognized in a manner consistent with expectations" (Parse, 1998, p. 47). Quiescent vitality, when conceptually integrated as powering, "is fundamental to being. It is the force of human existence and underpins the courage to be" (Parse, 1998, p. 47).

Quiescent vitality as powering is evident in the participants' descriptions of hope. It is the calming and quieting—yet enlivening, fortifying, and propelling—nature of hope. All the participants describe quiescent vitality when they speak about hope. One person believes "hope is quietly personal and it plays a part in daily life." Others say, for example, that hope is "an anchor [that] calms uncertainties," or that it is "the daily bread, a positive force, a spring that pushes you to continue to look ahead for satisfactions and calmness."

The findings from this current study are consistent with other literature in which hope has been described as an indispensable virtue inherent in being alive (Erikson, 1964) and as a dynamic life force (Dufault & Martocchio, 1985). Hope "gives human beings a sense of destination and the energy to get started" (Cousins, 1974, p. 5). It "comes close to being at the very heart and center of a human being" (Lynch, 1965, p. 31). Hope is viewed as a way to thrive amid life's day-to-day struggles. Many authors believe it is essential to survival (see for example, Bushkin, 1993; Cousins, 1979; Douville, 1994; Keith, 1991; Linge, 1990). The views of the participants from this present study are congruent with, and expand, this view of hope as an essential energizing force. Participants in this study contribute the understanding that hope can be energizing and calming, fortifying and quieting, propelling and solemn all-at-once. Amid their descriptions of the sustaining and energizing nature of hope, they also speak of it as "pleasant," "serene," "tranquil," and "calm." For instance, one person says, "Hope is a calm waiting. . . . It is part of being human," while another participant offers, "Without hope one would die. . . . It allows one to quietly go on," and another contributes, "Hope is an element of energy and a sense of serenity and tranquility."

Hope was conceptually integrated with the human becoming theory as powering in only one other Parse method study (Thornburg, 1993). In that study, parents of infants who had died from sudden infant death syndrome described moving on despite barriers. Thornburg structurally transposed moving on despite barriers as propelling through impediments and conceptually integrated it as powering. For the participants in Thornburg's study, the powering in hope is related to moving on despite impediments. Similarly, for the persons in this current study, powering relates to expectations and desires amid opportunities-restrictions that are energizing, yet quieting and calming.

The core concepts *expectancy amid the arduous* and *quiescent vitality* arose simultaneously with participants' explications of shifting views of their life situations. This reflects expanding horizons, the third core concept in the structure of the lived experience of hope.

Expanding Horizons

The third core concept, *expanding horizons*, was structurally transposed as *shifting familiar-unfamiliar*, and conceptualized as *transforming* (see Table 4). Transforming is one of three concepts connected with the third principle of the human becoming theory: "Cotranscending with the possibles is powering unique ways of originating in the process of transforming" (Parse, 1998, p. 46). Transforming is "the shifting of views of the familiar as different light is shed on what is known" (Parse, 1992, p. 39). It is linked to the continuous changes in life that accompany changing views of one's life situation. Expanding horizons, as transforming, captures the variety of ways participants speak about hope being integral to their shifting and changing views of life.

TABLE 4.
Third Core Concept as Evident in Propositions

Core Concept:	Expanding horizons
Structural Transposition:	Shifting familiar-unfamiliar
Conceptual Integration:	Transforming

1. expanding horizons
2. diversity . . . with confinement . . . expanding
3. fleeting apparitions of the obscure . . . metamorphosis
4. expanding possibilities
5. expanding horizons
6. uniquely . . . spirited possibles
7. expanding horizon
8. prolonged contemplation of possibles
9. expanding horizons . . . emerges with clarity
10. auspicious possibles . . . seclusion . . . unique convergences

For some participants, expanding horizons was linked to shifting views of hope itself. One participant says, "One's view of hope changes. . . . Its meaning and importance vary with the passing of years amid the vicissitudes of life" as the familiar is seen in a new light. When this participant was young, his hope "focused on the future." But, he says, "Maturity brings with it obligations, duties, and expectations, and hope becomes more concrete." As he grows older, he believes hope will "assume a renewed importance." Another person agrees, saying that her hope has changed as she has matured and her view of it has shifted. When she was young hope was for "things that did not exist yet. . . . Now it is for things concrete and reachable." Another person says, "Hope is very wide and can assume multiple meanings. . . . It has a thousand facets . . . like a ray of light that strikes a crystal and gets reflected in all different colors and shades. . . . Each person chooses a different way."

Other participants speak about the ways hope shifts their views of situations, people, and events important to them. They say, for example, hope is "changing things. . . . It is being able to create an illusion beyond reality"; "it helps a person believe in what he's doing, to look at life differently"; "to confront life with enthusiasm"; "it makes sense of life"; and it "offers a gleam of possible solutions."

Findings from two other studies (Parse, 1990b; Stanley, 1978) guided by the human becoming theory are congruent with findings from this current study. Stanley (1978) asked undergraduate students to write about situations in which they experienced hope. Stanley reported hope was characterized by a quality of transcendence. Also, Parse (1990b), in her study of the lived experience of hope for adults on hemodialysis, reported that participants spoke of hope as "unfolding a different perspective of an expanding view" (p. 15), which is similar to the way participants in this present study describe hope, for instance, as "a glimpsing of what can be," and "a new positive way of looking at things."

There are several other authors who have alluded to the transforming nature of hope. For instance, Moltman (1967) described hope as forward looking and moving, revolutionizing and transforming. Stephenson (1991) did a concept analysis and identified "a new perspective" as a consequence of hope. Still, the link between hope and shifting and changing views of life is not well articulated in other literature.

SUMMARY

This research study explored the lived experience of hope with ten persons who live in Italy. The structure that emerged is the lived experience of hope is expectancy amid the arduous, as quiescent vitality arises with expanding horizons. When conceptually integrated with the human becoming theory, the lived experience of hope is imaging enabling-limiting in the powering of transforming. The findings, along with those of the other studies reported in this book, expand understanding about the lived experience of hope and about the principles and concepts of the human becoming theory. Research and practice implications are discussed in the last chapter.

REFERENCES

Bloch, E. (1986). *The principle of hope* (N. Plaice, S. Plaice, & P. Knight, Trans.). Oxford: Basil Blackwell. (Original work published 1959)

Boyd, E. (1994). What makes a survivor? *Modern Maturity, 4–5, 72.*

Brunsman, C. S. (1988). *A phenomenological study of the lived experience of hope in families with a chronically ill child.* Unpublished master's thesis, Michigan State University, East Lansing.

Bushkin, E. (1993). Signposts of survivorship. *Oncology Nursing Forum, 20,* 869–875.

Casey, B. L. (1988). Hope, suffering, and solidarity: The power of the sabbath experience. *Dissertation Abstracts International, 50* (05), 1336-A. (University Microfilms No. AAG8914925)

Cousins, N. (1974, December 14). Hope and practical realities. *Saturday Review/ World. An Inventory of Hope* (Special Issue), 4–5.

Cousins, N. (1979). *Anatomy of an illness as perceived by the patient.* New York: Norton.

Douville, L. M. (1994). The power of hope. *American Journal of Nursing, 94*(12), 34–36.

Dufault, K. , & Martocchio, B. C. (1985). Hope: Its spheres and dimensions. *Nursing Clinics of North America, 20,* 379–391.

Erikson, E. H. (1964). *Insight and responsibility.* New York: W. W. Norton.
Godfrey, J. J. (1987). *A philosophy of human hope.* Dordrecht, The Netherlands: Martinus Nijhoff.
Keith, S. J. (1991). Surviving survivorship: Creating a balance. *Journal of Psychosocial Oncology, 9* (3), 109–115.
Linge, F. R. (1990). Faith, hope, and love: Nontraditional therapy in recovery
from serious head injury, a personal account. *Canadian Journal of Psychology, 44* (2), 116–129.
Lynch, W. F. (1965). *Images of hope: Imagination as healer of the hopeless.* Bal-
timore: Helicon Press.
Marcel, G. (1951). *Homo viator* (E. Craufurd, Trans.). Chicago: Henry Reg-
nery Co.
Mitchell, G. J. (1992). *Exploring the paradoxical experience of restriction-free-
dom in later life: Parse's theory-guided research.* Unpublished doctoral dissertation, University of South Carolina, Columbia.
Moltman, J. (1967). *Theology of hope.* New York: Harper & Row.
Parse, R. R. (1981). *Man-living-health: A theory of nursing.* New York: Wiley.
Parse, R. R. (1990a). Health: A personal commitment. *Nursing Science Quar-
terly, 3,* 136–140.
Parse, R. R. (1990b). Parse's research methodology with an illustration of the
lived experience of hope. *Nursing Science Quarterly, 3,* 9–17.
Parse, R. R. (1992). Human becoming: Parse's theory of nursing. *Nursing
Science Quarterly, 5,* 35–42.
Parse, R. R. (1998). *The human becoming school of thought: A perspective for
nurses and other health professionals.* Thousand Oaks, CA: Sage.
Staats, S. R. (1987). Hope: Expected positive effect in an adult sample. *Jour-
nal of Genetic Psychology, 148* (3), 357–364.
Stanley, A. T. (1978). The lived experience of hope: The isolation of discreet
descriptive elements common to the experience of hope in healthy young
adults. *Dissertation Abstracts International, 39* (03), 1212B. (University
Microfilms No. AAG7816899)
Steindl-Rast, D. (1984). *Gratefulness, the heart of prayer.* New York: Paulist
Press.
Stephenson, C. (1991). The concept of hope revisited for nursing. *Journal of
Advanced Nursing, 16,* 1456–1461.
Thornburg, P. D. (1993). *The meaning of hope in parents whose infants died
from sudden infant death syndrome.* Doctoral dissertation, University of
Cincinnati, OH. (University Microfilms International No. 9329939)
Wang, C. E. H. (1997). *Mending a torn fishnet: Parse's theory-guided research
on the lived experience of hope.* Unpublished doctoral dissertation, Loyola
University Chicago.
Wu, K. W. (1972). Hope and world survival. *Philosophy Forum, 12,* 131–148.

Chapter 7

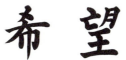

Kibou: Hope for Persons in Japan

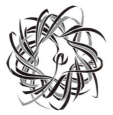

TERUKO TAKAHASHI

Japan is located off the east coast of Asia near the Korean peninsula and China. Japan consists of five islands: Honshuu (main island), Hokkaido, Shikoku, Kyushuu, and Okinawa. The total area of all these islands is roughly equal that of California. The population of Japan is 126 million, approximately half that of the United States. In 1995 the life expectancy of Japanese (*Japan As It Is*, 1997) was the highest in the world: (men: 76.38 years, women: 82.85 years); the elderly population in Japan is growing faster than in any other nation.

Japan is a homogeneous country with a traditional culture in spite of the technological developments. The Japanese history is characterized by two main points: (a) more than 10,000 years of cultural continuity and (b) the ability to adapt imported culture and technology to improve Japanese living standards. In comparison with Western individualism, the Japanese are characterized by groupism. The Japanese are oriented to family, company, and society, rather than the individual. Hayasaka (1984) pointed out that the Japanese prefer not to be singled out from the majority and prefer some ambiguity in their way of living, including interpersonal relationships. The Japanese people tend to dislike discussing close relationships and prefer not to make their situation clear. As a result, aggressive or very independent persons are rejected in light of the propagation of traditional Japanese values. Although these characteristics are slowly changing in the younger generation, the Japanese as a homogeneous nation unconsciously keep the traditional point of view.

PARTICIPANTS

Ten Japanese-speaking men and women representing every age group from 20 to 70 years, volunteered to participate in the study. They were all healthy persons living in the Tokyo area. The right to privacy, anonymity, and confidentiality were preserved. Each participant agreed to be audiotape-recorded.

DIALOGICAL ENGAGEMENT

The researcher-participant dialogical engagement began when the researcher invited each participant to reflect and describe the experience of hope in his or her life. The dialogues lasted from 20 to 50 minutes each and took place in participants' houses or offices or in the researcher's office.

EXTRACTION-SYNTHESIS

Takeshi's Story

Takeshi is 21 years old and a freshman in medical school. He failed the entrance examination to the medical universities three times before finally passing. When he was asked about the lived experience of hope, he immediately talked about his experiences taking the entrance examination to medical school.

When I took the entrance examination the first time, I had not seriously prepared for it. So I was not disappointed in my failure. Then, I really studied hard for three years, and during this time, I felt that I was walking in the dark without any light. I despaired of my future. Then I found a bright light in the darkness when I passed the entrance examination the fourth time.

Takeshi talked about similar experiences of finding a light in the dark. "When I talked with my girlfriend on the phone, I just felt that my love was going well because of her gentle responses. Although it was not clear how she felt, I was very happy and found a light of hope." Then Takeshi began to talk about painful experiences of childhood.

I was boisterous when I was little. In fourth grade, all my classmates did not tell me anything. Nobody asked to play with me. I was very sad. I never knew what to do. I made up my own ceremony. I just prayed every morning before going to school and I never gave up hope. I did not know why, but one day, one of my classmates spoke to me. I was really happy and felt that my prayers were a symbol of hope for me.

Essences: Participant's Language

1. Hope is about a time when the participant took an entrance examination after studying hard for three years. He said that when he passed the exam at medical university, he felt that he found a bright light in the dark.
2. Hope is when the participant knew that his love was going well.
3. Hope in the participant is the time when he was in fourth grade and all his classmates neglected him; he was very sad and prayed every morning before going to school. Eventually, one classmate spoke to him. He never gives up hope.

Essences: Researcher's Language

1. A radiance with accomplishment arises with steadfast devotion.
2. Confirmation of an affectionate affiliation surfaces with anticipation of what will be.
3. Contemplation with the sacred emerges with desired recognition amid rejection.

Proposition. The lived experience of hope is a radiance with accomplishment arising with steadfast devotion, as the confirmation of an affectionate affiliation surfaces with anticipation of what will be, while contemplation with the sacred emerges with desired recognition amid rejection.

Masahiko's Story

Masahiko is 33 years old and works at a university. His whole family graduated from a famous university. Therefore, when he could enter a junior high school of the university, which meant that he would be able to enter the university, he was very glad and relieved. At the university, he enjoyed student life:

> I organized a new sport club for me and for the younger students. I felt hope when I recognized reaching a goal. I sometimes worked hard to earn money as a manual laborer for the new club; I felt that I lived a full life every day.

Recently, Masahiko married and bought a new house. He talked about another experience of hope.

> I lived hope while my wife and I were going to buy a house. I was very happy whenever I even thought about it. For me, hope is to be realistic. If a dream is far from my real life, I can't feel hope. I feel hope when I recognize that something can become an actuality.

Essences: Participant's Language

1. Hope for the participant was reaching a goal when he organized a new sport group with very hard work.
2. Hope was present when the participant and his new wife were buying a house. He felt very happy and satisfied with life.

Essences: Researcher's Language

1. Inspired movement surfaces with desired accomplishments amid arduous liberation.
2. Realizing a desire emerges with joyful contentment.

Proposition. The lived experience of hope is inspired movement surfacing with desired accomplishments amid arduous liberation as realizing a desire emerges with joyful contentment.

Hisako's Story

Hisako is a 36-year-old homemaker with two children. She talked about her experience of hope as the time when she gave birth to her second child:

> My delivery occurred during the worst situation in my family. My mother was hospitalized for angina pectoris and was very seriously ill. My grandmother began to grow senile and was also hospitalized. I was in a hospital for the delivery. So my husband had to go to three hospitals to see us. The doctor told us that my mother was going to die. I could not even cry. Then I gave birth to my second child, who was the daughter that I wanted. Therefore, I just thought I passed through difficult times. I felt that I found a bright light. I was relieved and felt that I would be able to do anything in any situation.

Hisako continued to talk about hope as a new experience she had in Australia.

> Since my husband worked in Australia, I visited him and I really recognized the different circumstances in Australia. I lived comfortably there because I was free from social discipline. In Japan, I thought that I should follow what everybody else did. However, I came to know that it was only right that everybody has his or her own values and decides for him- or herself. After coming back to Japan, it was not easy to keep my new point of view. I know that I am told that I am a unique person, and I would like to keep the ideas that I learned in Australia.

Essences: Participant's Language

1. Hope for the participant is finding a bright light through difficult times like the time she gave birth to her daughter when her family was ill; she is relieved that she can do anything in any situation with hope.
2. Hope is living comfortably in another country where she can think and decide for herself.

Essences: Researcher's Language

1. Unburdening anticipation emerges with the radiance of realizing a desire amid adversity.
2. The novel surfaces with expanding possibilities.

Proposition. The lived experience of hope is an unburdening anticipation emerging with the radiance of realizing a desire amid adversity, while the novel surfaces with expanding possibilities.

Akira's Story

Akira is 41 years old and a psychiatrist at a university hospital in Tokyo. He was born and raised in a small town. His parents were very strict and they disciplined him. When he failed an entrance examination for a local university, he decided to go to Tokyo and was happy to get away from his parents. When he prepared for the entrance examination for another university, he felt hope:

> I felt that I could do anything almighty, like painting on a white canvas. In Tokyo, I encountered various kinds of people and felt that my world was getting bigger. I had a sense of freedom from the restraint of my parents. I was filled with great expectations and was bursting with energy.

Akira talked about his experience after becoming a psychiatrist:

> While I concentrate on studying, I experience hope because I feel that my work is worthwhile. Especially, since I know that nobody is investigating what we are studying, I have a sense of superiority and a

feeling of running at the top of the world. I am very satisfied and have a sense of freedom.

Essences: Participant's Language

1. Hope for the participant was when he went to Tokyo from his parents' house in a small town. He felt that he could do anything, like painting on a white canvas. He had a sense of freedom from restraint with great expectations and was bursting with energy.
2. While the participant concentrates on studying, he experiences hope that his work is worthwhile and he is very satisfied.

Essences: Researcher's Language

1. Liberation arises with the vigor of anticipation amid remembered restrictions.
2. Devotion to the prized emerges with contentment.

Proposition. The lived experience of hope is liberation arising with the vigor of anticipation amid remembered restrictions, while the devotion to the prized emerges with contentment.

Kumiko's Story

Kumiko is 46 years old and a faculty member in a school of nursing. She wanted to become a high school teacher, but she failed the entrance examination for the teacher's college where she sought admission. She decided to become a nurse, because nurses could work independently. She graduated from a diploma school of nursing. While she worked in a hospital, she learned conversational English and became a part-time student in a university. When she graduated, she was very happy and felt hope:

> I felt free from being restrained and came out of my shell. I acquired a license to be a school teacher. It meant for me that I could select my job—a teacher or a nurse. I have never felt such a sense of freedom and relief, and I relaxed. I felt that I could decide my life for myself.

Kumiko talked about her life after graduation:

> I was recommended and became a teacher nurse in a diploma school. Although it was not my first choice to become a nurse, I selected and decided to be a teacher nurse. I felt that I could demonstrate my ability. I just felt that I could live a full life. I was filled with hope that I could do what I wanted.

Essences: Participant's Language

1. Hope for the participant was when she graduated from a university; she felt free from being restrained and came out of her shell.

2. Hope is when the participant can demonstrate her ability; she is filled with the hope that she can do what she wants.

Essences: Researcher's Language

1. Unburdening liberation amid restriction surfaces with expanded possibilities.
2. Desired accomplishments emerge with the contentment of confident anticipation.

Proposition. The lived experience of hope is an unburdening liberation amid restriction surfacing with expanded possibilities, as desired accomplishments emerge with the contentment of confident anticipation.

Mamoru's Story

Mamoru is 54 years old and an editor for medical and nursing sciences in a publishing company. His company is the largest and most famous in these fields. When he graduated from the university, the Japanese economic condition was poor, so it was not easy to get a job as a journalist. Even so, he acquired the position as editor in this company. He appreciated working for the company because he had spent much time looking for a job. Throughout this experience, he felt that his hope would be not fulfilled. But, as he continued to work as an editor and took care of young writers, he gradually felt hope:

> I think that editors should be like backstage personnel. Since I think that the best magazine is the next magazine, I always try to promote the new ones. It is like planting seeds and cherishing them for bearing fruit. I supported and took care of young writers. When one of them was appraised as a good writer, I felt happy and hopeful. This means that my support bore fruit.

Mamoru continued, "When one project was successful in publishing many copies, I felt that my ideas were good. Hope for me is that I have achieved my wishes in business. I think that I would like to always publish good magazines."

Essences: Participant's Language

1. The participant experiences hope while supporting young writers after the restraint in his finding a job; he felt hope, happiness, and satisfaction.
2. Hope for the participant is when his ideas and projects are successful; it is achieving his wishes in business.

Essences: Researcher's Language

1. Inspiring contentment surfaces with liberating nurturing affiliations.
2. Visioned possibles arise with desired accomplishments.

Proposition. The lived experience of hope is an inspiring contentment surfacing with liberating nurturing affiliations, as visioned possibles arise with desired accomplishments.

Sawako's Story

Sawako is 58 years old and works at a city hall. She is divorced and has two children. Although she had a congenital dislocation of her hip joint, she lives an ordinary life. After her divorce, she acquired a license to be a kindergarten teacher. Several years later, she had pain in her leg. She tried to fulfill her obligation in her work. However, when she found out that fellow workers had told the union about her condition, she took a jaundiced view of the matter. Sawako said, "Although my boss supported me, I felt that I should leave my job. I lost my hope in my future. I was worried that I would not be able to walk. Then I decided to have an operation. When I was in bed, it seemed for me that everybody was bright and happy." Sawako continued to talk about her experience of hope after the operation. "When I could walk, I was very happy, because my life before the operation was too serious. I do not know how I can express my feelings in words. Hope for me is deep emotion at the moment I was able to walk." Sawako talked about her divorce:

> When I divorced, I had a sense of guilt because divorce was uncommon at that time. The divorce meant that a woman could not take care of her family and children. As a kindergarten teacher, especially, I did not tell anybody about my divorce. I worried that I was not appropriate as a kindergarten teacher. Several years later, some other divorced mothers talked with me about their divorces and appreciated me. Then, I felt hope that the painful experience would give me energy to keep my job. Recently, I met these mothers and expressed my appreciation to them.

Essences: Participant's Language

1. The participant says that she lost hope during difficult times, then experienced deep emotion at the moment she was able to walk.
2. Hope is when the participant recognizes that her painful experience gives her energy to keep her job.

Essences: Researcher's Language

1. An inspiring contentment amid the arduous emerges with the accomplishment of expanded possibilities.
2. Confirming the significance of suffering surfaces with liberation-restriction.

Proposition. The lived experience of hope is an inspiring contentment amid the arduous emerging with the accomplishment of expanded possibilities, while confirming the significance of suffering surfaces with liberation-restriction.

Yuji's Story

Yuji is 64 years old and retired from a famous broadcasting corporation. He was secretary to the president for several years and was vice president of a broadcasting museum before his retirement. Now he is working as an instructor of several seminars for businessmen. While he was working in the corporation, he was demoted to a local branch. He was very angry and felt desperate. One day, he saw the following words in blue on a girl's white T-shirt: "Get up with hope. Walk with joy. Sleep with thanks." He said, "Those words saved me from my disappointment. They encouraged and revitalized me. I felt that the sun suddenly came up, and I completely changed my feelings to look forward and I had hope. I think that hope is on the opposite side of despair and anxiety. I felt full of energy."

Yuji continued to talk about his experience of work. "When I found the meanings of my work, I felt full of energy and able to do anything that I wanted. I also felt that I was accepted and appreciated. I became gentle and trusted others."

Essences: Participant's Language

1. Hope is looking forward and being encouraged and revitalized by the words "Get up with hope. Walk with joy. Sleep with thanks"; he felt saved from a desperate situation.
2. Hope is found in the meanings of work; the participant felt accepted, appreciated, full of energy, and a trust in others.

Essences: Researcher's Language

1. Vivification with emancipation amid adversity surfaces with the inspiring utterances of anticipation of expanding possibilities.
2. Prized accomplishments emerge with the contentment of the vigorous certitude of reliant affiliations.

Proposition. The lived experience of hope is prized accomplishments emerging with the contentment of the vigorous certitude of reliant affiliations, while vivification with emancipation amid adversity surfaces with the inspiring utterances of anticipation of expanding possibilities.

Michiko's Story

Michiko is 67 years old. She was an editor for a publisher but left her job before retirement. She sometimes still edits books. When she was young, Michiko went to an acting school. She said, "I was filled with dreams and hopes. I felt that I had to do many things before becoming an actress. Whenever I earned money, I went to a play or a movie. I was absorbed in doing so. I did not care for food and clothing. I was just running toward my goal." Michiko continued to talk about hope and her new job:

> I began to work in a publishing company in order to earn money for my dream. Since I was involved in publishing a new journal on public health nursing, I met many nurses and was surprised to learn that they worked for people and not for themselves. It was a different experience from my dream of becoming an actress. This experience brought

me a new world and I found that editing was an expression of self, like acting. I was delighted and uplifted with my contribution to people and society through publishing a new journal.

Michiko talked about her child:

> When I was expecting a baby, I had a different kind of hope from that in my work. I felt that I had another life which was growing in my body. It was the happiest time and so filled with pleasure. When my son was 1 year old, he went to the house next door by himself and played for an hour. It was the first time that he left my side. I was really happy with such a simple event. It was hope itself that I saw in the child's smile and felt his growth.

Essences: Participant's Language

1. The participant said she was filled with hope as she became absorbed with running toward her goal.
2. Hope is being delighted and uplifted with finding a new world through the works of others to make personal contributions to society.
3. Hope is found in the participant's child's smile and in the pleasure of seeing her child grow.

Essences: Researcher's Language

1. Steadfast propulsion with the desired emerges with inspired submersion.
2. Rejoicing with expanded possibilities arises with the liberation of prized accomplishments.
3. Aspiration surfaces with the contentment of nurturing intimate affiliations.

Proposition. The lived experience of hope is steadfast propulsion with the desired emerging with inspired submersion, while rejoicing with expanded possibilities arises with the liberation of prized accomplishments, as aspiration surfaces with the contentment of nurturing intimate affiliations.

Fumi's Story

Fumi is a 77-year-old widow. She lost her husband when he was 35 years old. She raised three children by herself while she worked for a company. Now she lives alone near her sister's house. Fumi said:

> When I am asked about hope, I recall my husband's death. Although I was sad when he died, I felt it was God's will. Three days before his death, he was baptized. Then he quietly died in his sleep. After his funeral, I was also baptized. I believed that he went to Heaven. I tried to believe that my difficulties were given by the love of God. I found

pleasure in my difficulties without a hatred for my destiny. Therefore, hope for me is to believe in God.

Fumi continued, "I encountered many coincidences in my life. When I had a serious disease, I went to see several doctors. The last one was a Chinese physician and I think that I recovered by a miracle. I felt hope when I was saved and supported by something beyond human understanding." Fumi talked about her current life:

> Since I am not rich, I should devise everything for saving money. Now, I am making letter papers and bookmarks from old milk cartons. If I were rich, I would not have to make them and I could not understand others' suffering. I think that the rich do not always live wealthy. I felt hope because my poverty gave me new vision to enjoy my life.

Essences: Participant's Language

1. Hope is believing in God during her difficulties in life; she felt saved and supported by something beyond human understanding.
2. Hope for the participant is giving new vision in her poverty.

Essences: Researcher's Language

1. An unburdening with redeeming solace amid the arduous arises in accomplishments of divine faith.
2. A different view of the world brings anticipation of possibilities.

Proposition. The lived experience of hope is an unburdening, with redeeming solace arising amid the arduous, as accomplishments surface with divine faith, while a different view of the world brings anticipation of possibilities.

FINDINGS AND RELATED LITERATURE

The structure of the lived experience of hope follows: *hope is an anticipation of expanding possibilities, while liberation amid arduous restriction arises with the contentment of desired accomplishments.* The structure contains three core concepts that were central to all propositions and were uncovered in the extraction-synthesis process. (See Table 1.) The first concept of the structure, *anticipation of expanding possibilities,* incarnates *imaging transforming.* Imaging as knowing in the cocreating of reality structures the meaning of an experience, and transforming is the changing of change, coconstituting anew in a deliberate way (Parse, 1981). Imaging transforming, then, is cocreating the reality of an experience while changing the familiar-unfamiliar. Hope is envisioning the yet-to-be, transposing the unfamiliar to the familiar all-at-once. Participants confirmed this in their comments: "I was filled with hope that I could do what I wanted"; "I felt that I could do anything almighty, like painting on a white canvas"; "I felt full of energy and able to do anything that I

TABLE 1.

Progression of Abstraction of Core Concepts with Heuristic Interpretation

Core Concepts	Structural Transposition	Conceptual Integration
Anticipation of expanding possibilities	Envisioning the not-yet	Imaging transforming
Liberation amid arduous restriction	Struggling with opportunities and limitations	Enabling-limiting
Contentment of desired accomplishments	Emerging intended fulfillments	Valuing

Structure

Hope is anticipation of expanding possibilities, while liberation amid arduous restriction arises with the contentment of desired accomplishments.

Structural Transposition

Hope is envisioning the not-yet while struggling with opportunities and limitations in emerging intended fulfillments.

Conceptual Integration

Hope is imaging transforming in the enabling-limiting of valuing.

wanted." They imaged a bright future, although the future was unfamiliar. "Painting on a white canvas" means for the Japanese unlimited possibilities. These possibilities arise in multidimensional experience and shift the familiar-unfamiliar. This is imaging transforming.

The second core concept of the structure, *liberation amid arduous restriction*, incarnates the notion of *enabling-limiting*. Parse (1990) specifies that the structure of the lived experience is the paradoxical living of the remembered, the now moment, and the not-yet. When participants were asked to describe the experience of hope, they spoke of their struggling experiences of restriction and social discipline. They also described that they felt free from restraints and found opportunities to have different perspectives. One participant said, "I encountered various kinds of people and felt that my world was getting bigger. I had a sense of freedom from the restraint of my parents." Another said, "I lived comfortably there [in Australia] because I was free from social discipline. In Japan, I thought that I should follow what everybody else did. However, I came to know that it was only right that everybody has his or her own values and decides." According to Parse (1992), there are inherent opportunities and limitations with all decisions; one is enabled-limited by all choices. As participants chose their ways of living, they experienced hope. Therefore, hope for participants is an enabling-limiting experience.

The final concept of the structure, *contentment of desired accomplishments*, incarnates *valuing*. Parse (1981) described valuing as the human's process of confirming cherished beliefs, which are reflective of one's worldview. Participants described satisfaction with their studies and their businesses. One participant said, "While I concentrate on studying, I experience hope because I feel that my work is worthwhile. . . . I have a sense of . . . running at the top of the world." Another said, "When one project was successful in publishing many copies, I felt that my ideas were good. Hope for me is that I have achieved my wishes in business." Through contentment with their desired accomplishments in studying and conducting business, the participants confirm their beliefs. This is valuing.

The findings from this study are consistent with other qualitative studies on hope (Gaskinis & Forté, 1995; Parse, 1990). In Parse's study (1990), ten English-speaking persons on hemodialysis between the ages of 23 and 75 participated. In this study, ten Japanese-speaking participants in good general health between the ages of 21 and 77 agreed to describe hope. In spite of the differences between these groups, conceptual interpretation of the structure of the lived experience is very similar. The structure of hope in the Parse (1990) study is imaging the enabling-limiting of transforming. In the Japanese study, hope is imaging transforming in the enabling-limiting of valuing. Gaskinis and Forté (1995) pointed out that although the participants identified very personal sources of hope, the meanings yielded common themes, and the structure of the lived experience of hope could be universal in any situation.

Gaskinis and Forté (1995) also described the essential structure of hope as a positive emotion and response to a desired future situation experienced in the present. While their study was from a different perspective, this notion relates to the first core concept of the current study, anticipation of expanding possibilities. Stephenson (1991), also from a different perspective, defined hope as "a process of anticipation that involves the interaction of thinking, acting, feeling, and relating, and is directed toward a future fulfillment that is personally meaningful." This definition somewhat relates to all three core concepts arising in this study: anticipation of expanding possibilities, liberation amid arduous restriction, and contentment of desired accomplishments.

In a recent article, Kylmä and Vehviläinen-Julkunen (1997) suggested that hope research should be expanded to take in not only sick individuals but also healthy people at different stages of their lives. This study was conducted in light of this suggestion.

Implications for research and practice related to the findings of this study are discussed in the final chapter of this book, along with the findings from the other studies.

REFERENCES

Gaskinis, S., & Forté, L. (1995). The meaning of hope: Implications for nursing practice and research. *Journal of Gerontological Nursing, 21,* 17–24.

Hayasaka, T. (1984). Phenomenology of the Japanese self. In D. Kruger (Ed.), *The changing reality of modern man.* Cape Town: Juta.

Gakken (Ed.). 1997. *Japan as it is.* Tokyo: Gakken.

Kylmä, J. & Vehviläinen-Julkunen, K. (1997). Hope in nursing research: A meta-analysis of the ontological and epistemological foundations of research on hope. *Journal of Advanced Nursing, 25,* 364–371.

Parse, R. R. (1981). *Man-living-health: A theory of nursing.* New York: Wiley.

Parse, R. R. (1990). Parse's research methodology with an illustration of the lived experience of hope. *Nursing Science Quarterly, 3,* 9–17.

Parse, R. R. (1992). Human becoming: Parse's theory of nursing. *Nursing Science Quarterly, 5,* 35–42.

Stephenson, C. (1991). The concept of hope revisited for nursing. *Journal of Advanced Nursing, 16,* 1454–1461.

Chapter 8

Hopp: The Lived Experience for Swedish Elders

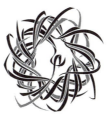

ANIA WILLMAN

Sometimes
I have dreams
about another change
without knowing
what it is

Ania Willman

The meaning of hope that surfaced in the following research is similar to the meaning of hope suggested in the poem above. In this study, the lived experience of hope emerges as *envisioning possibilities amid adversity, as persistent expectancy arises with nurturing affiliations.*

PARTICIPANTS

Eight women and two men between the ages of 74 and 91 from Malmö, Sweden, participated in the research. At the time of the research, the participants were residing on the same ward at the university hospital in the city of Malmö, a southern coastal city with 250,000 people—the third largest city in Sweden. Malmö has the highest percentage of elderly population of any city in Sweden; it is an old industrial area with a retired working-class population. The participants were on an acute care service for older adults for a variety of reasons; all were planning to return home.

DIALOGICAL ENGAGEMENT

Dialogical engagements took place in the hospital rooms of the participants.

EXTRACTION-SYNTHESIS

Ingrid's Story

Ingrid is an 88-year-old widow who was admitted to the hospital because of pulmonary disease. She wants to go home, but the doctors and nurses want her to stay for a period of three months for rehabilitation. Ingrid said that "people are always hoping, but for different things." She said that she had hoped for good and kind children and she got that. "Sometimes you have hope without knowing what you are hoping for." While in the hospital, she said she hopes "everything will turn out well, but you never can tell; you never know about that." She said that hope is significant and that her thoughts about hope will help "push her in the right direction." She also said that "you only fully know what your hopes were later on." Ingrid said that she hopes she will be a little bit better so that she will be able to go home, "but you never know about that." She sighs and says, "I will never give up hope"; she knows that, at other times in her life, hope was important, but she cannot remember exactly when. Ingrid said she "hopes for people, everyone, to be happy and to have happiness." Hope is difficult for her to describe, but she "hopes for a happy departure for everyone." She cannot explain this further. Ingrid said, "I am rather satisfied with life. I have nothing to complain about."

Essences: Participant's Language

1. The participant says that she is always hoping for different things even if she doesn't know what she is hoping for or how things will turn out. She has good and kind children.
2. Hope for the participant is significant; it pushes her in the right direction.
3. The participant says hope is difficult to describe, yet she knows it is there and important to hold on to even in difficult times.

Essences: Researcher's Language

1. Continuously envisioning novelties with benevolent affiliations.
2. Pivotal expectations surface with forging desirable paths.
3. The ineffable emerges with salient immanence amid adversity.

Proposition. The lived experience of hope is continuously envisioning novelties with benevolent affiliations, as pivotal expectations surface with forging desirable paths, while the ineffable emerges with salient immanence amid adversity.

Tor's Story

Tor is an 82-year-old widower. He is in the hospital because he fell at home. He does not always follow his physician's treatment plan. Sometimes he does not take his medication and he gets dizzy. When Tor was asked to talk about his experience of hope, he talked about his life's work. He started as a carpenter and a stonecarver. He said that in 1945 he got a job in Malmö as a bookkeeper. After ten years on that job, he started at a coal company because he got a higher salary. "When I started to work at the coal company, the manager told me that 90 percent of the men working there were 'drinkers.'" Tor said that in his view "90 percent of them did not drink." Several years later when the company closed, he was released, but the manager recommended him for a new job because, according to the manager, he worked well with the "drinkers." After that, Tor worked at an employment agency, again working with people who drank, this time together with the police. Tor said that he succeeded with the "drinkers" because he was not afraid and he "had hope for them." After Tor's wife died, he moved to a new flat in the same building because "it is important to know the same people as before." Tor said, "Today I am alone; I don't hear from my son. Sometimes I brood and feel hopeless. . . . It is important to know people; hope comes from knowing people." After his wife's death, a woman he knew from work phoned and told him that she had read about his wife's death in the newspaper. Now Tor and the woman are phoning one another "four, five times a day. It is important to have her to talk to," he says.

Essences: Participant's Language

1. The participant says he succeeded in his work with the "drinkers" because he had hope for them.
2. The participant says that it is important to have people to talk to because when alone and brooding, he feels hopeless, but hope is knowing people— the same people over time.

Essences: Researcher's Language

1. Envisioning possibilities with firm expectations arises with satisfying achievements.
2. Desired longing for uplifting togetherness arises amid despair.

Proposition. The lived experience of hope is envisioning possibilities with firm expectations arising with satisfying achievements, as desired longing for uplifting togetherness arises amid despair.

Allan's Story

Allan is a 79-year-old former sailor who is in the hospital with pulmonary disease. He is constantly coughing. He speaks Swedish with a Norwegian accent. Allan said, "Hope, hope . . . I hope to be better . . . at least . . . that is my first hope . . . that I hope to be better." He believes that it will take time to be better because he has had emphysema for a long time. He said that he knows that "it will never be as before" and that he hopes "to live and have health. That is most important. . . . My best time was at sea. I want to go back to that time. It is difficult to talk specifically about hope, but hope played a part of my life at sea. Now I am retired. . . . Hope is when you have positive thoughts about everything; you have hope that the way life turns out is the best way. It is not a good thing to be ill; hope is significant, more significant when you are cared for." Allan said that hopelessness "is when it is depressing and gloomy, and you must not allow yourself to be that way. . . . You have to look at it in a positive way. You must not think negative thoughts; sometimes it seems hopeless, but it will change and it will go the right way. It will work out the right way, and it depends on a lot of things. It depends on yourself and also on the circumstances." He said he knows "that hope is always there. You always have hope; if you stop hoping, things will not work out." He said that he thinks hope is necessary if you want to stay alive.

Essences: Participant's Language

1. The participant said his illness has changed his life; he hopes for health, and he recalled his life at sea as hopeful.
2. Hope for the participant is having positive thoughts about everything; even when things appear hopeless, life will turn out for the best.
3. The participant says hope is always there and it is significant, but more significant at times he is cared for.

Essences: Researcher's Language

1. Envisioning remembered vitality surfaces with the unalterable.
2. Inspiring contemplation amid despair arises with confidence.
3. Persistent expectancy emerges with nurturance.

Proposition. The lived experience of hope is envisioning remembered vitality surfacing with the unalterable, while inspiring contemplation amid despair arises with confidence, as persistent expectancy emerges with nurturance.

Maria's Story

Maria, 74 years old, is in the hospital with a medical diagnosis of anemia. This is her second visit to the hospital in three weeks. Maria thinks that it is difficult to talk about hope. When she starts to think about hope and about illness and treatments she says, "I am the kind of person who thinks that you have to take it, and that there is nothing you can do, but you hope for the best." Maria has confidence and trust in God. Maria says that hope is significant and "if you give up hope then . . . there is nothing to . . . keep you up." Maria said, "I have had a good life, marriage, and a daughter, but this last period of life is not so good, but I have to take it anyhow." Maria said that there have been no troubles. "Life goes on, and you look forward and you yourself can do nothing about it. You have to take each day at a time. You know hope by how things work out; when some situations turn out well, then you have hope." Maria was worried about a medical test, and she sobbed and said, "You hope it will turn out well, but you have to take it." It was the work in the congregation and her friends and acquaintances that helped her during the time of her husband's death seven years ago. She sobs and says that it was a hard time, because her husband died so suddenly. He died at the summer house, in midsummertime, and she thought of selling the house, but she still has it. Maria said that the first year after her husband's death was very hard. "If you do not have hope, then you are not alive; you waste away." She said it was because of her previous work in the congregation that they asked her to return and help out. She said, "Then you think you have something to pass on." She became sad and said that she hoped to be well for a few more years. She hoped that her illness would be a small thing, "but you never know." She thinks it is good not to be confused and to see that your own activity is important. "Yes, to be active, to keep going, that is important."

Essences: Participant's Language

1. Hope is when you think you have something to pass on; it is important to keep going even if there is nothing you can do.
2. You are not alive, you waste away, if you do not have hope, and if situations turn out well, you have hope that someone helped, and she trusts in God.

Essences: Researcher's Language

1. Contemplating a legacy arises with persistent endurance despite doubts.

2. Vitality amid potential vanquishment surfaces with expectant confidence in divine intercession.

Proposition. The lived experience of hope is contemplating a legacy with persistent endurance despite doubts, as vitality amid potential vanquishment surfaces with expectant confidence in divine intercession.

Elna's Story

Elna, age 84, has been in the hospital for three weeks. When not in the hospital she lives alone in a flat. When she was asked to talk about hope, Elna's first comment was "Hope! Yes. I feel it sharply! I think that it cures me and that I will be able to go back home again." She says that every time she is in the hospital she thinks, "I give myself up to the doctors and I hope that it will turn out well, and so far it has worked! I am well in spite of the illness. I am well because I am strong; hope makes you willing to stay alive longer." Elna thinks that one reason for her willingness to stay alive is her brothers and sisters and their children. They are important to her, and she looks forward to their letters and seeing them, particularly the children. She talked about the last time she was in the hospital: "I felt hope the last time I was here; I wished to return home, and I did!" Elna said that she has a lot of friends who help her. One woman washes for her, and a boy vacuums, cleans, and does her shopping. She says that it is her own decision to accept this help, and that this is a good thing, because it helps her stay home. She says that she thinks of the words faith, hope, and love. "You hope for the best, but you never know. You never know what your hope is; when you get bad, maybe then you will want to waste away." Elna thinks that her attitude makes a difference. "Your own activity . . . matters. . . . You help the physicians . . . to get you well again." She talked about an episode that past summer. It was hot and she lost all her energy. She feels she has not recovered yet. "Maybe I will get my energy back," she says. She thinks that she is a strong and active person. She makes plans for this summer. "I want to go home, and I do not want to make visits. I want to be by myself, in my own home." She says that hope is "always the same experience. Hope now is like it was before."

Essences: Participant's Language

1. The participant hopes for the best; she is strong and makes plans for the following summer, but she thinks that if things get worse, she might change her mind and want to waste away.
2. Hope is always the same, a sharp feeling that keeps you alive.
3. Hope can cure, but attitude and activities matter; one needs energy and helpful friends and relatives.

Essences: Researcher's Language

1. Envisioning possibilities surface with potential vanquishment.
2. Piercing expectancy arises with vitality.

3. Personal commitment with nurturing affiliations emerges with desired remedies.

Proposition. The lived experience of hope is envisioning possibilities amid potential vanquishment, as piercing expectancy arises with vitality, while personal commitment with nurturing affiliations emerges with desired remedies.

Elly's Story

Elly is an 81-year-old widow who has been in the hospital for ten days. She plans to go back home to her own flat within two days. While talking, she became short of breath and could not complete her sentences. Elly talked about hope: "Well, I am always optimistic, *always*, and I would rather laugh than cry." She described her situation as rather difficult and she preferred not to talk about it. "It hurts to make wounds bleed anew." She then began to sob and said, "I have had a little bit of trouble with my husband, but hope has helped me. If you do not have hope and if you do not look forward, then it is hopeless." She thinks that hope is "the thing that makes you go on." Elly said that during the years, there have been many difficult situations for her. "My daughter was killed in an accident. That was a very hard time in my life. I pushed that memory away by being active. I sewed rugs and pictures, and I crocheted. I was active all the time and I read books to occupy my brain." She said that she is not the kind of person who sits down and broods, because that does not make anything better. "You have to look forward and keep yourself healthy and eat well."

Elly said that it is difficult to define hope with words. "Hope is something you feel within yourself. If you are a happy person in your soul and heart, you are full of hope." She said hope is when she thinks it will be better the next day, and when it is not, then she thinks it will be better the day after. Elly thinks that some people are pessimists; they are dull and they make it dull for themselves and others. "If you have troubles, figure it out the best way you can, and try to disperse dull thoughts. Every person should think of not making it dull for their fellow creatures."

Essences: Participant's Language

1. The participant says that she is an optimist, full of hope; hope is when you disperse the dull thoughts and think the next day will be better.
2. Hope is the thing that makes you go on and look forward in difficult situations. You can push hard times away by participating in activities like reading and crocheting. Hope is something you feel within yourself.

Essences: Researcher's Language

1. Confident expectancy emerges with determined contemplation of new possibilities.
2. Persistent envisioning amid adversity arises with personal commitment to engaging affiliations.

Proposition. The lived experience of hope is confident expectancy emerging with determined contemplation of new possibilities, as persistent envisioning amid adversity arises with personal commitment to engaging affiliations.

Asta's Story

Asta is 77 years old and has been in the hospital for four days. She plans to go back home in a few days. She lives alone, was never married, and has no living brothers or sisters. When asked to talk about hope, Asta laughed and said, "You do not mean jumping?" (The word is the same for both in Swedish.) She giggles. "You mean hope about the future, don't you? When you grow old, you have less and less hope. You get frail and you are not able to do what you want. Then you get depressed." Asta said that she does not have much hope for the future. She said that hope is connected to health: "It is the alpha and the omega; you cannot buy your health with money." Asta talked about her parents and her brother. She said, "I hoped for my parents—that they should have a long life—but they went so quickly. Both my parents died and I had hoped to keep them for a long time." She said her brother died ten years ago. "He was two years younger than me. It was hard for me when he died; I was hoping that he would survive me." She said that after he died it went downhill for her. Asta said that her brother's wife lives far away, in Stockholm, and that she has no other relatives.

> I am lonely. I have lost hope. Parkinson's disease can't be cured; it only gets worse. At the end you can do nothing; you get stiff and eventually can't talk. Now I need help to put my clothes on and to take them off, and I need help with my washing and cleaning. It is hard for me to find hope. I do not know what to have hope for; maybe life. I feel hopeless-ness, actually; but it could be worse. All people say that. But I feel it gets worse all the time; well, you try to do the best with the situation anyhow. I am rather lucid; I am happy about that. The worst thing would be to be unclear. But, I cannot say that I have much of a future.

Asta said that she used to solve crosswords and that she reads, but everything takes time and the day is so short.

Essences: Participant's Language

1. When you grow old you have less and less hope, you get frail and you are not able to do what you want, and you get depressed, but you try to do your best with the situation.
2. Hope is connected to your health and family, the alpha and the omega. You cannot buy health with money. She says she is happy that she is still lucid.

Essences: Researcher's Language

1. Envisioning forebearance amid potential vanquishment arises with a persistent expectancy.

2. Promise surfaces with familiar affiliations in the joyful contentment of accomplishment.

Proposition. The lived experience of hope is envisioning forebearance amid potential vanquishment, as the persistent expectancy of promise surfaces with familiar affiliations in the joyful contentment of accomplishment.

Esther's Story

Esther is a 91-year-old widow who was in the hospital for a few days with chest pain. When asked about hope, Esther was silent but eventually said, "They thought I had pneumonia. I am lost. I want to go home, home to my own place." She said that she has hope she will go home, but she wonders how it will work out. "The ambulance has to pick me up and drive me home. . . . I do not know . . . if I will go home tomorrow. . . . We will have to see about that. . . . It is good here. I have lots of help from the kind girls here." Esther says she needs help to dress, to make her bed, and to cook. "I do some crocheting and knitting and I sit and stare at the walls. You have to do that too," she says and giggles. "I have been alone for many years; I have been a widow since 1934." Esther tells that she raised two children without much help. "I did well. You have to say that, when you think of it . . . when you think back." She said she did not feel hopeful or hopeless. "You have to take what comes and work."

Essences: Participant's Language

1. Hope is taking what comes; the participant says that she has been alone since 1934 and had to work hard to raise her two children.
2. Hope is wanting to go home to her own place even though she wonders how it will work out, since she needs help from kind others. She does not feel hopeful or hopeless.

Essences: Researcher's Language

1. Promise arises with forebearance amid adversity.
2. Yearning for the nurturance of the envisioned familiar surfaces with vexing expectancy.

Proposition. The lived experience of hope is promise arising with forebearance amid adversity, while yearning for the nurturance of the envisioned familiar surfaces with vexing expectancy.

Ruth's Story

Ruth, an 84-year-old widow, has been in the hospital for two weeks and was planning to return home soon. When asked about hope, Ruth asked, "Do you mean if I feel inclined to live?" She brought out photos and talked about her life, her daughter, and her family in the United States. She said that her daughter's husband had died, and she began to sob and said her husband had died also—both from smoking. Ruth said, "Hope, what is hope? I have always had hope for the future . . . and I have willpower. I have been to the United States every second year and my daughter has been here . . . and I had part-time work." Ruth said that some years ago she had been told she had cancer, but she was grateful that her children were grown up. "This was the only thing I was thinking of, how wonderful that they will manage. My daughter was 20 years old and had a job and my son was 16. I was thinking of my husband and of my children. I was not afraid of death. Now I have hope to see my daughter and my grandchild again. I am happy about that. They have ordered tickets and will come and visit me this summer. I have hope that I will survive until August," she says and laughs. "Yes, I have hope. . . . I have this hope. I hope that I will manage. . . . I will go home soon." Ruth thinks that hope is significant for her "inclination to live. It is very significant . . . if you look forward and you can see a future. It is important not to dig yourself down even if it is a hard time. I have been through difficult situations, very difficult. I have been down in a very deep valley, but at that time my mother was alive, and I have to say she was a great help." Ruth said that her mother comforted her. She began to sob and said, "It was a very hard time for me when I was between 40 and 50 years old. I was depressed and my mother helped me. It is important if you have a person who understands and pays attention to your feelings. That is for sure." Ruth thinks it is important to be positive. She has faith in God and believes that her faith has helped her. "I think that people must have something to believe in. I have been a member in a group for needlework and I have good friends and much fun. It is important to have friends and fun." Ruth says that hope can be interpreted in many ways. "You can say that you must live on your hope." She laughs. "This is about the future. . . . It is bright . . . that it will be bright. That is important. We all know life is not forever, we all know . . . that is the only thing to be sure of . . . that we shall pass away and if you have that feeling . . . that feeling of hope if you have something to trust in, then it is not so dark."

Essences: Participant's Language

1. Hope for the participant is knowing that her family can manage without her; it is to be with friends, to have fun, and to have a person who understands and pays attention to her feelings.
2. The participant says she has always had hope and willpower. She connects it with a will to survive and the inclination to live.
3. Hope is something to believe in and trust in; then it is not so dark when you look forward, even if it is hard times.

Essences: Researcher's Language

1. An inspiring promise surfaces with benevolent reverent engagements.
2. Persistent expectancy arises with a fortifying vitality.
3. Confident reliance emerges with envisioning possibilities amid adversity.

Proposition. The lived experience of hope is an inspiring promise surfacing with benevolent reverent engagements, while persistent expectancy arises with a fortifying vitality, as confident reliance emerges with envisioning possibilities amid adversity.

Lisa's Story

Lisa, an 82-year-old widow, is in the hospital because she had a fall at home. She lives in her own flat and plans to go back there. Lisa finds it hard to explain hope.

> Hope is when you think . . . you want . . . events and things to happen. It is when you wish for the best of everything. I have had a lot of illnesses, and I have been alone for so many years, but I have always been full of hope. I have always looked forward. I have never been sad. I have always thought that things straighten themselves out. People have said to me that I have had a difficult time, but I say that you have to take it and undergo it. I have never been sad in life even if it has been very, very troublesome at times.

Lisa talked about her husband and their four children. She had been married for twenty-three years and she had four children in five years. She and her husband where happy about the children even though they lived in poverty. She says that it was difficult to live, but they were able to look forward, and they had a saying, "Tomorrow is another day." Lisa continued:

> I have had my misfortunes, but they are there to overcome; it is easier to live if you can think . . . in a straight way . . . and think there will be a new tomorrow. I have always been hopeful; I was never sad and complaining . . . that is not my way of being. I cannot complain. I am satisfied with my life. There have been some misfortunes, but it should not be too easy for you. There ought to be days with sunshine but also some dark days. Otherwise you will not find your life valuable.

Today Lisa hopes to get well. "I never give up. I always think it could have been worse." She talked about her seven grandchildren and she thinks about them a lot. "My health is not so good, but I have hope to go back home . . . for a little while." Lisa says that hope is important for health. "It is important to be happy and not brood and brood; it depends on yourself." Her own future is gloomy now, she thinks, "but it is my happiness to follow the grandchildren as they grow up." She has photos and she values them. "I am *very* satisfied with life."

Essences: Participant's Language

1. The participant says that she has always been full of hope, always able to look forward; she never gives up and believes that there ought to be both

sunny and dark days; otherwise, you will not find life valuable. Even with great difficulties in life, she believes in a new day tomorrow.

2. Hope is when you want events and things to happen, when you wish for the best. The participant wants to go back home and continue to watch her grandchildren grow up, and she thinks of them often.

Essences: Researcher's Language

1. Buoyancy with the promise of new possibilities arises with gleaming anticipation amid dismal adversity.
2. Contemplating desires surface with yearning for familiar nurturing engagements.

Proposition. The lived experience of hope is a buoyancy with the promise of new possibilities arising with gleaming anticipation amid dismal adversity, as contemplating desires surface with yearning for familiar nurturing engagements.

FINDINGS AND RELATED LITERATURE

Table 1 shows the essences from the propositions that the researcher used to derive the three core concepts. Table 2 shows the core concepts and their progression across levels of abstraction. The core concepts comprise the structure: *The lived experience of hope is envisioning possibilities amid adversity, as persistent expectancy arises with nurturing affiliations.* Structurally transposed, the lived experience of hope is *envisaging the will-be amid the disheartening, as resolute prospectivity arises with propitious involvements.* With conceptual integration, hope is *imaging the powering of connecting-separating.*

The finding of this study was that the lived experience of hope is envisioning possibilities amid adversity as persistent expectancy arises with nurturing affiliations. Each core concept reflects extracts from the dialogues. The first concept, *envisioning possibilities amid adversity,* is an essence of the lived experience of hope. Each participant described this in a unique way. Ingrid said, "Sometimes you have hope without knowing what you are hoping for," and Asta, who has Parkinson's disease, said, "I am rather lucid; I am happy about that. The worst thing would be to be unclear."

The second extracted concept, *persistent expectancy,* can be described as living a particular way, while not knowing all that is yet-to-be. For example, Allan, the former sailor, said, "You have hope that the way life turns out is the best way." In the human becoming theory, change is a continuous, unitary human-universe process. Within this process, persons coparticipate in change choosing meaning, in relationship with others, and reaching to what is not yet while pushing-resisting with resolute expectancy (Parse, 1987, 1992).

The third core concept, *nurturing affiliations,* can be viewed as propitious involvements and connecting-separating. This concept was described in unique ways by each participant. Tor said, "It is important to know people; hope comes from knowing people." Maria said that because of her work in her congregation,

TABLE 1.
Core Concepts and Underlying Essences

Core Concept 1:   Envisioning possibilities amid adversity

1. envisioning novelties . . . amid adversity
2. envisioning possibilities . . . amid despair
3. envisioning remembered vitality . . . amid despair
4. contemplating . . . potential vanquishment
5. envisioning possibilities . . . amid potential vanquishment
6. persistent envisioning . . . amid adversity
7. envisioning forebearance . . . amid potential vanquishment
8. forebearance amid adversity . . . envisioned familiar
9. envisioning possibilities . . . amid adversity
10. promise of possibilities . . . amid dismal adversity

Core Concept 2:   Persistent expectancy

1. pivotal expectations
2. firm expectations
3. persistent expectancy
4. expectant confidence
5. piercing expectancy
6. confident expectancy
7. persistent expectancy
8. vexing expectancy
9. persistent expectancy
10. gleaming anticipation

Core Concept 3:   Nurturing affiliations

1. benevolent affiliations
2. uplifting togetherness
3. remembered vitality . . . with nurturance
4. legacy . . . divine intercession
5. nurturing affiliations
6. engaging affiliations
7. familiar affiliations in the joyful contentment of accomplishment
8. yearning for the nurturance
9. benevolent reverent engagements
10. familiar nurturing engagements

TABLE 2.
Progression of Abstraction for Core Concepts

Core Concepts	Structural Transposition	Conceptual Integration
Envisioning possibilities amid adversity	Envisaging amid disheartenment	Imaging
Persistent expectancy	Resolute prospectivity	Powering
Nurturing affiliations	Propitious involvements	Connecting-separating

Structure

Hope is envisioning possibilities amid adversity, as persistent expectancy arises with nurturing affiliations.

Structural Transposition

Hope is envisaging the will-be amid the disheartening, as resolute prospectivity arises with propitious involvements.

Conceptual Integration

Hope is imaging the powering of connecting-separating.

they asked her to return and help out, and that gave her hope. "Then you think you have something to pass on," she said. Lisa says that in spite of her gloomy future, it is her happiness "to follow the grandchildren as they grow up." Statements from all ten participants show that the concept nurturing affiliations encompasses significant relationships among persons alive today, loved ones from childhood, and persons who are dead.

Implications for further research and practice based on these findings are discussed in the final chapter of this book, along with findings from other studies.

REFERENCES

Parse, R. R. (1987). *Nursing science: Major paradigms, theories, and critiques.* Philadelphia: Saunders.

Parse, R. R. (1992). Human becoming: Parse's theory of nursing. *Nursing Science Quarterly, 5,* 35–42.

Chapter 9

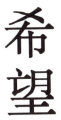

He-Bung: Hope for Persons Living with Leprosy in Taiwan

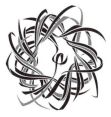

CHING-ENG HSIEH WANG

He-Bung is a phonetic representation for the word hope, since there is no Taiwanese written language.

Yearning

I want a site with trees and stream—
Near some majestic mountain scene—
On which to build a little home;
A place to call my very own.

Betty Martin (1959)

This poem written by Betty Martin (1959) depicts hope as a living paradox fraught with the mysteries of human experience and spurred by resolute choosing from moment to moment in everyday life. She went to Carville, Louisiana, at age 19, where she married Harry, also a patient, and stayed for the next twenty years. Carville, a U.S. leprosarium, was founded as the Louisiana Leper Home in 1894. It is now the Gillis W. Long Hansen's Disease Center, where about 140 residents still live today (Parascandola, 1994).

Betty reflected her lived experience of hope as a living paradox and a chosen way of imaging what is not-yet. The little poem houses a season of hope that mysteriously interlaces with despair. The imaginary home, a comfortable dwelling place of her own, is like an invincible summer living in the midst of harsh winter, as depicted in Martin's (1959) writing:

> Harry and I knew that dream house of ours so well we might actually have lived in it for twenty years, and in a sense we had, because our years in Carville had been made bearable by that imaginary home where Harry and I spent much of our secret lives. (p. 21)

To pursue their dream together outside the sheltered life of an institution, the couple left Carville, struggling against fear, rejection, and countless devastating setbacks. After three hard years, they finally bought a place of their own, a cheerful little house in the foothills of California.

Like Betty and Harry Martin, ten male residents of a Taiwanese leprosarium who participated in the qualitative research study on hope shared similar stories of dreams, struggles, fear, despair, and courage. The findings of the study show that hope is *anticipating an unburdening serenity amid despair as nurturing engagements emerge in creating anew with cherished priorities.* The following are remarkable stories of hope told by the participants. A brief description of Taiwan and the leprosarium where they have lived since they were young is also included.

TAIWAN AND THE LO-SENG LEPROSARIUM

Taiwan is approximately the size of West Virginia and the home of about 21 million people. Centuries ago, Malay-Polynesian tribes settled on Taiwan. In the sixteenth century, Chinese settlers started migrating to Taiwan. From 1895 to 1945, Taiwan was under Japanese colonial rule. Most of the participants were born during this era.

Taiwan Provincial Lo-Seng Leprosarium (now called Lo-Seng Sanitorium), built in 1930, is situated in Hsin-Chuang City, about 14 kilometers (8.75 miles) from Taipei, Taiwan. This institution has about 170 employees, including thirty-four nurses and twelve physicians. In 1994, there were 579 residents, 459 men and 120 women. The average age of residents was 67 and many were designated as disabled. When the institution was under Japanese administration from 1930 to 1945, leprosy was classified as incurable and contagious. People with leprosy were forced to leave their homes and were incarcerated in the sanitorium. Policemen were dispatched to capture escaped patients, who were then detained in jail for weeks. After the Chinese administration took over, the human condition remained the same. The residents had no right to vote and were required to be sterilized if they planned to get married.

Persons with leprosy used to be called *tai-ger* in the Taiwanese language. This word means "unclean" or "dirty" and is a derogatory term meant to demean those with leprosy. Over the years, many groups, such as missionaries and student clubs from nearby universities, have come to work with the residents. Today, segregation of those with leprosy is no longer compulsory in Taiwan. The residents receive about US$200 a month from the government, have the right to vote, and may leave the facility at will.

PARTICIPANTS

The participants in this study were ten men between the ages of 59 and 80 living in the leprosarium.

DIALOGICAL ENGAGEMENT

Dialogical engagement took place in the dwelling places of the participants.

EXTRACTION-SYNTHESIS

Ah Tim's Story

When Ah Tim arrived at age 16, his hope had been to cure leprosy and to return home quickly. He dreamed of launching a career and having his own family. Now, at the age of 59, still a bachelor, still living at Lo-Seng with both legs gone and hands contracted, he has ceased to dream but works tirelessly to lead the residents fighting for their benefits. When Ah Tim talks about his hope, he says:

> Now I have come to terms with myself that cure is impossible. . . .
> I hope for being free of pain and illness . . . to live my life day by day.
> . . . Although I do not have any more hope in this world, I hope for an

afterlife . . . after death, I will not have any more tears, pains, and illnesses to torture me in Heaven. In the past, we were deserted and rejected by society. The outsiders glanced at us with terror. . . . But now, things have changed. Many people from society are concerned about us. . . . They bring us joy and warm feelings. . . . I hope that they will keep coming and bring more people along.

After surgery failed to correct his clubbed hands, Ah Tim "began to pursue other interests." He says, "I made efforts to learn how to read . . . how to read music notes." (See Figure 1.) "I am able to sing a song. . . . I can write a letter for myself or help others write. I feel I have achieved some of my hopes."

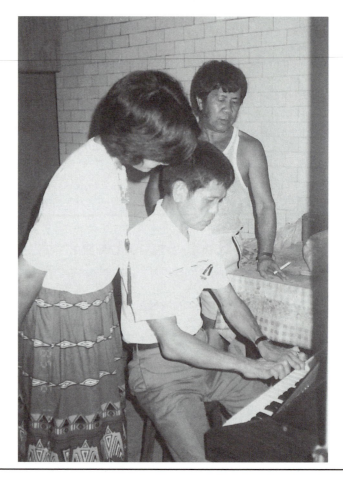

FIGURE 1.
Ah Tim plays the organ to entertain friends.

Essences: Participant's Language

1. The participant says he knows he cannot be cured of leprosy and his dreams are shattered, but he hopes to be pain-free and for a future in Heaven as he lives day to day.
2. The participant says he cannot have a worldly career, but he loves music and literature, has learned to read and write better, can play music with just his knuckles, and works for the welfare of residents in spite of difficulties.
3. Feeling deserted, isolated, and rejected by society and receiving little money from the government, the participant is hopeful, comforted, and very happy with the love and concern of outside people, and he hopes for many more contacts.

Essences: Researcher's Language

1. Unfulfilled wishes surface with anticipating an unburdening serenity.
2. Shifting cherished priorities arise with possibilities despite adversity.
3. Nurturing engagements surface with the delightful contentment of anticipating togetherness amid spurnful aloneness.

Proposition. The lived experience of hope is anticipating an unburdening serenity amid unfulfilled wishes, as togetherness with spurnful aloneness surfaces with the delightful contentment of nurturing engagements, while shifting cherished priorities arise with possibilities despite adversity.

Ah Fu's Story

Ah Fu, an 80-year-old man, had hoped, initially after contracting leprosy, to "keep working in society while receiving treatment." However, he lost jobs as a bookkeeper of a Japanese store and as a clerk in a post office because of leprosy. "Hopeless, jobless, and broken," Ah Fu went back to his hometown, Penghu, an archipelago in the Taiwan Strait. At age 26, he was forced into quarantine. He refers to the period of waiting for shipment to mainland Taiwan as "the most dreadful time of my life."

Speaking of his hope, he says, "After the war was over, I went back to Penghu. . . . My parents looked down on me, even though I was their son. They put me in separate quarters to live so that I did not have to mingle with my family. After one or two miserable years, I was once again forced back into the hospital." He changes the tone of his voice:

> My second trip was quite different. . . . Mrs. D—, an American missionary, came. . . . She initiated a food and clothing drive for us. . . . She gave us new hope and expectation. . . . I felt that our society was still caring. . . . I had hope . . . felt like I was reborn. I worked in the brick factory, just like people working in society. . . . I was very happy to work there since the work made me feel like an ordinary person

> working in society day after day. The money I made was used to buy extra food. During that time, food money was $20 a month. You could only buy one small dry fish with that amount. Life was harsh.

In the end, he says:

> A cure is impossible. There is no more hope for me in my hometown . . . in society. All I want is to live my life here day by day until the one day the Lord comes to summon me. I hope I do not have any more illnesses, which I cannot afford, and any more pain. . . . My hope is to wait for my Lord to summon me to heaven.

Essences: Participant's Language

1. The participant says he used to hope to stay in society, but he was disappointed and felt hopeless at every turn, and now he knows it is impossible; he hopes his remaining days will be free of suffering while preparing and waiting for the Lord to summon him to Heaven.
2. The participant had many hardships in pursuing the treatment of leprosy, and to supplement his income, he has tried many things. He worked with pleasure in a brick factory, since he felt like an ordinary person.
3. The participant's parents and townspeople rejected and belittled him, but a caring American missionary cared for him, helped him survive, and gave him hope through difficult times, which made him feel like he was reborn.

Essences: Researcher's Language

1. Despairing disillusionment emerges with anticipation of an unburdening serenity.
2. Joys and sorrows arise with new ventures while striving for cherished priorities.
3. Nurturing engagements amid spurnful contempt surface with new aliveness.

Proposition. The lived experience of hope is anticipating an unburdening serenity amid despairing disillusionment as joys and sorrows arise in striving for new ventures with cherished priorities, while nurturing engagements despite spurnful contempt surface with new aliveness.

Ah Ming's Story

Sixty-two-year-old Ah Ming, a former steel mill worker and the father of two grown children, is living in small quarters shared by two other residents. He is wheelchair-bound, with both of his legs amputated. The focus of the lived experience of hope is his family:

> Coming to Lo-Seng, I left my father, wife, and two young kids behind. Although it was difficult for my wife, who was a housewife, to work as

a manual laborer, she could not help but work very hard to support the family. My eldest brother was very kind. . . . He helped me look after my wife and kids. When she worked during the day, he kept two kids and fed them. . . . She was determined to take up my responsibility of caring for my father, no matter how hard the life would become. To help support my poor family, I worked as an aide to take care of chickens. Working with only one leg, I cleaned chickens' litter, fed them, and swept chicken coops. My leg got injured—covered with blisters— it had to be amputated. . . . Now, my children are grown up. My son is a fine young man. I do not have to worry about them anymore. . . . I can rest easier here day by day. My children want to take me home. I gave that deep thought. What's it for? I would have to stay inside the house. Society is still afraid of persons with leprosy. People turn away from us. . . . I used to hide when reporters came to interview me. . . . Some reporters might have taken my picture and showed it on television screens. My family and neighbors might have seen it. People would have whispered, "So and so's father is a leper." This would hurt my son's reputation. I lose face; so does my son.

Ah Ming tries very hard to make a living here:

> There is no way out. I complain to myself that if I had not suffered from this disease, I would not have to depend on the government for a living. I could have happily lived with my wife and children every day. I can no longer earn any money. The only thing I can do is save. To live here, you cannot help but save for rainy days.

Essences: Participant's Language

1. The participant said he was sad, complained of his lot in life, and wondered why he could not have lived with his family, yet he declined his son's invitation to return and says after deep thought that he is not sorry to depend on the government for a living but they should provide more.
2. The participant avoids interviews and going to restaurants with his family in the hope of protecting his family's name, as he rests in the leprosarium peacefully, while hoping for a good death.
3. Even with one leg, the participant cared for chickens to help support his poor family. Now, in spite of inadequate income, he saves and says he keeps healthy in his own way to make life secure.
4. The participant remembered the love and kindness of his brother and wife in caring for the family in a time of hopelessness, and he says now he does not have to worry, since his children have grown up fine.

Essences: Researcher's Language

1. Careful deliberation emerges with the feasible amid regretful resentment.

2. The refuge of willful disguise arises with anticipation of an unburdening serenity.
3. Cherished priorities surface with fortifying insurances creating anew despite adversity.
4. Recollections of nurturing engagements during despair surface with an unburdening contentment.

Proposition. The lived experience of hope is anticipating an unburdening serenity with careful deliberation of the feasible amid regretful resentment, while the refuge of willful disguise surfaces with fortifying insurances of cherished priorities in creating anew despite adversity, as recollections of nurturing engagements during despair emerge with contentment.

Ah Li's Story

The room is dark and plain, with a stereo and a karaoke system standing by a small bed. Next to the room is a small garden. Ah Li, age 64, sits in his bed, singing a song he has written, his face marred with scars, ears deformed, and fingers clawlike.

The Song

Those young men with a good heart are like light shining in
 the dark
The light shining on darkness of the road illuminates us
We are so thankful for the love and true happiness you bring
 to us
We appreciate you all who are forever in our hearts
We are always missing you, the passionate students who care
 so much about us.

Besides singing, he spends a great deal of time on landscaping, gardening, and collecting empty cans and wine bottles to decorate this garden. Ah Li says nurses frequently show his garden to visitors and that is the source of his pride and accomplishment. "The flowers I grew would bring the joy of happiness to people." Becoming a flower farmer had been 17-year-old Ah Li's dream:

> But this dream was crushed as I contracted leprosy. . . . I felt myself so worthless. Being broken in pride, I was hopeless. But after my arrival, a head nurse at Lo-Seng consoled me and treated me very kindly. Her attitude made me realize that not everyone in society was terrified of this disease. . . . A feeling of warmth welled up within me . . . a feeling of hopefulness. Yes, there was still hope in my life. I had the courage to live on against all odds. As I get older, I grow flowers and make many friends and we take care of one another. At present, growing flowers is

a kind of hope for me. . . . Although I still live with an incurable disease, I live happily and courageously. . . . I always hope myself being capable of memorizing the words of every song I sing. I have achieved this hope that I have memorized many songs. . . . The only thing I ask for is to be peaceful. As long as I am healthy, everything . . . then I do not have worries and afflictions. This is my greatest hope. (See Figure 2.)

Essences: Participant's Language

1. The participant says he is satisfied with what he has received through the years, and he does not hope for anything greater than a peaceful life without worries and ailments as he lives happily.
2. The participant says he feels thankful for people visiting and caring about him with loving kindness at the times of dark hopelessness, especially a head nurse who made him feel warm and hopeful, and encouraged him to live on against all odds.
3. The participant says contracting leprosy early in life prevented him from becoming a flower farmer or receiving a good education, but now he grows flowers, which are a kind of hope for him to keep his spirits up, and he has memorized the words of every song he sings with happiness.

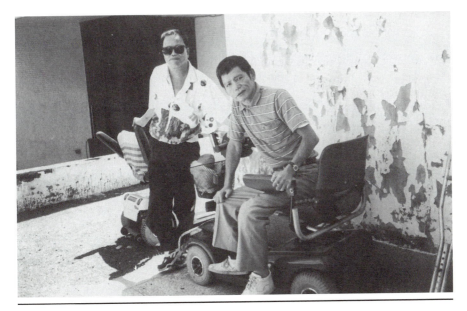

FIGURE 2.
Ah Ai (right) hopes for a peaceful life.

Essences: Researcher's Language

1. Blissful contentment surfaces with anticipating an unburdening serenity.
2. Gratitude for nurturing engagements amid despair emerges with deliberate fortitude.
3. Shifting cherished priorities arises anew with uplifting merriment.

Proposition. The lived experience of hope is anticipating an unburdening serenity with blissful contentment, as gratitude for nurturing engagements amid despair surfaces with deliberate fortitude, shifting cherished priorities that arise anew with uplifting merriment.

Ah Ping's Story

Ah Ping, aged 65, a wheelchair-bound man, has lived at Lo-Seng for forty years. As a member of a rich family, Ah Ping didn't necessarily have to earn a living; he had "a good life." Life was never the same after he came to Lo-Seng, "a long journey with horrifying pains."

> When I first arrived, this institution was experimenting with DDS (dapsone). "A lone bird even with wings cannot fly away" after travelling through a thousand mountains. Not only could I not escape but the pains along with contracted hands made me feel that life was meaningless. Life and death made no difference to me. No one dared to try the drug. I volunteered. . . . This medication made me very weak and caused arthritis and nerve pain. I was bedridden. The old-timers came over to see me and to help me out with medication and chores. . . . I was getting better.

Ah Ping's legs and arms were injured from a car accident. Over a six-month period, he spent ten days in the hospital, then went home for the rest of the month. He explains:

> For ten hospital days, it costs me two to three thousand dollars. There is not much left for me after I pay it in full. Thus, I discharged myself after ten days. I waited and was readmitted to the hospital after I received another monthly check. . . . Sometimes, I am lying in bed and hoping for miracles that my arms are healed spontaneously and I could use crutches to help me walk again . . . my only hope. I think a lot. Even if I strive to survive, there is no road; but, if I desire to die, there is no door either.

But he has conspired to live his hope:

> My hope is to get through day by day without any trouble. "A person without trouble feels like a god." I try very hard to live on what I have received from the government. . . . I hope for getting through my old age without the suffering of pain and illness. . . . An old Taiwanese

proverb says, "Requesting for good birth and good death." It would be a blessing for me if I could die sooner to escape all sufferings.

Essences: Participant's Language

1. Feeling that life was meaningless with no way to escape and no difference between living and dying, the participant volunteered for an experimental treatment and became very ill, but he was helped and cared for by other residents and got better.
2. The participant says even if he wants to survive, there is no road, but, if he wants to die, there is no door either, and he hopes for peace of mind, free of trouble like a god, and a good death to escape all sufferings.
3. Even with the injury to his arm and leg, the participant wants very much to move around freely, but with barely enough income and the red tape, he feels he might have to bow to fate and dream of miracles, yet he has tried what he can to deal with his disability.
4. The participant wrote letters and spoke up for a better standard of living for the residents, which led to some improvement; now he supports others who work to achieve this aim.

Essences: Researcher's Language

1. Nurturing engagements arise with afflictions amid despairing agony.
2. Truncated possibilities emerge with anticipating unburdening deliverance.
3. Desire for expanding possibilities surfaces with yielding to what is feasible amid adversity.
4. Cherished priorities emerge with beneficial endeavors.

Proposition. The lived experience of hope is anticipating an unburdening deliverance amid truncated possibilities, as a desire for expansion surfaces with yielding to what is feasible in adversity, while nurturing engagements emerge with the afflictions of despairing agony, as cherished priorities arise with beneficial endeavors.

Ah Fan's Story

Ah Fan, aged 62 and married, is a representative and an organ player at the Catholic church located in the leprosarium. He wears prostheses, dresses in a black Catholic uniform, and is very hopeful, confident, and articulate. In fact, he often leads visitors on tours and addresses a wide range of audiences. (See Figure 3.) He describes his hope as "growing out of hopelessness through many dark years" of his life. After acquiring leprosy at age 12, he was confined to his home for the next ten years. Feeling like "the living dead," he attempted suicide many times. Yet he says, "Now I have a peaceful mind. . . . Peace has been within me since I had faith. . . . I have nothing to say about leprosy which is still with me. . . . I live year by year until the day I stop breathing. I feel hopeful." Then with enthusiasm he goes on to describe what would happen after death: "They will

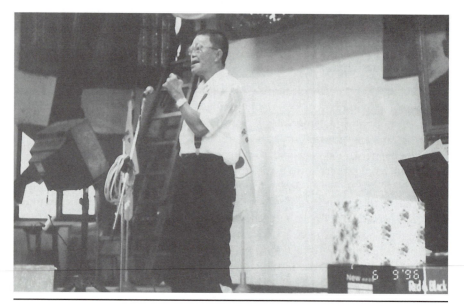

FIGURE 3.
Ah Fan addresses a large audience.

take my body to church; my coffin will be nailed down with a cross. When my body is ready for cremation, Father will come to bless me. Then I will be on my way to Heaven. . . . What I am hoping for is heaven." It seems Ah Fan has found his hope in life. It does not come easily.

Essences: Participant's Language

1. Feeling hopeless, like living in a dark prison, the participant attempted suicide many times during his ten-year confinement at home. Finally he decided to leave because he thought there still might be hope out there, although he did not know where or how.
2. The participant went through a lot to treat his disfigured looks and leprosy, but knowing that this will not change, he does not care anymore. Instead, he devotes his life to volunteering as a representative of the Church and as an organ player.
3. The participant says that during bouts of hopelessness, the love, care, and encouragement of Catholic fathers and sisters and his wife have helped him regain hope in life. Now he does enjoyable things, feeling peaceful and self-respecting, and hopes for an afterlife in Heaven.

Essences: Researcher's Language

1. Destructiveness with despairing restrictions arises with the uncertainty of resolute change.

2. Shifting cherished priorities in adversity emerges with newly committed resolve.
3. Nurturing engagements surface with the prospects of delightful undertakings while anticipating an unburdening serenity with pride.

Proposition. The lived experience of hope is anticipating an unburdening serenity with pride amid the destructiveness of despairing restrictions, as nurturing engagements surface with the prospects of delightful undertakings, while shifting cherished priorities in adversity emerges with newly committed resolve in the uncertainty of change.

Ah Jin's Story

Ah Jin, aged 70, is a volunteer librarian and the father of an adult, married daughter. A graduate of Taipei Industrial Junior College, he speaks fluent Japanese and is a former teacher and a Japanese soldier. Speaking of his hopes and dreams, he at first strived for a bright future by taking many exams, but that ended after he came to Lo-Seng. Later, his priority changed to surviving the hardship within the institution:

> Life was extremely hard in the past. . . . If you desired a better life then, you had to be able to use a plow . . . to cultivate a land. If you could cultivate, you could grow yams. Then you could use leaves of yams to feed rabbits. . . . You can eat both yams and rabbits. . . . I had never used a plow before. I tried to use it but my hands were covered with blisters each time I used it; I couldn't do it. Since I could not do that, I had to climb up the mountain to gather twigs for a living.

But after the birth of his daughter, he gave priority to supporting family. He says, "To bring up my child, I used to do a chick business. I bought baby chicks, right after they hatched, from other merchants, then kept them warm by using plastic bags as incubators for two weeks. When the chicks were mature enough, I packed them up and rode a bicycle to Wulai [a mountain place inhabited by the Atayal aborigines] to sell them." Now all he wants is to "do meaningful things" through working as a volunteer librarian for the Presbyterian Church.

Essences: Participant's Language

1. Hoping to serve his country, the participant took many exams to become a civil servant, but later, in order to raise his child, he sold chicks to the remote village, travelling by bike and on foot, and to get the highest pay he worked with hot bricks that injured his hands.
2. When he felt no hope and did not care about himself, the participant says the love of God and the care of a missionary changed his view toward life and gave him courage to live on. Now he feels peaceful and hopes to devote his life to doing meaningful things.

3. The participant recalled that his daughter was insulted by others and at that time "even if he wanted to cry, there were no tears," but he told her to study hard and now he is pleased with the successes of youngsters born in the leprosarium.

Essences: Researcher's Language

1. Shifting cherished priorities arises with new ventures despite harmful adversity.
2. Nurturing engagements amid despair emerge with beneficent prospects in anticipating an unburdening serenity.
3. Sorrowfully recollecting scornful moments surfaces with a joyful pride in fulfillments.

Proposition. The lived experience of hope is anticipating an unburdening serenity amid despair that emerges with beneficent prospects, as sorrowfully recollecting scornful moments arises with joyful pride in fulfillments, while nurturing engagements surface with shifting cherished priorities with new ventures despite harmful adversity.

Ah Ding's Story

Ah Ding came to the leprosarium at age 21 and has stayed for more than forty years. He has held jobs as a barber and a member of the Lo-Seng band, in which he plays a saxhorn for funeral processions. Ah Ding says that his hope to return to society was so fierce in the early years that he would stop at nothing to go for it. "We had to escape, since [getting] passes to leave the place was quite difficult. We often hid on the hilltop at midnight, then climbed over the mountain to run away. However, once back, we were put in jail," he says. He explains that fears of rejection by society had prevented him from pursuing this path further. This is no longer important to him. He has found "good health" and "helping others" as "my hope for my life." He says, "In the past, our shop had five to six barbers. Everyone except me was reluctant to cut the hair of the one resident who had a strong odor . . . the entire body covered with unhealed wounds. I went. My happiness . . . helping others can bring me comfort." Ah Ding also expresses gratitude to a former director. He says, "We could not vote and had no human rights before. The director championed and lobbied for our rights to remove the stigma. His message was 'Leprosy is not dreadful.'"

Essences: Participant's Language

1. The participant says he risked going to jail when running away from the leprosarium, but fears and other considerations had prevented him from staying at home. Now he is too old to leave but lives here day by day, hoping for peace and good health.
2. Being satisfied with what he has, the participant says to be able to help others with difficulties is his hope in life. He cuts hair for disabled people

who are refused by others or live in the inaccessible area, and in spite of difficulties, that brings him happiness and comfort.

3. When there was no hope of freedom and human rights in the leprosarium, the participant says a former director to whom he still owes thanks cared and helped him to gain rights to vote and dispel the horror linked with the disease.

Essences: Researcher's Language

1. Calm acceptance surfaces with anticipating an unburdening serenity amid the daunting struggles of dissonance.
2. Shifting cherished priorities arises with joyful contentment despite obstacles.
3. Recollecting nurturing engagements amid dreadful deprivation emerges with gratefulness.

Proposition. The lived experience of hope is anticipating an unburdening serenity amid the dreadful deprivation of the daunting struggles of dissonance, while recollecting nurturing engagements with gratefulness surfaces as shifting cherished priorities arises with joyful contentment despite obstacles.

Ah Zin's Story

Ah Zin, aged 77, stutters and walks with a waggle. His home is a small cubicle furnished with a chair and a bed with a mosquito net in a ten-bed living quarter. A small kitchen and bathroom are located next to the living area. Ah Zin uses the phrase "no hope" over and over to describe his hope. After contracting leprosy at age 18, he was brought here by policemen, despite his protest. To pursue freedom, he escaped and was put in jail three times. He describes one incident:

> I escaped to home. The local policemen tracked me down. I refused to leave. . . . A Japanese policeman knocked on my father's head. . . . I broke a long wooden bench, grabbing a leg to fight. . . . "I am a patient, not a convict. What right do you have to handcuff me?" He released my handcuffs and walked away.

Although Ah Zin says "no more hope" and that "living here for me is as if I were incarcerated in a prison, a life sentence," trips with students have brought him hope and pleasure. "I had been here for a long time, but never had gone out for fun. After being here for so many years, I now have opportunities to go out with students; otherwise, I have no hope."

Essences: Participant's Language

1. Seeing no hope to cure his leprosy if he stayed in the leprosarium and not wanting to be treated as a convict with handcuffs, the participant escaped and was jailed three times.

2. Feeling hopeless and as if he had been serving a life sentence in Hell, the participant says he has more freedom now, but he still cannot walk to the outside world. Yet with the help of the students, he has opportunities to take trips for pleasure.
3. The participant does not dream anymore and knows he cannot work, but he wishes he could still make money to supplement his income while praying to Buddha and hoping to keep living well until death.

Essences: Researcher's Language

1. Questing for liberty amid despair surfaces with cherished priorities.
2. Joyful journeys arise with nurturing engagements while enduring an eternal immurement.
3. Disillusioning resignation emerges with anticipating serenity in faith.

Proposition. The lived experience of hope is anticipating an unburdening serenity in faith amid the disillusioning resignation of despair, as questing for liberty surfaces with the cherished priorities of nurturing engagements while enduring an eternal immurement.

Uncle Jim's Story

Uncle Jim, aged 80, lives with his wife and youngest son, who is close to age 40 and, according to Uncle Jim, mentally retarded. His greatest anguish was parting with his mother to come here sixty years ago. In a very sober tone, he says, "Looking back, even now I am still feeling very sad." Living in the leprosarium has not been easy for Uncle Jim. He works very hard to prepare and sell animal feeds and "the money was saved up penny by penny . . . to buy a house for my son . . . later on . . . for my son's wedding." In that way, Uncle Jim says, "I have achieved my hope more or less, so to speak." But he could not find dentists willing to fix his dentures. He feels that the institution neither made enough effort to solve their problems nor treated them nicely. In comparison, he recalls "much more compassionate care during the Japanese era. When a patient passed away, all the hospital's employees, from the director down, came to the funeral held at an auditorium. . . . The patient was part of this family." Although he does not see any more hope, he says, "I only hope not to have any pain and suffering. . . . I wish the government could have built nicer housing for us to live in and could have sent someone to assist our living. I cannot see very well. I wish there were someone to help me clean, cook, and do the laundry."

Essences: Participant's Language

1. The participant has lost faith in the system that does not deliver compassionate care, yet he always hopes to be well cared for by the government as he lives a pain-free life through his old age.
2. The participant says he knew it was impossible to accomplish a great career but now hopes for a better future for his family and for his own health, and he has done many things to achieve this in spite of difficulties.

3. Feeling unkindly treated, the participant recalled his dear friend's death and parting with his mother and says there used to be more compassion in the days when nurses lovingly hung mosquito nets for patients, employees attended patients' funerals respectfully, and a missionary kindly cared for the sick.

Essences: Researcher's Language

1. Disillusionment emerges with anticipating an unburdening serenity.
2. Shifting cherished priorities arises with varied ventures despite adversity.
3. Memories of nurturing engagements surface with tenderness amid the hurtfulness.

Proposition. The lived experience of hope is anticipating an unburdening serenity that emerges with the disillusionment of hurtfulness, as memories of nurturing engagements surface with tenderness, while shifting cherished priorities arise with varied ventures despite adversity.

FINDINGS AND RELATED LITERATURE

Propositions from the ten participants revealed three core concepts. Through heuristic interpretation these were taken up levels of abstraction to the theoretical level (see Table 1).

The first core concept, *anticipating an unburdening serenity amid despair*, is the rhythmical pattern of envisioning freedom from the hopelessness of turmoil, pain, and suffering. This concept was described by participants as looking forward to the peace and easiness of a time beyond while living the day-to-day existence in the leprosarium. They also spoke of a serene life after death in the context of personal struggles and disappointments, hopelessness, and anguish. Many participants depicted their past and present lives as hopeless while looking beyond the boundaries of life as the ultimate hope.

The conceptualization of anticipating an unburdening serenity amid despair provides additional scientific evidence for a view of hope as a living paradox, rather than as an opposite of hopelessness (Stotland, 1969), as a continuum (Kast, 1991), or as a dialectic between hope and hopelessness (Farran, Herth & Popovich, 1995). These latter views pervade and dominate the extant hope literature. No participants fragmented the experiences of hope and despair into two distinct, linear entities at a point where one ends and the other begins. Rather, they shared a vision of being at peace at last while glimpsing the despairing moments. As such, hope and hopelessness coexist and interplay in a rhythmical process, going beyond the boundary of spacetime to multiple realms of the universe in what was, is, and will be all-at-once.

Additionally, anticipating an unburdening serenity amid despair specifies the hope experience as a unitary, changing phenomenon. It is neither reducible to a discernable, fixed element nor an enduring "good" element for life causally associated with survival, coping, maintaining, regaining, or augmenting one's health. This is particularly evident in various participants' descriptions of living

TABLE 1.
Progressive Abstraction of Core Concepts of Hope with Heuristic Interpretation

Core Concepts	Structural Transposition	Conceptual Integration
Anticipating an unburdening serenity amid despair	Envisioning the unencumbered amid desolation	Imaging
Nurturing engagements	Attentive involvements	Connecting-separating
Creating anew with cherished priorities	Inventing the treasured	Originating valuing

Structure

The lived experience of hope is anticipating an unburdening serenity amid despair, as nurturing engagements emerge in creating anew with cherished priorities.

Structural Transposition

The lived experience of hope is envisioning the unencumbered amid desolation, as attentive involvements arise with inventing the treasured.

Conceptual Integration

The lived experience of hope is imaging the connecting-separating in originating valuing.

and dying, as they related the experience of hope. The participants made comments like "there is no difference between living and dying," and living is "a life sentence," "a hell," "a joy," or "contentment." They also named death as "a blessing" and a way "to escape all sufferings." Life after death was called "the ultimate hope." Many ardently said that they "did not worry about death" and were "waiting for that day." For the participants, living was both terror and awe; so was dying. In essence, living is not necessarily more hopeful or better than dying. It is a matter of how meanings are related to situations and how persons choose to live their lives. These findings support Parse's (1992) notion that "the human is a living unity continuously coconstituting patterns of relating" (p. 38). As the meanings of experiences change, the ways of being with living and dying are also changed. In fact, the participants assigned a peaceful meaning to their experience of hope in both life and death. As such, the experience of hope is an ever-changing process of the unitary human's becoming.

The second core concept, *nurturing engagements*, is the lived pattern of experiencing being loved and cared for by others, which kindles new meaning for surviving through predicaments. These loving persons had *jing* and were identified by the participants as missionaries, nurses, doctors, other residents, family members, and "outside people." *Jing* in the Taiwanese language refers to a special affection in caring and helping relationships. Some persons helped and took care of the participants when they were ill or provided them with necessities. Others simply offered kind words and concerned looks and treated them as fellow human beings. Participants said that important others helped them continue their lives with a sense of hope, joy, warmth, happiness, comfort, encouragement, revival, appreciation, and gratitude, even though their realities were still filled with the experiences of hopelessness, rejection, and isolation from the wider society, some of which involved their own family members.

Nurturing engagements as a core concept of hope is congruent with Marcel's (1949/1969) notion of availability (Bollow, 1984) and Buber's (1970) doctrine of I-Thou. To be available is to be open to others without expectation and calculation. As with availability, I-Thou is togetherness without greed, purpose, and expectation in a web of genuine human interconnection. Nurturing engagements in many ways are resonant with the descriptions of availability and I-Thou. Every word by the participants shows a profound human relatedness at the heart of hope, which is what Marcel (1951/1978) says: "I hope in thee [you] for us" (p. 60).

Nurturing engagements is not a source or a strategy of hope. Hope-inspiring strategies and sources have been receiving increased attention in the nursing literature as studies of hope proliferate (Cutcliffe, 1995; Herth, 1990; Miller, 1991). Nurse scholars use various terms to describe patterns of nurturing engagements, and the phrasing is different in their studies on hope. For instance, Herth (1990) listed interpersonal connectedness as a hope-fostering strategy and suggested that nurses foster hope through a caring relationship. In a similar vein, Miller (1991) described a caring relationship as a hope-inspiring strategy. Cutcliffe (1995) postulated an integrated theory of hope inspiration to explain the process of how a nurse inspires a patient's hope. All participants in this study stated in their descriptions of hope that special relationships were significant; none described hope as a strategy. Nurturing engagements as emergent in this study are integral to the experience of hope, but are neither a source nor a strategy, from the human becoming viewpoint.

The last core concept emerging from the participants' descriptions is *creating anew with cherished priorities*, which relates to the lived pattern of inventing unique ways to accomplish what is prized, against the backdrop of institutionalized life. All participants spoke of cherished priorities as what was important to them at the moment and beyond. They cherished helping others, supporting family, pursuing their own interests, and surviving. Some explicitly indicated that what was important before had become unimportant on their new paths. Others expressed that to achieve what they valued was difficult; yet they found their own way to strive for it against enormous adversity. The ways created to enliven hope were unique for each person.

In comparing these findings with the literature that views hope as merely the cognitive process of goal-directed expectations (Snyder, 1989; Stotland, 1969), creating anew with cherished priorities provides a fundamentally different view. It offers insight into the complexity and depth of patterns of living hope rooted in personal choices and values accompanied with struggles and challenges in pursuit of what is dear and feasible in daily life. In contrast, the cognitive-based view does not illuminate the process of hope itself; instead, it simply reduces hope to a rational appraisal of the importance and probability of attaining a goal. More importantly, the meaning of hope to a person is lost in the reductive process. Hence, creating anew with cherished priorities differs in depicting the hoping process without judging a person's reality.

Implications of these findings for further research and practice are discussed along with findings from other studies on hope in the final chapter of this book.

REFERENCES

Bollow, O. F. (1984). Marcel's concept of availability. In P. A. Schilpp & L. E. Hahn (Eds.), *The philosophy of Gabriel Marcel* (pp. 177–199). La Salle, IL: Open Court.

Buber, M. (1970). *I and Thou* (W. Kaufmann, Trans.). New York: Charles Scribner's Sons.

Cutcliffe, J. R. (1995). How do nurses inspire and instill hope in terminally ill HIV patients? *Journal of Advanced Nursing, 22,* 888–895.

Farran, C. J., Herth, K. A., & Popovich, J. M. (1995). *Hope and hopelessness: Critical clinical constructs.* Thousand Oaks, CA: Sage.

Herth, K. (1990). Fostering hope in terminally-ill people. *Journal of Advanced Nursing, 15,* 1250–1259.

Kast, V. (1991). *Joy, inspiration, and hope.* College Station: Texas A & M University Press.

Marcel, G. (1969). *The philosophy of existence* (M. Harari, Trans.). Freeport: Books For Libraries Press. (Original work published 1949)

Marcel, G. (1978). *Homo viator: Introduction to a metaphysic of hope* (E. Craufurd, Trans.). Gloucester, MA: Peter Smith. (Original work published 1951)

Martin, B. (1959). *No one must ever know.* Garden City, NY: Doubleday.

Martin, B. (1963). *Miracle at Carville.* Garden City, NY: Image Books.

Miller, J. F. (1991). Developing and maintaining hope in families of the critically ill. *AACN Clinical Issues in Critical Care Nursing, 2,* 307–315.

Parascandola, J. (1994). The Gillis W. Long Hansen's Disease Center at Carville. *Public Health Reports, 109,* 728–730.

Parse, R. R. (1992). Human becoming: Parse's theory of nursing. *Nursing Science Quarterly, 5,* 35–42.

Snyder, C. R. (1989). Reality negotiation: From excuses to hope and beyond. *Journal of Social & Clinical Psychology, 8*(2), 130–157.

Stotland, E. (1969). *The psychology of hope: An integration of experimental, clinical, and social approaches.* San Francisco: Jossey-Bass.

Chapter 10

The Lived Experience of Hope with Persons from Wales, UK

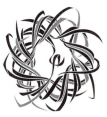

F. BERYL PILKINGTON
BRIAN MILLAR

To Hope

When by my solitary hearth I sit,
And hateful thoughts enwrap my soul in gloom;
When no fair dreams before my "minds eye" flit,
And the bare heath of life presents no bloom;
Sweet Hope, ethereal balm upon me shed,
And wave thy silver pinions o'er my head.

John Keats (1884)

PARTICIPANTS

In this chapter, a study on the lived experience of hope that was conducted with persons living in Wales is presented. Wales is the smallest country in the United Kingdom, with a population of 5 million. Participants were ten adults (seven women and three men) whose ages ranged from 30 to 75 years. One participant was recovering from a severe head injury, one was living with the side effects of surgery to remove a brain tumor, five were family members who were currently caring for a person with a head injury in their homes, and one was a nurse who worked in trauma care. Two others were women with cancer who expressed a strong desire to share their experiences of hope. Interestingly, the persons who survived the head injuries were all men, and the caregivers were mostly women; all participants were white and living in their own homes. Many had strong family networks. All of the participants were able to understand, read, and speak English and were willing to share their lived experiences of hope with the researcher. Their stories were real-life expressions of the above poem written by the poet John Keats (1884).

The selection of these participants ensued from Brian Millar's involvement with Headway, a head injury support group in Cardiff, Wales. The two women with cancer were professional acquaintances of his. Because of the effects of a serious injury or illness on their lives, the subject of hope was of special importance to these participants. As many as 170,000 people in the UK are currently suffering the long-term consequences of a severe head injury resulting from an accident, sports injury, industrial accident, or street violence (Headway National Association of Head Injuries, 1997). The estimated total number of survivors of severe head injury in Wales is 4,300. This incidence may not appear large; however, disabling head injuries have a substantial impact upon family, friends, spouse, and workmates, as well as on those injured. The prevalence of head injury demonstrates the ability of medical services to save and extend the lives of severely injured persons; at the same time, many of those hospitalized with head injury each year will have symptoms that interfere with their daily living, and a number of them will be unable to return to independent living, which creates substantial, often indefinite, long-term needs and responsibilities. The incidence of head injury peaks between 15 and 25 years of age (Office of Health Economics, 1992; Rose & Johnson 1996; Stratton & Gregory,

1995); thus, at a time when individuals are usually beginning to assert their independence, the person with the head injury typically experiences disability and dependency (Headway, Cardiff and District Report, 1995).

While a head injury signifies a personal tragedy for many young people and their families, cancer causes 25 percent of all deaths in England and Wales (Welsh Health Planning Forum [WHPF], 1990). In Wales, almost one of every five persons has a diagnosis of cancer, and half of them are below the age of 65 (Office of Population Census and Surveys [OPCS], 1992). For Welsh women, the death rate from cancer—especially of the breast and lung—is among the worst in Europe (WHPF, 1990).

DIALOGICAL ENGAGEMENT

After the researcher explained the purpose of the research to the participants, they were asked to talk about their experiences of hope. All of the dialogical engagements were audiotaped and transcribed. The dialogues lasted from 30 to 75 minutes.

Andrew's Story

Andrew is a nurse who works with people with a variety of injuries and disabilities. He sees hope "as being all about this inner strength" that people find in "devastating" situations. It's like "a light . . . [at the other end of] a dark hole," he says. "People need to hang on to some hope, whatever is happening." While "an inner thing," hope is affected by "human relationships . . . whether it be family or . . . whoever you talk to." Also, hope has to be "hope for something . . . whether you're hoping that thing for yourself or for another person." It can begin as a wish for "something small" and then become "a stronger thing" that you really hope and "pray for. . . . [It] seems to be the start of other things that keep you going," and it gives "strength and courage."

Andrew thinks that "hope can mean different things at different times, depending on what you're going through or heading for." For example, in "a traumatic situation, [one] really hope[s] that the outcome isn't going to be the worst outcome." However, if "whatever it is that you're hoping for is not achieved by having that hope," or the "drastic event . . . doesn't turn out for the best . . . then hope must be turned into something else," for instance, "doing the best you can to make those days or weeks left into something positive." Hope is "important" in that it inspires you "to do something that is in your control . . . or gives you the inspiration to go forward."

Andrew describes himself as "optimistic." He always has "some hope for something," for instance, "wanting the world to be a better place." He also hopes for things for the future and adds that "usually [one] hopes that certain things will get better." Andrew says he would not want to be "going down a track" that is without hope; and so, "maybe you hang onto hope to stop veering off in other directions." In his view, "It's all related to aspirations." Although he does not know where he will be in five years, he hopes he will still be "working closely with people . . . in a job [he] enjoy[s] and living in an area where [he'd] like to live." Andrew feels it is sometimes difficult "to stop what you are doing in your life" in order to think about things like hope. His way of "taking a step back" and reflecting on hope is to take walks in the country. This helps him "clarify and re-look at" situations and "decide some of the pragmatics." It is a time "of looking at scenarios that make things more hopeful for the future."

Essences: Participant's Language

1. Hope is an inner strength that gives the inspiration to go forward or to keep going in traumatic situations, but it can be influenced by family and others.
2. Hope is related to aspirations for something and someone, and it means different things at different times. If whatever is hoped is not achieved, or doesn't turn out for the best, then hope must be turned into something else. Sometimes the participant steps back with the aim of looking at scenarios for a more hopeful future.

Essences: Researcher's Language

1. Persevering with enlivening fortitude amid adversity arises with the persuasion of close alliances.
2. Yearning for the cherished emerges in diversity with immersion in confident anticipating.

Proposition. The lived experience of hope is persevering with enlivening fortitude amid adversity, with the persuasion of close alliances, while yearning for the cherished emerges in diversity with immersion in confident anticipating.

Pete's Story

Pete says that "hope played a big part [in] the traumatic experience [he has] been through." His son, Jeff, was seriously injured in an accident, and the physicians painted "the blackest of pictures." Nonetheless, Pete says, he kept hoping for Jeff "to get back to normal. . . . In those circumstances . . . [hope for the future is] very important," as it keeps one going. For Pete, to hope is "to wish, to desire" something to happen: "It's really a wish for a positive outcome. Without hope, it's very difficult to carry on." He remembers starting out each morning "with a renewed hope for the future," believing that "something that day was going to happen, to give that something to latch on to—courage for the future; and very often, it did. A very small thing would give [him] that hope . . . [but] toward the end of the day, [his] hope would wane," and he would feel "depressed." Then he and his wife "had to remind each other about those little positive things that kept [them] on the road of hope—of believing that there was a future for Jeff."

For Pete, it was "helpful to share [his] experiences with . . . people in a similar situation." He says they were able to "comfort each other and give each other hope" by looking for "positive things," which "encouraged or maintained the hope." Also, "seeing that things could be worse . . . gives you hope." According to Pete, "The more positive things that happened to improve Jeff's recovery, the more hopeful [they] became . . . of a better future."

He adds that presently, Jeff is "doing things [he] never dreamt he would do. . . . In the beginning . . . you're afraid to hope for too much," he said, "but on the other hand, we've made big strides—so perhaps there's nothing wrong with maintaining that hope." Pete and his wife have hope that Jeff "will succeed."

According to Pete, we all hope "all the way through life . . . for as normal and as good a life as we can have. Your hopes change, obviously, as you move into adulthood." For instance, "as a child, [one] hopes for everything [one] wants," whereas in adulthood, "hoping for normality in one's life . . . [is] a desire that is with you." Pete says he looks forward "to the better things, the positive things in life, that are going to happen to [him]. . . . That just helps you lead your life, that keeps you going," he adds. Without hope, Pete suggests, one gets "deeper and deeper . . . into despair . . . [until] you see no way out. . . . Hope is a part of recovery from [depression]. You've got to feel that there is light at the end of the tunnel."

Essences: Participant's Language

1. Hope is feeling that in traumatic circumstances there is light at the end of the tunnel. When their son was seriously injured in an accident and the picture was blackest, the participant and his wife comforted each other and others with whom they shared experiences. Reminding each other about positive things kept them believing in a future for their son and gave them courage to keep going each day.
2. Hope is looking forward to better things, the positive things, that are going to happen; it changes as you move through life. As an adult, the participant hopes for a normal life, and, whereas he had hoped for his son to get back to normal, now he hopes that he will succeed in life.

Essences: Researcher's Language

1. Anticipating the alleviation of adversity with benevolent affiliations arises in persevering with assurance.
2. Anticipating cherished possibilities emerges with the diversity of life's vicissitudes.

Proposition. The lived experience of hope is anticipating the alleviation of adversity with benevolent alliances while persevering with assurance, as anticipating cherished possibilities emerges with the diversity of life's vicissitudes.

Twila's Story

Twila says she had not thought much about hope before her son John's accident. "In the early days immediately after his accident," she recalls, she and her husband felt as though they could not "afford to hope at all . . . but deep down" they were hoping for a better outcome, "hoping for some sort of recovery for John." Twila "still feel[s] angry . . . [that the professionals] tried to take that hope away from [them]." She adds that they did not want to be given "false hope," but they would have liked "to be treated as sensible people and given . . . the possible outcomes right across the board." Instead, she recalls, they were told that "the chances of any good outcome from [the situation] were nil." She and her husband were "very aware of the possible outcomes," she asserts; thus, it was not "wishful thinking" that made them want to have "all the knowledge made available. . . . We should be given the possibilities, we should be given the range—at least to have [a] little bit of hope left intact," she maintains. "I think it is wrong to try and strip it away."

Twila feels that "talking together" with family and friends helped her and her husband muster "that little bit of hope" to see things "as better" and to "hang in there." Cupping her hands together as though gently supporting something, Twila talks about how they were "really held" by a whole network of family and friends who were "rooting" for them. She and her husband "drew strength" from them and "started to pin [their] hopes on better things. . . . I think it just gave us strength to have some hope," she explains. Twila says that she is not religious, but she remembers someone telling her about "the prayers [being] said" and the "positive energy being directed towards John and the family"; this, in her view, is "part and parcel of the same thing. It's a positive outlook."

Noting that the dictionary defines hope as a combination of expectation and desire, she questions whether "it's as easy as that—it goes far deeper," she asserts. "And I think it [is] essential, because it's the thing that keeps you positive. . . . That [is what] helps people through an ordeal or through a trauma. . . . [Being positive means that] you can't take a step back," Twila explains. "You've got to think forward."

Essences: Participant's Language

1. Hope is having a positive outlook and thinking forward; that is essential to help you through an ordeal. Even though the professionals tried to take their hope away, the participant and her husband were hoping for a better outcome and some sort of recovery for their son, and that kept them going.

2. Hope is drawing strength from close family and friends who are "rooting" for you. Through talking together and with others, and knowing that prayers and "positive energy" were being directed toward them, the participant and her husband "hung in there" and started hoping for better things.

Essences: Researcher's Language

1. Confidently anticipating cherished possibilities emerges with persevering amid adversity.
2. Fortitude arises with benevolent affiliations.

Proposition. The lived experience of hope is confidently anticipating cherished possibilities while persevering amid adversity, as fortitude arises with benevolent affiliations.

Rena's Story

Rena describes her experience of hope in relation to her son's serious accident six years ago. She remembers that she and her husband "were told [their son] would be totally brain damaged and paralyzed, and [they] were given no hope at all." Still, she feels that "[their] faith gave [them] hope, [and they] never gave up that hope—[they] always felt [they] could not let him down, that [they] had to be in there fighting with him, for him." Rena talks about being at the hospital constantly for three months, and then "he just woke up and regained consciousness."

She believes it is true that "where there's life, there's hope . . . [and so, never] give up, however bad you feel the circumstances are, and whatever . . . you're being told by the medical profession. . . . There is always light at the end of the tunnel." Rena says that there could not have been a "blacker picture painted." Still, had someone suggested "switching the machine off" she does not think she could have gone along, "because . . . there is an awful lot they don't know." She suggests that others in similar circumstances should "just go with [their] gut feeling. Although everybody is very supportive, at the end of the day, it's down to you."

For Rena, hope is "connected with [her] faith, which has increased "ten-fold now," because at the "darkest times of your life when you feel the chips are really down, there's still somebody or something there with you . . . that's sort of pushing you on . . . and guiding you." She feels "that God was with [them]," adding "I couldn't have coped if I didn't believe. . . . [I would have wondered,] 'What have I got to hang on to?'" Their rector helped them, also: "Just his presence there was hope, you know, because he was so good. He just seemed to know what to do."

Rena emphasizes how "all important" it was to her and her husband to have spent "every waking hour" with their son. Accepting the staff's invitation "to do something to help" actually "helped [them] as much as it helped [their] son," in that it gave them "hope" and "meaning" to feel as though they were doing something "constructive." She stresses how it was also "tremendously important" that the nurses "never showed that they felt that . . . there wasn't much of a chance" for their son. "That gives you hope, because you feel that they're there with you," Rena explains. "If people around you are positive . . . [and] supportive," she adds, "that sort of inspires you; I think your hope just grows."

Rena believes that "hope and faith . . . get you through these terrible situations." At present, she says, "All I hope and pray is that [my son] will be able to be independent and look after himself. . . . That's all, really, that I want."

Essences: Participant's Language

1. Hope is connected with believing that there is somebody or something there with you, pushing you on and guiding you through the darkest

times of your life. When their son had a serious accident, being there fighting with and for him gave the participant and her husband hope, as did God's presence, their rector's presence, and feeling the support of positive people, which is inspiring.

2. Hope is being patient and never giving up, knowing that miracles do happen and there is always light at the end of the tunnel. The participant and her husband stayed with their son constantly, never giving up hope for him; now, she hopes and prays that he will be able to be independent and look after himself.

Essences: Researcher's Language

1. Assurance of benevolent affiliations arises with enlivening solace amid adversity.
2. Persevering with devotion emerges with the diversity of anticipating cherished possibilities.

Proposition. The lived experience of hope is the assurance of benevolent affiliations arising with enlivening solace amid adversity, as persevering with devotion emerges with the diversity of anticipating cherished possibilities.

Debbie's Story

Debbie discovered she had breast cancer several years ago. She remembers being "optimistic" that it would be curable, even when she had a small recurrence. She thinks that it was possible to remain optimistic because she had "a lot of other things going on in [her] life, so [she] didn't need to dwell on [or] worry about this disease."

When she had a major recurrence of the cancer, Debbie recalls being "absolutely scared stupid" at the thought that "this thing is not controllable." She told herself to "stick with optimism, because if you're pessimistic and down about things you just feel worse." She explains that she did not feel the need to hope, because in her view, "hope is about investing trust [in] someone else or something else, and abdicating responsibility for dealing with the situation." However, she "[doesn't] want to rely on anybody else, because people let you down."

When the cancer came back again, Debbie says it "was a complete shock. . . . I couldn't believe that I had gone through all those things . . . trying to live better, eat better, [and] do all the things that I felt were positive, and I'd been let down. . . . I suddenly realized [that] . . . I couldn't just rely on myself. . . . I just felt the need to allow myself to hope that things would work out." Even then, it "wasn't really comfortable" to hope, but a counselor helped Debbie "to work through that."

Debbie now realizes that "there is no escape, and that [she] can't expect to live for more than another few years." In that sense, she feels "resigned" and "hopeless"; and yet, she does not feel "hopeless" in the sense that she feels "lost," "incredibly sad," or "distraught." As Debbie sees it, she has "still got some good life to live" and "some experiences to have. . . . I'm tending to invest my energies in finding ways of surviving comfortably as long as I can," she continues. "All I can hope for . . . is a good quality of life until I finally drop." Debbie shares that she wants to take "control" and "make choices." She "[does] not want to go down hill slowly"; rather, she wants to "pop off [her] perch one morning—bonk dead!" She still does things like "visualization" and "meditation," since she believes that "the mind can conquer disease"; however, "deep down inside," she does not believe that she can "beat this disease." Nor has she "found something else" that will give her "the ability to relinquish control and invest in that hope, and trust in it."

For Debbie, hope is "all tied up" with "what one expects from life [and] what one hopes to gain." When one is faced with the "uncertainty" of "an unknown amount of time," she explains, "[it makes] hoping . . . and wishing for the things you want very difficult. . . . You have to re-prioritize . . . [and] re-examine everything that you expect from life." One's values and expectations "are all completely thrown up in the air and mixed up." While it is "very difficult [to adjust]," Debbie sees herself "getting to . . . acceptance." That, she thinks, is allowing her to move towards using other sources of support . . . like allowing herself "to hope for better things."

Essences: Participant's Language

1. Hope is about trusting someone or something else, something with which the participant is not really comfortable, but she realizes she cannot just rely on herself in her battle with cancer. Seeing a counselor helped her with that, and now she is getting to an acceptance and is moving toward using other sources of support.
2. Hope is investing energy in surviving comfortably with a good quality of life until she dies. The participant very much hopes to take control and make choices.
3. Hope is tied up with what you expect and want from life. Faced with the uncertainty of an unknown amount of time, the participant has had to re-prioritize her values and expectations, which allows her to hope for better things.

Essences: Researcher's Language

1. Acquiescing in the disquieting impotence of affliction surfaces with consoling alliances.
2. Laboring for enduring solace arises with yearning for sovereignty.
3. Anticipating cherished possibilities amid the ambiguous emerges with aspirations for new opportunities.

Proposition. The lived experience of hope is acquiescing in the disquieting impotence of affliction surfacing with consoling alliances, as laboring for enduring solace arises with yearning for sovereignty, while anticipating cherished possibilities amid the ambiguous emerges with aspirations for new opportunities.

Linda's Story

Linda believes that hope is more than a desire or a wish: It is a "deeper feeling . . . something that you really feel in your heart." Linda's son, Lyndon, was involved in a motorbike accident. She remembers being told, "If he lives through the month, he may well survive. It [would depend] on the length of time he was unconscious or in a coma. . . . For four months, every day I visited him, I hoped he would wake up that day," she continues. "The feeling of hope was with me all day and every day." Linda's hope for Lyndon to get well "was hand in hand with faith," which was based partly on her religion and partly on Lyndon and his "willpower." Her faith and her hope "stayed with [her] right up until he did wake up."

It was over a year until her son actually woke up, Linda recounts, and then she was told there was a possibility that he would never speak or walk. "But I just kept on hoping that he would. . . . I wasn't believing what people were telling me." In her view, her hope and faith were "greater than what they were telling [her]. . . . [She] just knew things to be different. . . . Without that hope, [her] determination would have faltered." Moreover, Linda doubts that "[Lyndon] would have survived . . . without my determination and motivation. . . . I hoped things would be better, and that feeling of hope overcame everything everyone else said." Lyndon survived, and he can now walk and talk. Linda acknowledges that her "hope is fading . . . [that] he's going to improve any more." Lyndon's lack of interest in continuing his therapy "is forcing [Linda] to give up hope . . . but it's still there. . . . [She] still hope[s] he will continue." Linda shares that during the time Lyndon was in the hospital, her husband left her. She says, "I thought it was only a temporary thing, and I hoped and hoped he would come back." Now, that hope "has faded," she admits, but "not because I'm not hoping enough. I haven't got the faith that goes with it." She believes that hope, faith, and love go together: "In my hope for Lyndon's well-being, there was a lot of love given as well. . . . With the love, you give your whole being." Linda thinks that "there's a lot more to us than we know—that we can transmit those feelings." When the person feels the love, hope, and faith "that you're putting in them," s/he "reciprocates." Linda says she has no faith in her husband and she knows he does not love her, so he isn't going to return.

Other hopes of Linda's are that her daughter's two children will grow up happily, that the world will improve, and that life will be better for them—"but that's wishing," she says, "rather than hoping."

Essences: Participant's Language

1. Hope is a feeling in your heart that is deeper than a desire or a wish. The participant hopes that her badly injured son will continue to improve, and that her little grandchildren will grow up happily, in a better world.
2. Hope, faith, and love are feelings that go hand in hand; they are transmitted with your whole being, and if the recipient receives them, s/he reciprocates. The participant's hope, based in her religious faith, love, and faith

in her son, overcame doubts about his recovery; without it, her determination and motivation would have faltered.

Essences: Researcher's Language

1. Ardent yearning for the cherished emerges with dreams of the preferred.
2. Assurances with devoted alliances arises with fortifying commitment amid adversity.

Proposition. The lived experience of hope is an ardent yearning for the cherished emerging with dreams of the preferred, as assurances with devoted alliances arises with a fortifying commitment amid adversity.

Martin's Story

Martin had a boating accident six years ago in which he received a head injury. He thinks that his experiences of hope "might well be tainted a little bit by some of the trauma [he's] gone through for five years following [his] accident, because [he's] had a legal battle over it, and it was not at all a pleasant experience."

Many of the effects of his injury only became apparent after he left the hospital, when he remembers starting "to feel the differences" in himself, which others noticed as well. For instance, he was getting "a little bit irrational, hotheaded—so much so that a doctor was called," who put him on medication. Martin could see that the medication made a "slight difference," but "everything was slowing down about [him]," and that "annoyed" him. He thought he had a "serious mental problem" or "was defective," and he "could see no light at all." Now he is on a new medication, but he says his "number-one objective in life" is to "not need medication of any sort. . . . [He's] always got to have something positive to look forward to, [and that gives him] hope." Martin hopes to go back to work, in "a job that has some responsibility . . . [although he knows his] short-term memory probably limits that. But [he's] got to push [him]self along the fact [he's] going to one day find a job." For Martin, "hope is [linked] with motivation. . . . The hope, with me," he continues, "was in my sport, that I'd do well. . . . [If] you believe in yourself, then you've got a chance." Describing his involvement in playing badminton, Martin says he "stayed at it for about three years. . . . I'd tell myself 'I'm going to get that much better,' . . . and the hope factor was always there," he adds.

Martin thinks he has changed since his accident. He realizes that "with what I've come through, there must be something inside me worth bringing out. . . . Sometimes you get feelings deep inside yourself," he continues, "[a] tremendous . . . warm feeling . . . that you've done well." That is "really invigorating" to Martin, and when he looks back, it "heartens" him that he has "jumped so far forward." Nonetheless, what happened to him has given him a "distaste" for "the whole legal system," even for "humanity as a whole." And yet, people like Princess Diana, "who do things for people who need someone to help them," give him "hope for humanity." When people step in and show that they care, "that gives me hope for life in general," he adds.

He shares that he has "down moods" when he has "just a totally black outlook [and] can't think of anything positive. . . . [Without] hope for life in general," Martin says, "I'd probably switch off myself in one way or another. . . . I've got to have hope," he declares.

Essences: Participant's Language

1. Hope has to do with motivation and having something positive to look forward to. The participant looks forward to not needing any medication, having a responsible job one day, and doing well in badminton; it is hope that pushes him along, although he knows he is limited.
2. Hope comes through believing in yourself, and then you have a chance. Looking back, the participant feels warmed and heartened that he has come so far.
3. Hope is seeing people do caring things for those who need help. The participant feels he must have hope for humanity, because in a down mood, he has a totally black outlook and can't think of anything positive. Without hope, he would probably switch himself off in one way or another.

Essences: Researcher's Language

1. Anticipating cherished possibilities emerges in perseverance with restrictions.
2. Assurance arises with the encouragement of successful opportunities.
3. The enlivenment of compassionate affiliations surfaces amid deadening despair.

Proposition. The lived experience of hope is anticipating cherished possibilities emerging in perseverance with restrictions, as assurance arises with the encouragement of successful opportunities, while the enlivenment of compassionate affiliations surfaces amid deadening despair.

Beverly's Story

Beverly says that her life has been "fairly traumatic" in the last ten years, starting when her husband left her alone with a 2-year-old; then her mother died. Still, she thinks she has always been "quite a hopeful person"; hence, she was determined not to let it "get her down." Not until she was diagnosed with inoperable cancer did Beverly experience a "rock bottom . . . hopeless feeling," and that was when she began to realize the meaning of hope.

She explains, "You've got to see hope in the context of despair. . . . It's like two sides of a coin; . . . you [cannot] understand one until you have experienced the other." On the "desperate day" that she learned she was terminally ill, Beverly recollects being "really scared." She had a "sinking feeling," as though she had "no power over" what was happening to her, and "there was nothing she could do to help [her]self." She said to a nurse who was there at that time, "I don't want to die in pain!" and remembers him replying, "We're going to get you on some treatment. There's nobody [who] knows what the future is going to bring." That nurse gave Beverly "something to hang on to. . . . He in some ways restored my equilibrium a bit," she says.

For Beverly, hope is "not being in despair . . . and that means taking control." She remembers becoming very angry at the thought of dying, and telling her father and her friends, "I want to fight this as much as I can." The fact that everyone was upset and sympathetic made her even more determined not to "lay down and die." When she "got busy" finding out "more about the disease and about the support that was available," she "started to feel empowered that [she] could just do something about it [her]self." Beverly describes the things that she did: for example, taking vitamins, eating a vegan diet, practicing meditation, and using aromatherapy, all the while hoping that she "was going to get better. [And] it seemed to be coming true." She "started feeling well," and was "very buoyant . . . very excited," as though she had been "given a second chance."

Beverly goes on to relate that she has since found a malignant lump on her neck. "As far as hope is concerned," she says, "it's just a question of . . . thinking, 'This is my lot in life . . . and I've got to make the best [of the situation].' . . . Acceptance is part of it as well," she adds. For Beverly, "hope is the feeling that you're able to go on and . . . enjoy your life despite limitations." "[Life is] much more precious to me now," she reflects, then continues, "You've got to nurture your hope . . . [and] find ways to overcome desperate moments." For instance, "there has to be something to look forward to—and you can give yourself that, even if it's thinking . . . [about what you will do] this weekend."

At the moment, Beverly's hope "[has] become more of a short-term thing." She knows there "might come a point where they can't do anything more to help [her] . . . but even then there is a quality of life to be had." Having "a religious faith" helps Beverly to believe that "there is something better—this is just a transition. There is something there that we're going to. This is not the end of things."

Essences: Participant's Language

1. Hope is being determined not to let traumatic experiences get you down. On the desperate day that she learned that she was terminally ill, the participant felt hopeless and powerless; then she got angry and decided to fight it, and felt empowered that she could take control and help herself.
2. Hope is nurtured by giving yourself things to look forward to, so you can overcome desperate moments. Having religious faith helps the participant think about something better that we're going to; also, turning to family, friends, and others for help and support helps restore her equilibrium.
3. Hope is accepting what you've been given in life, making the best of it, and enjoying life, despite limitations.

Essences: Researcher's Language

1. Ardent resolve emerges with assurance amid impotent desolation.
2. Anticipating cherished possibilities with consoling affiliations emerges with tranquility.

3. Yielding with vicissitudes arises with enlivening opportunities with constraints.

Proposition. The lived experience of hope is an ardent resolve that emerges with assurance amid impotent desolation, as anticipating cherished possibilities arises with the tranquility of consoling affiliations, while yielding with vicissitudes surfaces in enlivening opportunities with constraints.

Bernice's Story

Bernice says, "It was not until my husband was diagnosed as having a progressive disease that I thought about hope. . . . Suddenly the bottom fell out of our world." One of her first thoughts was "to hope he would get better." For the next ten years, Bernice and her husband lived "with the hope that [the disease] would burn out eventually," but when that didn't happen, they "had to look for some other way of thinking."

For instance, Bernice's hope shifted "to carrying on with life" in spite of her husband's illness. She recalls reading a magazine article in which "something was brought home to [her] about hope." The article was about "people who are in hospital and terminally ill [and yet they] still have hope—that they can see the flowers, the trees, and everything about them, and for them, life still goes on. They have hope that someone, somewhere, will help them on the way."

Bernice speaks about her experiences working with elderly and mentally ill people. Helping them was "one way of bringing hope back into [their lives]," but it also taught her "the value of living from day to day. . . . It was sort of a healing process for both of us," she remembers; "I was able to come back to my husband and family with a fresh outlook."

She goes on to say that when her husband suffered a head injury, "[It] really took us to the depths of despair." Once you realize that it is "really happening," Bernice says, "then you start hoping that your future will be better than expected. . . . That's the way life goes on, every time you get a setback. There must be something, which maybe is hope, which sets you on another path to put your life back into perspective again."

Bernice and her husband joined a group for "head-injured persons" and their families, "[who] gave [her] hope that there was something to work towards." They were "very supportive" and Bernice found hope just "to be with them" and watch "the improvement" in their own and others' lives. Now that she and her husband are getting older, Bernice hopes "that [they] can both go on the way [they] are now, until [they] are called to wherever [they] are going after this life. . . . But as long as there's life . . . there's always hope. . . . [Hope] gives you a sense of contentment, in many ways," Bernice says. "It is a flame within us that is always [there] and always burning; and even when you're at your lowest ebb, something or someone comes along, who helps you and gives you hope to carry on." Hope lets you "see ahead . . . [that] there is a light shining somewhere which is for you, and helps you on your way." Bernice describes how you can go to bed at night feeling "very low," but when you look outside in the morning and see the beauty in nature, "that makes you feel better, and if you feel better," she says, "you have hope . . . [that] today is going to be a good day. . . . It's invigorating, it lifts you up. . . . What I look forward to," Bernice affirms, "is to find the good side of every day."

Essences: Participant's Language

1. Hope is having something to look forward to and work toward when you're at your lowest ebb, and that's the way life goes on. Whenever the participant gets a setback that takes her to the depths of despair, hoping that her future will be better and making plans in that direction sets her on another path, and puts her life back into perspective again.
2. Hope is seeing that there is a light shining somewhere that is for you; it is having something or someone come along to help you carry on. The participant got hope in helping others and through joining a group where she and her husband could watch the improvement in their own lives and those of others around them.
3. Hope is a flame within that is always burning, as long as there is life. It gives you a sense of contentment in many ways, it is invigorating, and it lifts you up. The participant hoped that her husband would get better; then her hope shifted to carrying on with life in spite of his illness; now she looks forward to finding the good side of every day and going on the way they are until they are called to another life beyond this one.

Essences: Researcher's Language

1. Anticipating cherished possibilities amid devastation emerges in persevering with new visions.
2. Personal solace arises with benevolent affiliations.
3. Enduring ardor surfaces with the serene enlivenment of diversifying aspirations.

Proposition. The lived experience of hope is anticipating cherished possibilities amid devastation while persevering with new visions, as personal solace arises with benevolent affiliations, while enduring ardor surfaces with the serene enlivenment of diversifying aspirations.

Tony's Story

Tony is a 42-year-old who had surgery to remove a brain tumor two years ago. He shares that since the surgery "[he] can't walk, [he] can't talk, [he] can't eat properly, [he] can't see properly, [he's] deaf, and [his] family is going through hell." Tony begins talking about hope by saying that before his surgery he "never really used the word hope" the way he does now. He used to think of it as "achievable expectations—something that could be done," but now he "has no expectations; what [he] expected to achieve before, [he] now hope[s] to achieve." He adds that "it seems very easy for life to go on and to say 'c'est la vie,' [but] in the back of [his] mind [he'd] love to be able to get up and walk, [he'd] love to be able to speak properly," and sometimes he even thinks he would rather that they had let him go than have let him "live a life like [he's] living at this moment." Tony says that "every morning when [he] wake[s] up the first thing that comes into his head is 'oh dear . . . another day stuck in the wheelchair' and then there's that hope that things might get better."

Tony adds that he "admits . . . it has gotten better. Hope has fulfilled itself—but only in very small degrees." He remembers that in those early weeks he hoped to be able to get from the wheelchair into an armchair and to get into his bed upstairs. He can do both of those things now—yet at the time he did not expect it since "nothing in [his] condition is guaranteed." Tony now hopes "to achieve as much as [he] can, to get to as near normal as [he] can."

Tony believes "hope is a necessity" that is "increased or amplified when your needs are great." When one's "needs are not satisfied, [one] turns to hope." Tony says his "whole being, [his] whole existence . . . is hope because . . . nothing can be expected or guaranteed." When he "was fit," Tony recalls he "did not need much hope" because "things that [he] needed or wanted— [he] was in the business of making happen. Now that [he] can't [make things happen], hope is all there is at the end of the day." He says he spends most of the time he is on his own "thinking about something [he's] hoping for."

Tony also talks about his sense of humor. He says he has it and hope, and since "they're working together, [he's] just about getting by." He thinks "if hope is in your system . . . it keeps you going forward."

Finally, Tony describes his love and his hope for his family. He thinks his hope for his wife and his child "increases [his] hope for [himself]. It . . . makes [him] feel stronger." Tony also believes hope is related to "determination."

Essences: Participant's Language

1. Hope is wanting things to get better but having no expectations of achievement, because things can only be hoped for and nothing can be expected or guaranteed.
2. Hope is a necessity and it makes one feel stronger. It is one's whole being, one's whole existence, and it keeps one moving forward. It is all there is at the end of the day.
3. Hope is related to determination. It is increased when one loves and has positive hopes for others. It is also amplified when one's needs are great. One turns to hope when one's needs are not met.

Essences: Researcher's Language

1. Anticipation of the cherished arises with unsure possibilities.
2. Requisite inspiriting surfaces with propelling fortification.
3. Tenacity with benevolent affiliations emerges with ambitions amid the arduous.

Proposition. The lived experience of hope is anticipation of the cherished arising with unsure possibilities, as requisite inspiriting surfaces with propelling fortification, while tenacity with benevolent affiliations emerges with ambitions amid the arduous.

FINDINGS AND RELATED LITERATURE

Through dwelling with the propositions from the dialogues with participants, the following core concepts were identified: *anticipating cherished possibilities, persevering amid adversity,* and *benevolent affiliations.* These core concepts were joined to form the following structure of the lived experience of hope for the Welsh participants in this study: *The lived experience of hope is anticipating cherished possibilities while persevering amid adversity with benevolent affiliations.* Transposed to more abstract language, this structure became *assuredly envisioning the prized as pushing-resisting in tribulation arises with uplifting communion.* This was conceptually integrated with the human becoming theory as *imaging valuing in the powering of connecting-separating* (see Table 1). In the following sections, each of the core concepts will be explained and considered in relation to the relevant theoretical and research literature, in order to enhance understanding about the lived experience of hope.

TABLE 1.
Progressive Abstraction of the Core Concepts of the Lived Experience of Hope

Core Concepts	Structural Transposition	Conceptual Integration
Anticipating cherished possibilities	Assuredly envisioning the prized	Imaging valuing
Persevering amid adversity	Pushing-resisting in tribulation	Powering
Benevolent affiliations	Uplifting communion	Connecting-separating

Structure

The lived experience of hope is anticipating cherished possibilities while persevering amid adversity with benevolent affiliations.

Structural Transposition

The lived experience of hope is assuredly envisioning the prized as pushing-resisting in tribulation arises with uplifting communion.

Conceptual Integration

The lived experience of hope is imaging valuing in the powering of connecting-separating.

Anticipating Cherished Possibilities

Anticipating cherished possibilities indicates looking forward to something important with a deep desire. In describing their experiences of hope, participants used phrases suggesting that they were already enjoying what they were anticipating; for instance, they said "you start hoping that your future will be better than expected because you have made plans in that direction"; "giving yourself things to look forward to"; and "looking at scenarios. . . [to] make things more hopeful for the future." For six of the participants, the possibilities that they were anticipating related to a loved one's recovery. In two cases, the participants anticipated thier own recovery, from either a head injury sustained in an accident or surgery to remove a brain tumor. For two women who were terminally ill with cancer, anticipating cherished possibilities pertained to hope for a cure or for a good quality of life until they died. While the dialogues with these participants centered on anticipating a positive outcome for their current difficulties, they also touched on other cherished possibilities, like looking forward to "the good in everyday life," to "success" for themselves and family members, and to "a better life" in this world and in the hereafter. For another participant, a nurse who worked with patients on trauma and orthopedic units, anticipating cherished possibilities related to his work, and to "wanting the world to be a better place."

Anticipating cherished possibilities reflects the sense of assurance with which participants were looking forward to something, in that they linked hope with faith, belief, or expectation, as well as deep desire and love. As one participant stated, "I feel [faith and hope] go hand in hand, and the third virtue to go with that is . . . love." Those participants whose family members had serious head injuries recounted that they kept looking for signs of recovery, as they were "hoping for a better outcome" than that proffered by the physicians. And as one man said, "You'd start off in the morning . . . with renewed hope for the future—something that day was going to happen . . . and very often it did; a very small thing would give you that hope." As a number of participants observed, hope changes with circumstances and with passage through life; so too, did the cherished possibilities that they were anticipating. For instance, one woman, who was terminally ill with cancer, tied hope "with . . . what you [want and] expect from life." Therefore, she had had "to re-prioritize . . . [and] re-examine everything that [she] expected from life," because she was uncertain about her remaining time.

Appearing in every proposition, anticipating cherished possibilities was associated with picturing what one ardently desires with faith and love, which led to its structural transposition as assuredly envisioning the prized; this was conceptually integrated with the theory as imaging valuing (see Table 2), concepts from Parse's first principle.

Principle 1 addresses the theme of meaning: "Structuring meaning multidimensionally is cocreating reality through the languaging of valuing and imaging" (Parse, 1981, p. 42). It specifies how humans are continuously constructing the meaning of lived experiences at many realms all-at-once, thus cocreating reality. Personal reality is expressed "through speaking–being-silent

TABLE 2.
First Core Concept as Evident in Propositions

Core Concept:	**Anticipating cherished possibilities**
Structural Transposition:	**Assuredly envisioning the prized**
Conceptual Integration:	**Imaging valuing**

1. yearning for the cherished . . . confident anticipating
2. anticipating cherished possibilities
3. anticipating cherished possibilities
4. anticipating cherished possibilities
5. ardent yearning for the cherished
6. anticipating cherished possibilities
7. anticipating cherished possibilities
8. anticipating cherished possibilities
9. confidently anticipating cherished possibilities
10. anticipation of the cherished . . . possibilities

and moving–being-still" (Parse, 1998, p. 39), the paradoxical rhythms of languaging. Valuing is choosing, prizing, and acting on one's priorities (Parse, 1981) and unfolds as "confirming–not-confirming cherished beliefs in light of a personal worldview" (Parse, 1998, p. 38). Imaging refers to the personal knowing that happens at explicit and tacit realms all-at-once. Through imaging, humans picture and realize events and experiences (Parse, 1981, 1994, 1998).

The construct imaging valuing, as interpreted in this research, signifies assuredly envisioning the prized. The participants made real their situations as they pictured, with love and faith, the possibilities that they deeply desired; for instance, recovery from injury or illness, or having a good quality of life until they died, or having a better life in the hereafter. The envisioned possibilities were chosen from among other options for their worthiness and personal importance. The participants knew, at explicit and tacit realms, that what they hoped was both possible and real. Prizing these possibilities meant that participants acted on them; in other words, hope was a lived value priority, even in the midst of circumstances that challenged the viability of hope.

Three phenomenological studies of hope have been conducted (Brunsman, 1988; Parse, 1990; Stanley, 1978). Findings from each of these studies have both similarities and differences with findings reported here. For instance, Stanley (1978) reported that "the lived experience of hope is confident expectation of a significant future outcome accompanied by comfortable and uncomfortable feelings, characterized by a quality of transcendence and interpersonal related-ness, and in which action to affect the outcome is initiated" (p. 1231). The theme expectation of a significant future outcome has some similarity with the core concept anticipating cherished possibilities. The 100 participants in Stanley's (1978) study, all undergraduate students, described their belief in a pos-itive outcome despite feelings of comfort and discomfort. Brunsman's (1988) study of families with a chronically ill child reported that "hope is a process that arises as one anticipates the future in the day-to-day struggle of living opportuni-ties and limitations and creating a different view of the situation" (as cited in Parse, 1990, p. 16). Parse (1990) used the Parse methodology to study the lived experience of hope for ten adults with end-stage renal disease undergoing hemo-dialysis. The reported structure of the lived experience was "hope is anticipating possibilities through envisioning the not-yet in harmoniously living the comfort-discomfort of everydayness while unfolding a different perspective of an expand-ing view" (Parse, 1990, p. 15).

Persevering Amid Adversity

Persevering amid adversity reflects the participants' descriptions of hope as helping them to keep going in difficult and disheartening circumstances. Each one described moments of deep despair contrasting with moments of real hope. "You've got to see hope in the context of despair," one woman sug-gested; "It's like two sides of a coin, and I don't think you can understand one until you have experienced the other." Without exception, the participants spoke of their need to "hold onto hope" and recounted how they kept hoping, in spite of being confronted with reasons not to hope. For example, a mother whose son had a head injury stated, "I would always hope one day [he would awake]—you know, miracles do happen." Another woman, when she discov-ered that she was terminally ill with lung cancer, recounted feeling "shock," "really scared," and "distraught"; but then, she "became very angry" and decided to "fight it." Another participant with recurrent breast cancer said that she knows "there is no escape," and so she feels "quite resigned." However, she said she doesn't feel "hopeless," "lost," or "distraught" about her life. She explained, "What I'm tending to do is invest my energies in finding ways of surviving comfortably as long as I can, rather than thinking about beating the disease."

Those whose family members had head injuries felt as though medical per-sonnel had tried to "strip away" their hope. They experienced medical profes-sionals' reluctance to talk about hope as injustice and insensitivity at a time of personal suffering, and yet they tenaciously hoped for "a better outcome." One woman's persevering amid adversity appears in the following quote:

> The senior professionals . . . tried to take that hope away from us. . . . I think it just gave us strength to have some hope; because we were very sensible of, you know . . . the possible outcomes. . . . It wasn't

just wishful thinking. . . . I think [hope] is essential because it's the thing that keeps you positive, and . . . that helps people through an ordeal or through a trauma.

Present in every dialogue, persevering amid adversity involved an effort to resist or overcome the challenges presented by disconcerting circumstances. (See Table 3.) This core concept was structurally transposed as pushing-resisting in tribulation and was conceptually integrated with the theory as *powering*, a concept from the third principle.

Principle 3 elaborates on the theme of transcendence, that is, "reaching beyond with possibles—the hopes and dreams envisioned in multidimensional experiences" (Parse, 1998, p. 30). Principle 3 states: "Cotranscending with the possibles is powering unique ways of originating in the process of transforming" (Parse, 1981, p. 55). Citing Tillich (1952), Parse (1981) describes powering as "the force of human existence [which] underpins the courage to be" (p. 57). More specifically, "powering is the pushing-resisting process of affirming–not affirming being in light of nonbeing. . . . Pushing-resting patterns . . . are present in every human engagement, creating tension and sometimes conflict" (Parse, 1998, pp. 47, 48).

As elucidated in this research, powering is the energizing force underlying hope. Interestingly, some participants actually used words suggesting an energizing force, such as "a burning flame" or "a shining light" to describe hope.

TABLE 3.
Second Core Concept as Evident in Propositions

Core Concept:	**Persevering amid adversity**
Structural Transposition:	**Pushing-resisting in tribulation**
Conceptual Integration:	**Powering**

1. persevering with enlivening fortitude amid adversity
2. devastation emerges in persevering
3. an ardent resolve that emerges . . . amid impotent desolation
4. the disquieting impotence of affliction . . . laboring for enduring solace
5. a fortifying commitment amid adversity
6. perseverance with restrictions . . . amid deadening despair
7. anticipating the alleviation of adversity . . . while persevering
8. adversity, as persevering
9. amid devastation while perserving
10. tenacity . . . amid the arduous

Others tellingly commented that "as long as there's life, there's hope." One eloquent description of hope that reflects powering is as follows:

> [Hope is] an inner strength which people find. . . . Hope gives you the inspiration to do something that is in your control and you can do something about, or gives you the inspiration to go forward . . . [like] some sort of shining warm light. . . . [It is] the start of other things that keep you going . . . [such as] strength and courage.

Powering was manifested as a pushing-resisting rhythm creating tension and conflict, as participants experienced difficult situations; for example, when they were presented with "worst-case scenarios" for their own or their loved one's future. For some, conflict surfaced as a lingering anger at the professionals who painted "the blackest of pictures," seemingly intent on taking away their hopes. With the participants diagnosed with cancer, tension and conflict appeared as "getting angry and fighting" the disease, and as "investing energy" in having a good quality of life, as long as it lasted. One man, who had endured a long legal battle after being head-injured in an accident, said that that had given him "a totally black view on the world." His hope grew with believing in himself—that he could "improve"—and striving toward that "target." For every participant, hope flourished with pushing-resisting amid severe challenges and obstacles, enlivening them with inspiration, courage, and strength to persevere.

Participants in this study described a new awareness of hope after experiencing severe difficulties. For example, one person said:

> Before my accident I didn't really think about hope. It was something I took for granted. When people used to say to me "I hope you do well" or "I hope you get the job," I didn't really pay any attention to it. . . . Hope like that is not the same as the hope I have since my accident.

The struggles of the participants and their intensive efforts to overcome limitations and to persist with living despite times of serious despair have been identified as a theme in the philosophical literature. Marcel (1951) points out that to hope is to recognize the limitations in situations, while believing that opportunities also exist. Fromm (1968) contends that hope is paradoxical. He describes hope as being linked with faith, which is the knowledge of real possibility, and with fortitude, which is the capacity to resist the temptation to compromise faith and hope. Oliver (1974), too, describes faith and hope as inseparable. Hope, according to Oliver (1974), provides continuity between past and future; it gives power to find meaning in the worst adversity. The participants in this study talked of their intense struggles with everyday living, and the will to carry on despite everything. Wu (1972) asserts the necessity of life for world survival. He goes on to suggest that hope arises out of suffering; it is a creative pull between the now and the future.

Benevolent Affiliations

The third core concept, benevolent affiliations, represents relationships with others, which participants described as very important to their hope, in that they provided comfort, support, and encouragement. For example, most of the participants described their family and friends as being "supportive." Five participants with family members who had head injuries belonged to the Headway support group. For them, being with others who were going through a similar situation gave them "hope to carry on" by providing opportunities to share their experiences and witness "the improvements" in their own and others' lives. These participants recounted how being present with their loved one also nurtured hope. The entwining of love and hope is seen in the following passage from a dialogue with a mother whose son had been in a prolonged coma:

> I believe that [love is] tied up with [hope] as well . . . because there again, in my hope for [my son's] well-being, there was a lot of love given as well, and I think with the love you give . . . your whole being. . . . When he was unconscious—I feel there is a lot more to us than we know, that we can transmit those feelings, and the recipient receives the love, the hope, and the faith that you're putting in them. And if they're feeling it, they reciprocate.

One woman shared that participating in her son's care gave her and her husband hope: "We felt, I think, that we were doing something constructive. . . . We felt as if we were trying . . . with the staff to do anything and everything, really." For her and others, God was a comforting presence, even if they "weren't religious." "At the darkest times of your life," said this mother, "there's still somebody or something there with you. . . . You know, God really walked with us. . . . You just know that He's there for you, He's guiding you." Some related that relationships with professional caregivers strengthened their hope. For example, the same woman told how their clergyman "just was there. Just [in] his presence there was hope, you know, because he was so good. . . . He just seemed to know what to do." She found that "everybody was really supportive," and "[if] they felt that there wasn't much of a chance, they did not show it. That, I think, gives you hope," she explained:

> because you feel that they're with you and that everybody's on the same side. I think having support in a situation like that is tremendously important, even if you've got tremendous faith. . . . If people around you are positive, then it sort of inspires you.

Some found hope in helping others. For instance, one participant, whose husband had a progressive illness as well as a head injury, took jobs in which she helped others; this, she found, "took [her] out of [her] own environment and into another one . . . [and gave her a way] to come back to [her] husband and family with a fresh outlook." One man shared that he has "down moods" in which he has "no hope for humanity"; however, seeing people like Princess Diana who help the "downtrodden" gives him:

> . . . hope for humanity itself, which I've got to believe in. If I don't believe in that, then I just see trouble, and that's not something I just could deal with. . . . If I had no hope for life in general, I'd probably switch off myself in one way or another.

The core concept benevolent affiliations represents hope-enlivening relationships with others who are beloved, or compassionate and understanding. This core concept was structurally transposed as uplifting communion and was conceptually integrated with the theory as connecting-separating (see Table 4), a concept from the second principle.

Principle 2 centers on the theme of rhythmicity. It states, "Cocreating rhythmical patterns of relating is living the paradoxical unity of revealing-concealing and enabling-limiting while connecting-separating" (Parse, 1981, p. 50). According to Parse, human becoming is a reality that is lived at multidimensional realms and that emerges in rhythmical patterns of relating with the universe. Basic to everyday living (Mitchell, 1993; Parse, 1981, 1994, 1998), these rhythms are paradoxical and unitary in nature; that is, they are apparent

TABLE 4.
Third Core Concept as Evident in Propositions

Core Concept:	Benevolent affiliations
Structural Transposition:	**Uplifting communion**
Conceptual Integration:	**Connecting-separating**

1. persuasion of close alliances
2. benevolent affiliations
3. consoling affiliations
4. consoling alliances
5. devoted alliances
6. compassionate affiliations
7. benevolent alliances
8. benevolent affiliations
9. benevolent affiliations
10. benevolent affiliations

opposites that coexist. At any moment, one side of the rhythm is in the fore, while the other is in the background of one's becoming. Connecting-separating is a rhythm in which humans are "with and apart from others, ideas, objects, and situations all-at-once" (Parse, 1998, p. 45).

In this study, participants' descriptions of benevolent affiliations were brought to light as connecting-separating. Every participant described important connections with family members, friends, others going through similar situations, and/or God. These connections, which they believed strengthened their hope, were experienced in another's presence, or through the "felt presence" of prayers or "positive energy" being "directed toward" themselves and loved ones. As well, some participants spoke of connecting with oneself in ways that contributed to hope. For instance, one woman sought counseling so that she could begin to "trust" and hope. Another participant spoke about motivating himself to improve through involvement in "his sport," badminton. Still another, a nurse who worked on a trauma care unit, described how he sometimes "steps back" to contemplate "scenarios for a more hopeful future." In connecting with persons, ideas, and situations that fortified hope, participants were also separating from others, which made them "distraught" and "depressed"; for example, "the everyday mad rush of the world," an unpleasant legal battle, or the hopeless prognoses given to themselves or their loved ones by professionals whom they described as insensitive.

Several authors have alluded to hope in ways consistent with the ideas captured by the core concept of benevolent affiliations. Their writings support the notion that connections with important others are linked with one's hope. For instance, Vaughan (1991) wrote about intersubjectivity, saying that hope depends on one's loving and being loved in relationships. Several participants in this study speak about the interconnectedness of love and hope. One participant, who talks about his love and his hope for his family, thinks his hope for his wife and his child "increases [his] hope for [himself]. It . . . makes [him] feel stronger." In addition, Artinian (1984), Herth (1990), Jacobson (1992), and Miller (1989) suggest that supportive relationships are a factor linked with hope. This current study contributes details about the participants' hope-enlivening relationships with others. It illuminates that the participants believed that some relationships provided comfort, support, and encouragement that they felt, for example, when helping others and through being with loved ones, others in similar situations, or God.

SUMMARY

This study on the lived experience of hope was conducted with persons living in Wales. Participants were six caregivers (including five family members) of persons with serious head injury, one person recovering from a head injury, one person recovering from the removal of a brain tumor, and two women seriously ill with cancer. The structure that was generated is *the lived experience of hope is anticipating cherished possibilities while persevering amid adversity with benevolent affiliations.* At the theoretical level, the structure is *imaging valuing in the powering of connecting-separating.* These findings expand Parse's theory of human becoming with disciplinary knowledge about the lived experience of hope. Research and practice implications are discussed in the final chapter.

REFERENCES

Artinian, B. (1984). Fostering hope in the bone marrow transplant child. *Maternal Child Nursing Journal, 13* (1), 57–71.

Brunsman, C. S. (1988). *A phenomenological study of the lived experience of hope in families with a chronically ill child.* Unpublished master's thesis, Michigan State University, East Lansing.

Fromm, E. (1968). *The revolution of hope.* New York: Harper & Row.

Headway, Cardiff and District Report. (1995). *Needs of head injury persons and their families in the community.* Cardiff, Wales: Headway.

Headway National Head Injuries Association. (1997). *Headway National Head Injuries Association Homepage* [http://www.headway-national.demon.co.uk/#A].

Herth, K. (1990). Fostering hope in terminally ill people. *Journal of Advanced Nursing, 15,* 1250–1259.

Jacobson, A. (1992). Hope and AIDS. *Dissertation Abstracts International, 52* (11), 6086-B.

Marcel, G. (1951). *Homo viator* (E. Craufurd, Trans.). Chicago: Henry Regnery Co.

Miller, J. F. (1989). Hope inspiring strategies of the critically ill. *Applied Nursing Research, 2* (1), 23–29.

Mitchell, G. J. (1993). Living paradox in Parse's theory. *Nursing Science Quarterly, 6,* 44–51.

Office of Health Economics. (1992). *Office of Health Economics: Compendium of health statistics.* London: HMSO.

Office of Population Census and Surveys (OPCS). (1992). *General Household Survey 1990.* London: HMSO.

Oliver, H. H. (1974). Hope and knowledge: The epistemic status of religious knowledge. *Cultural Hermeneutics, 2,* 75–88.

Parse, R. R. (1981). *Man-living-health: A theory of nursing.* New York: Wiley.

Parse, R. R. (1990). Parse's research methodology with an illustration of the lived experience of hope. *Nursing Science Quarterly, 3,* 9–17.

Parse, R. R. (1994). Quality of life: Sciencing and living the art of human becoming. *Nursing Science Quarterly, 7,* 16–21.

Parse, R. R. (1998). *The human becoming school of thought: A perspective for nurses and other health professionals.* Thousand Oaks, CA: Sage.

Rose, D., & Johnson, D. (1996). Brian injuries and outcome. In D. Rose & D. A. Johnson (Eds.), *Brain injury and after—towards improved outcomes.* Chichester: John Wiley & Sons Ltd.

Stanley, A. T. (1978). The lived experience of hope: The isolation of discreet descriptive elements common to the experience of hope in healthy young adults. *Dissertation Abstracts International, 39* (03), 1212-B. (University Microfilms No. AAG7816899)

Stratton, M. C., & Gregory, R. J. (1995). What happens after a traumatic brain injury: Four case studies. *Rehabilitation Nursing, 20* (6), 323–327.

Tillich, P. (1952). *The courage to be.* New Haven, CT: Yale University Press.

Vaughan, S. B. (1991). Intersubjectivity as the ground of hope: Psychoanalytic and theological perspectives. *Dissertation Abstracts International, 52* (3), 970-A.

Welsh Health Planning Forum (WHPF). (1990). *Protocol for investment in health gain: Cancers.* Welsh Office NHS Directorate, Cardiff, Wales.

Wu, K. M. (1972). Hope and world survival. *Philosophy Forum, 12,* 131–148.

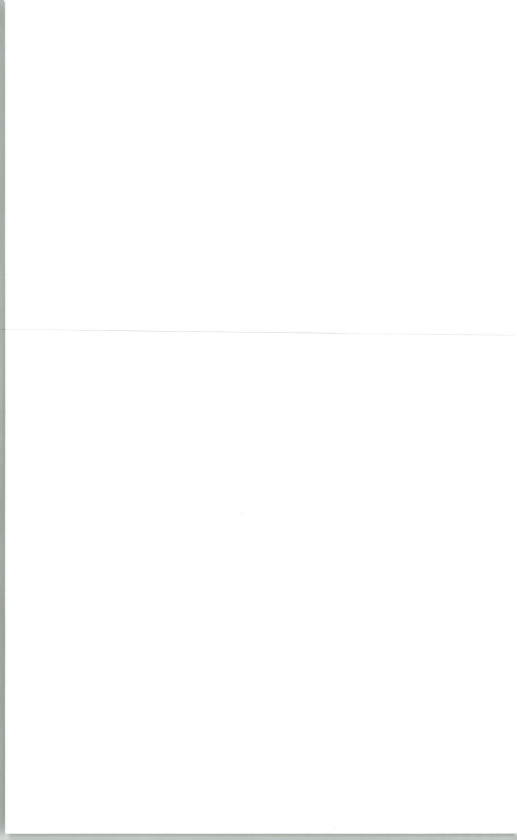

Chapter 11

The Lived Experience of Hope: Children in Families Struggling to Make a Home

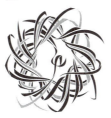

STEVEN L. BAUMANN

Historically and transculturally, children have been seen as symbols of hope. Like hope, they represent possibilities and challenges. Providing for children requires a long-term commitment and self-renunciation, on the part of families and societies. Listening to children requires time and a belief in the inherent worth of all human beings. The purpose of this study, guided by Parse's theory (1981, 1992, 1995, 1998) was to investigate the meaning of hope for children in families struggling to make a home. Making a home is seen here as a challenge that all families face. This chapter is a report of what has been uncovered about the meaning of the lived experience of hope for ten children in families struggling to make a home. In this study the lived experience of hope emerges as *the envisioning of nurturing engagements while inventing possibilities.*

PARTICIPANTS

All of the families in this study have turned to the government and private agencies for income and housing assistance. The children were in families living in a shelter, a motor lodge, or an apartment provided by a transitional housing program in New York. They were all African American or Latina/Latino children between the ages of 4 and 13. None of them were residing with their fathers.

DIALOGICAL ENGAGEMENT

After obtaining consent from the participants' mothers, the children were invited to draw and talk about hope. The children were told that they could draw and talk with the researcher even if they did not want to participate or talk about hope. The mingling of their drawings and verbal descriptions provided greater access to the child participants' ways of cocreating meaning, and it offered creative ways of relating to what was, is, and may be related to hope. The participants from the shelter and the transitional housing program met with the researcher either alone or with a sibling. After drawing for some time, each participant had a one-to-one dialogical engagement with the researcher to describe the meaning of his/her drawings. At the motor lodge site, the researcher met with a small group of participants several times, asking them to draw pictures about hope. During or after the group meetings, participants at the motor lodge met with the researcher in one-to-one dialogical engagement to describe the meaning of their drawings about hope. All of the dialogical engagements were audiorecorded, and the researcher asked to borrow participants' drawings in order to photocopy them. Most of the children gave the original drawings to the researcher.

EXTRACTION-SYNTHESIS

LaTania's Story

LaTania, an 8-year-old girl, is living in an apartment that is part of a transitional housing program, with her younger brother, her older sister, and her mother.

Her oldest sister is living elsewhere. She is the third child in a family of four children, all of whose photographs hang in the living room. LaTania says it makes her sad to look at the pictures because her oldest sister lives somewhere else. The family has use of the apartment under a program run by a nonprofit organization, where participating families are required to meet with a social worker once a month and the parents are required to attend school or be in job training. The coordinator of the transitional housing program who had worked with LaTania's family sees the family as one of their most successful families. LaTania's mother is expecting to graduate with an associate's degree at the end of summer, after a field placement as a legal secretary. Only weeks after their participation in this study, a photograph of LaTania, her brother Michael (also a study participant), her mother, and her older sister was in the local newspaper. The newspaper article emphasized that this was a mother who was working her way off of welfare. The published photograph showed LaTania's sister (aged 13) helping her with her homework, as LaTania's mother was helping her brother with his.

The researcher explains the project and invites LaTania and her brother to draw and talk about hope, or start with drawing anything they want. LaTania is eager to participate and draw. She says, "Hopeful is good surprises." She then says and writes the words, "I like to help eveyone [*sic*] who need [*sic*] help." Unsure whether LaTania is talking about help or hope, the researcher asks, "Is this about hope?" "Yeah," she replies and then says she loves to help her teacher. (See Figure 1.)

LaTania starts another drawing and says, "This is also about hope. It has lots of colors; it's a rainbow." She fills the paper with parallel lines of varying colors and says, "I've never seen a rainbow, but I know it has lots of colors. I saw a sunset—it had lots of colors. I love sunsets." The researcher asks if there is anything else about hope that she can talk about and LaTania says, "People. I like school and people. I like doing the times table, if they are not too hard," she adds.

Essences: Participant's Language

1. Hope is giving a friend a good surprise, and the participant sees hope as helping people, like her teacher, and doing school work, as long as it is not too hard, and doing things, like when mothers help children when they get hurt. [She drew herself helping someone, and wrote that she liked to help everyone who needed help.]
2. Rainbows are about hope; even though the participant had never seen one, she said they were like the colorful sunsets that she loved. [She filled a piece of paper with parallel lines of various colors and said it was a rainbow.]

Essences: Researcher's Language

1. Contributing to the unexpected arises with nurturing engagements.
2. Fashioning of an uplifting array of hues surfaces with the remembrances of cherished vespers.

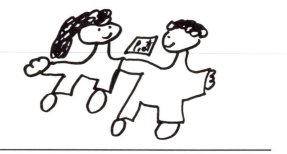

I like to Help eveyone who need Help

FIGURE 1.
LaTania, age 8

Proposition. The lived experience of hope is the fashioning of an uplifting array of hues surfacing with the remembrance of cherished vespers, as contributing to the unexpected arises with nurturing engagements.

Michael's Story

Michael is a 6-year-old boy living in an apartment (part of a transitional housing program) with two of his older sisters and his mother; his oldest sister lives elsewhere. He is the brother of LaTania. He is the youngest member of the family, and for three years the only male in the family. After the researcher explains the project, Michael begins drawing figures fighting. He says, "This is a Ninja Turtle. His name is Michelangelo. This is a terminator. These are my brothers; they like to beat the butts of bad guys." He draws the figures and writes "good guys" and "bad guys" over them. Then he says, "Remember when Rafael was eating an apple and they were beating him up? It was funny, right?" The researcher asks him if he can talk about hope. Michael says, "These are the good guys and the bad guys, and the good guys always win, like the time they saved April, the girl this guy goes out with." Then he says, "We got two sisters."

Michael says, "Hope is like when they showed the cops picking on the Black guy on TV. They just kept beating him, but he said 'I love you.'" Then Michael draws a house with a rainbow, calls it a "rainbow house," and says, "That's a hopeful picture for everybody." Michael copies his sister and says, "Hope is helping somebody. . . . I twisted my leg once and I had to see the nurse . . . when you get hurt and someone helps you."

Essences: Participant's Language

1. Hope is the cartoon guys who do things like protect their girlfriends and fight bad guys. The participant said they always win because they are the good guys. [He drew the good guys and bad guys fighting and labeled them.]
2. The participant talked about hope as seeing the police on TV beating a Black guy and stated that the guy then said, "I love you." [He described his drawing as a rainbow house for everyone and said doing things together was about hope.]
3. Hope is being hurt and getting help from a nurse. Hope is when you say something and go to jail; then you go somewhere else and you press the button and you get hit.

Essences: Researcher's Language

1. Contemplating valor arises when emulating significant others.
2. Envisioning harmonizing hues surfaces with regard-disregard all-at-once.
3. Discomfort-comfort emerges with forging new prospects.

Proposition. The lived experience of hope is envisioning harmonizing hues that surface with regard-disregard, while contemplating valor arises when emulating significant others amid the discomfort-comfort of forging new prospects.

Rachel's Story

Rachel is a 9-year-old African-American girl living at a motor lodge with her mother and two siblings, an older sister and a younger brother. They share a room with two beds and a bathroom at a rundown motor lodge in an industrial area of Long Island, New York. The presence of a large number of children and few cars suggests that most, if not all, of the people staying at the motor lodge, like Rachel's family, have been placed there by the local Department of Social Services. One of the few child-oriented aspects of this living situation is that one of the rooms has been converted into a classroom that houses an after-school tutoring program. For two hours each school day afternoon a Catholic nun, who is a retired school teacher, and a volunteer help children do their homework. Unfortunately, because of the number of interested children and the small space, each child is allowed less than half an hour to do homework and eat a snack so the next child can use the room. Most arrive in small groups. In the back of this makeshift classroom, the researcher has set up a small table to meet with the participants.

Rachel is happy to draw and talk about hope after she finishes her homework. She likes to draw and says her drawing is about hope. She says, "These are clouds, the sky, the sun, and an angel. . . . This is a brown bird and whales." (See Figure 2.) She says her drawing is about hope because "angels go up to Heaven and to God." She says she likes to think about such things. Rachel then says she is done and she wants her snack. The following week, she asks if she won. The researcher says it isn't a contest and explains the project again. Rachel says she still wants to participate. Rachel then does a drawing but does not like the way it is coming out. She says, "This is the boy, this is the girl, and that's the baby." Then she does a drawing she likes and says it is of a bird, trees (one is labeled "pineapple" and the other "cherry"), clouds, and sky. She says, "This branch sticking out is for the bird." She says there is grass and a hole in the tree "for an owl to live in." Rachel explains that "the bird shows hope, because birds can fly south when it's cold and they lay eggs. . . . Trees are hopeful too, because they give paper, fruit, and oxygen, things we need." She repeated, "Trees are home for birds."

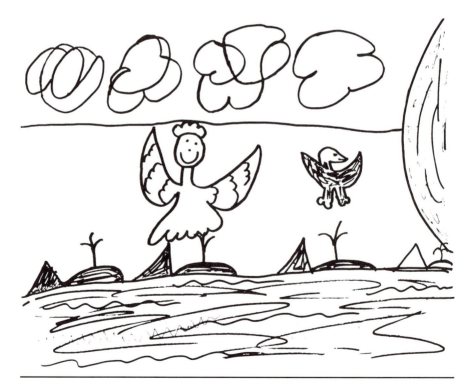

FIGURE 2.
Rachel, age 7

Essences: Participant's Language

1. The participant talked about hope as angels because they go to Heaven and to God, which she likes to think about. [She drew an angel and a bird flying over a sea with whales.]
2. The participant did another drawing about hope and said, "I did it. This is the boy, this is the girl, and that's the baby."
3. The participant said a bird was about hope because birds can fly south when it's cold and birds can lay eggs, and she said a fruit tree is about hope because it gives us many things we need, and it provides a place for birds to rest and to live. [She drew a bird in a cherry tree.]

Essences: Researcher's Language

1. Envisioning the strengthening presence of the divine arises with pleasure.
2. Inventing amid sustaining emerges with new possibilities.
3. Nurturing interconnections emerge with the comfort of reflecting on nature's providence.

Proposition. The lived experience of hope is envisioning the strengthening presence of the divine while inventing amid sustaining with new possibilities, as nurturing interconnections emerge with the comfort of reflecting on nature's providence.

Robert's Story

Robert, aged 8, an African-American boy, is living with his mother and two sisters in a room at a motor lodge. He is the brother of Rachel. He is also the youngest member of his family and the only male. He likes to draw and to do what his friend (Jamey, aged 10) is doing. Robert's first drawing includes two stick figures in front of several trees, a couple of large raindrops, and clouds. One of the figures is holding a black object. Robert describes his picture: "This is a boy. He has an umbrella. This is a girl. She is sneezing. The boy is saying 'hi,' and he is giving her some medicine to make her feel better." The researcher asks, "Is this about hope?" Robert says, "Yes. You see the trees makes this stuff, and she is allergic to the stuff from the trees, and when she came next to them, she sneezes. It is worse when it rains. He [the boy in his drawing] is not allergic to anything, you know, so he came to give her some medication, which helps her feel better." Robert says the boy is holding an umbrella. He points to the raindrops and says, "See the raindrops."

In Robert's second drawing about hope, he draws two dark-skinned male figures facing each other with their mouths open, as if talking. On the top of the paper Robert writes, "I Hope all have firends [friends] and peplo [people]." Under this he draws a small globe with tiny stick figures around it, similar to what his friend had done. Under this, he writes "all peplo [people]." Robert says, "Hope is people talking, like these two guys; they are good friends." Then he tells a story: "You see these two men? One is a old man and one is a young man. The old man is saying to the young man, 'What are you going to be when you grow up?' The old man is saying these hopeful things. I hope all have friends and people, all around the world."

Essences: Participant's Language

1. Hope is a boy helping a girl who is sneezing because she is allergic to trees. The participant says the boy is trying to help her feel better by giving her medicine for her sneezes. He has an umbrella because it is raining. [He drew a boy handing something to a girl. The boy was saying "hi."]
2. Hope is people talking to each other, like an older man saying hopeful things to a young man and asking him what he is going to do when he grows up.
3. Hope is people all over the world having good friends. [He drew the earth with tiny figures holding hands.]

Essences: Researcher's Language

1. Attention to comfort surfaces with nurturing engagements.
2. New possibilities emerge while participating in generational interchanges.
3. Visions of interconnections arise when contemplating global unity.

Proposition. The lived experience of hope is the attention to comfort that surfaces with nurturing engagements, as new possibilities emerge while participating in generational interchanges, while visions of interconnections arise in contemplating global unity.

Roy's Story

Roy is a 6-year-old African-American boy who is living with his mother and older sister in a room at a motor lodge. He visits the makeshift classroom at the motor lodge with his sister (age 8). Roy comes up to the researcher and sits next to him. Roy's first drawing is "a turtle and a box of ooze." He says the drawing is the Ninja Turtle Michelangelo, "who is very funny, and says, 'Carabonga.'" At that moment another boy comes in and says to Roy, "Your mother never shows up!" Roy does not respond. He draws a fish with a big smile and lots of raindrops and zigzag lines representing lightning. He says, "This is a river and a happy shark jumping up." The researcher asks him if this is about hope. He says, "Yeah." The researcher asks, "Can you talk more about your drawing or about hope?" Roy says, "Hope means like, I hope she'll get hurt and stuff like that. . . . Like when I hope that whenever we have no place to go, that we will go to my grandma's house. I like it there, because she takes me out to the movies. I like to think about that."

The following week, Roy draws a figure wearing a striped shirt and hat with his arms outstretched, saying, "I got a big dog." When asked about his drawing, Roy says, "This is about hope, because he wants the dog to grow up and be a mean dog. I want a mean dog, to protect me." Then he draws a smaller figure next to the first with the letter R on the figure's shirt. The second figure has outstretched arms and is kicking.

Essences: Participant's Language

1. As the participant was beginning to draw a picture about hope, another boy said to the participant that his mother never shows up. The participant drew a smiling shark jumping out of the water on a rainy day, and he said it was about hope, like when people say, "I hope she gets hurt and stuff like that."
2. Hope is thinking about when the participant has no place to go and he gets to go to his grandma's house, which he likes because she takes him to the movies.
3. Hope is when someone gets hurt, and when he gets a big mean dog to protect him.

Essences: Researcher's Language

1. Inventing surfaces with emancipating possibilities.
2. Envisioning the pleasure of nurturing engagements arises amid tribulation.
3. Fears arise with thoughts of heartening allies.

Proposition. The lived experience of hope is inventing that surfaces with emancipating possibilities while envisioning the pleasure of nurturing engagements amid tribulations, as fear arises with thoughts of heartening allies.

Jamey's Story

Jamey is a 10-year-old African-American boy living with his mother at a motor lodge. He is the boy whom Robert likes to copy and do things with. Jamey says that he was living at his grandmother's house before he came to the motor lodge and that he gets mail there and keeps some of his things there. Jamey's drawing of a figure begins with little triangles which turn out to be ears. He carefully draws a shirt that is zippered up to the neck of an older-looking male with short neat hair and detailed facial features. The following week he asks for the drawing back so he can color it in. He makes the skin brown and the shirt green. On the top of the drawing he writes, "I hope that All colors and Races Be together and don't fight and I Hope for world peace." He draws a small globe and on it, tiny stick figures holding hands. He says that he likes to think about world peace. When asked to talk about his drawing, he says it is himself; he reads the message of world peace from the top and says it is about hope. (See Figure 3.) Later Jamey draws a figure playing basketball. He brings it to the researcher and says it is himself and that he likes to play basketball. The researcher asks him if it is about hope, and Jamey says it is because he is making a shot, and then he adds, "I hope to be able to dunk it someday."

Essences: Participant's Language

1. The participant hopes that people of all colors and races will be together and that they will stop fighting. He says he hopes that there will be world peace. [The participant drew and later colored in a neatly dressed man and said it was a drawing of himself.]

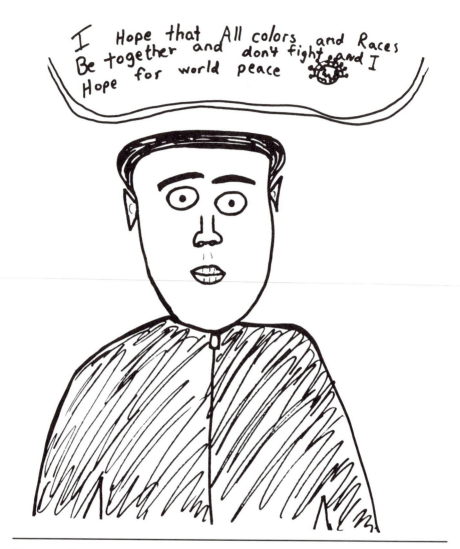

FIGURE 3.
Jamey, age 10

2. The participant likes to play basketball and wants to be able to dunk the ball someday. [He drew a figure dunking the ball.]

Essences: Researcher's Language

1. Anticipating genial interconnections arises with envisioning universal harmony.
2. Dreams surface with thoughts of prized activities.

Proposition. The lived experience of hope is anticipating genial interconnections while envisioning universal harmony, as dreams surface with thoughts of prized activities.

Anthony's Story

Anthony is a 6-year-old African-American boy who has been living with his older brother (aged 11) and mother in a shelter for about six months. He has a 2-year-old brother living elsewhere. The shelter is an old boarding house that has been converted into an emergency shelter in a nearly all-Black suburb of New York City. It is owned and managed by the same nonprofit organization that owns the transitional housing unit where LaTania and Michael live. Six-month stays are unusual for this shelter. Anthony is excited because he is going to visit his father for the next few days, something he has not done since he arrived at the shelter.

At first Anthony says he cannot draw, and therefore he does not want to participate. But with a little encouragement from his mother, he changes his mind completely. He starts several drawings but does not like how they are turning out, so he crumples them up and starts again. The first drawing that he likes and is willing to share with the researcher includes a woman and man, two trees, a house, a green front lawn, and a walkway leading to the house (see Figure 4). The figures are standing next to each other but not touching. They are both smiling and wear

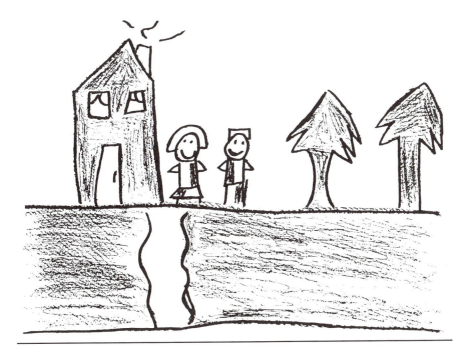

FIGURE 4.
Anthony, age 6

matching clothing. As soon as he finishes this drawing, Anthony takes it to show his mother and the shelter's evening coordinator. He is excited to tell them that it is a picture about hope. He soon returns to the researcher and says, "I hope my mom gets a place, like everybody else." He points to his drawing and says, "This is a house, with my dad." He says the trees are coconut trees and he smiles. He says his mother and father are both in his hope drawing and they are happy.

Anthony does several drawings with houses and trees. In one of them he makes the front of the house look like a face. He says this is his brother's house. He says his oldest brother lives in his own house. He again says, "I hope for a house with Dad. I hope my whole family has got a house. Just a regular ordinary house." The following week when the researcher visits the shelter, he is told that Anthony and his brother have gone to their father's and have not returned, and that his mother has joined them, even though it means they can no longer return to the shelter.

Essences: Participant's Language

1. Hope is for the participant's mother to find a place and for his whole family to live together in a house and be happy; he wants a regular ordinary house, like other people. [The participant did several drawings of houses, one with his mother and father together.]
2. Hope is how the participant likes thinking about and making things and how excited he is showing his drawings about hope to his mother.

Essences: Researcher's Language

1. Joyful longings arise with visions of harmonious living.
2. Resourceful constructing surfaces with the contentment of buoyant engagements in novel thinking.

Proposition. The lived experience of hope is a resourceful constructing surfacing with the contentment of buoyant engagements in creative thinking, while joyful longings arise with visions of harmonious living.

Matthew's Story

Matthew is a 5-year-old Latino boy who is the oldest of three children. He has a 4-year-old brother, Danny, also a participant, and a baby sister. The three of them and their mother have only recently moved into a second-floor apartment that is part of the transitional housing program. The apartment has new rugs and was recently painted, but there are few pieces of furniture or wall decorations. One of the items that Matthew's mother shows the researcher is the new answering machine, given to them by the social worker, to assure that they receive and return her phone calls. The apartment is in a mixed-race suburban neighborhood on the south shore of Long Island, New York.

Matthew comes to the researcher's car to greet him and check out his car. His mother is sitting on their neighbor's porch. Matthew helps himself to a box of crayons from the researcher's bag and says he wants to draw a dinosaur.

After the project is explained, he begins another drawing and says, "I hope my buddy is a cop, I hope my buddy." The researcher asks if he can talk more about that. Matthew says, "I hope my buddy becomes a cop; he wants to be a cop when he grows up." He draws shapes. He says his drawing is about hope and it has a boat, a house, and a dog. He says, "I hope for a doggie." Matthew says that his daddy told him that his doggie died. He adds that his friends said it was too bad. He repeats that his drawing is about hope and that it "has a big house and a little house, and a boat down here."

Matthew begins another drawing of objects and shapes and says, "Hope is my other buddy, my mother's buddy. . . . My other buddy doesn't live here. He lives over there [pointing out the window]. He can come over here. He's down by the ocean." The researcher asks Matthew whether there is anything else he wants to say about hope. Matthew says, "I hope I get a job, I hope I make a big job. I got my working job; my Daddy's got a job." He says, "Hope means when you get up and go to work. When I work I will get a car—a fat car—my Daddy has a fat car. I like cars. My father cleans over there. He's got a big car and a little car." Matthew holds up his drawing to show his mother and says, "This is a house and another house. No, this one is my apartment; it's down here. This is my boat and the water." Matthew says he needs his job. His mother says that he goes to a learning center and that he is going to start kindergarten in September (it is early August). When the researcher is getting in his car, Matthew comes over to his car and helps him open the door.

Essences: Participant's Language

1. The participant talks about hope as his buddies, referring to various others, and he hopes that his buddies will become what they want to be, like cops.
2. Hope is things the participant wants—a house, a boat, a doggie, and a car—and about getting up in the morning and going to work at a big job, like his daddy and so he could get a car like his dad's. [He drew colorful shapes that he said represented these objects.]

Essences: Researcher's Language

1. Nurturing interconnections surface with the excitement of shared dreams in desiring the mutual successes.
2. Envisioning desired possessions arises with the uplifting anticipation in illustrating an array of hues.

Proposition. The lived experience of hope is the excitement of shared dreams in nurturing interconnections while desiring mutual success, as envisioning desired possessions arises with the uplifting anticipation in illustrating an array of hues.

Danny's Story

Danny is the 4-year-old brother of Matthew (also a participant). He is not as articulate as his brother but just as active and free-spirited. He, his older brother, Matthew, their baby sister, and their mother have recently moved into an apartment that is owned by a nonprofit transitional housing program on Long Island, New York. Danny begins drawing as soon as he sits at the living room table, where the art supplies are. He draws rectangles, ovals, and triangles. After the researcher asks Danny whether he can draw or talk about hope, he says, "That's not a lot of colors." He draws a shape, and says, "This is a star." His brother comes over and says that it isn't a star. Danny says, "I said so; this is a star!" His brother moves back to the other side of the table.

Even though it is a hot and sunny day, Danny looks at his drawing and begins talking about Santa Claus. "This is a sky, where Santa comes from; I'm happy to think of Santa Claus coming down; I hope for Santa Claus. Christmas time of year is a pretty time." Danny then says, "Tap, tap, tap, crocodile" (reminding the researcher of the Peter Pan story). Danny makes a hand gesture of a crocodile biting the researcher's hand. The researcher asks if he has anything else to say about hope. Danny says, "Making colors," as he points to all of the crayons in front of him. Then he says, "Making everything." Matthew comes back over to his brother's side of the table and says, "He makes trouble." Danny says, "I hope that I eat lots of food. . . . I like soda. . . . Hope is when I sleep a lot. When I sleep, I dream."

Essences: Participant's Language

1. Hope is many colors, like the participant's drawing of a star that prompts him to think about how much he likes it when Santa Claus comes and how pretty things are at Christmas-time.
2. Hope is having lots of food to eat; the participant likes soda.
3. Hope is like the dreams he has when he sleeps a lot.

Essences: Researcher's Language

1. Fashioning an array of nature's uplifting hues surfaces with reminders of wonderful engagements.
2. Pleasing reflections arise with thoughts of abundant provisions.
3. Visions of anticipation emerge in moments of slumber.

Proposition. The lived experience of hope is the pleasing reflections that arise with thoughts of abundant provisions, while fashioning an array of nature's uplifting hues surfaces with reminders of wonderful engagements, as visions of anticipation emerge in moments of slumber.

Jose's Story

Jose is a 13-year-old Latino boy who is living with his mother and two sisters, aged 18 and 7. His older sister is about to start college and live there. The family has a second-floor apartment that is part of the transitional housing program in a small coastal city. Jose lived in a housing project in south Chicago until he was 9. His family relocated to the East Coast after his mother got in trouble with the law. Later, she had to return to Illinois to serve a very short sentence, and Jose's father came to live with them while his mother was in jail. This family had been in a shelter for nine months. About two months before Jose's participation in this study, he had been in the hospital. The social worker said that Jose had been talking about suicide at school. Jose has long black hair and skin that is darkened by a suntan. These features, and his size, make him look older than 13. His mother is entertaining two men in the living room, while Jose and the researcher sit at a small table in the next room.

It takes several minutes before Jose thinks of what he wants to draw. He draws a neat and clean older-looking man sitting at a school desk, thinking. On the desk in front of him is a piece of paper with the words, "What do you want to be when you grow up?" Over the figure's head is a thought bubble with the image of a basketball player making a dunk shot. (See Figure 5.) When asked about the drawing, Jose says, "He's a guy in school and his assignment is to write down, 'What do you want to be when you grow up?' This guy likes basketball, so he's thinking about himself playing basketball; he wants to be a basketball

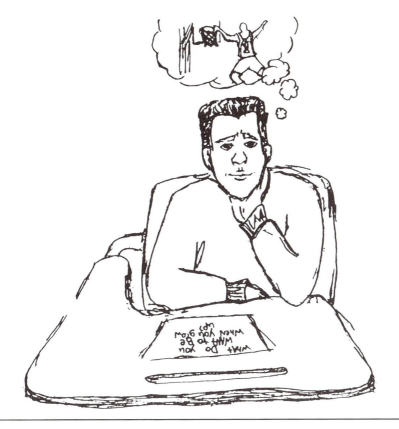

FIGURE 5.
Jose, age 13

player." When asked if he has anything else to say about the picture or about hope, Jose says, "He's just any guy; it makes him feel hopeful because he wants to be a basketball player. . . . I don't know where I got the idea from. I was trying to draw hope." Jose says he wants to be an actor. The researcher asks whether he wants to draw or say anything else about hope. He says, "No, that's about it. I had a little trouble thinking about this." He says he likes basketball and going to school.

Essences: Participant's Language

1. The participant says he has trouble thinking about what to draw about hope, but hope is thinking about places he likes to go, such as school and the basketball court.
2. The participant talks about hope as a guy at school who is asked to write about what he wants to do when he grows up. [He drew a man with a mustache sitting at a desk with a thought bubble of a man playing basketball, but the participant said he wanted to be an actor.]

Essences: Researcher's Language

1. Contentment arises in struggling with remote reflections of the joyful.
2. Inventive renderings of dreams surface amid diverse engagements.

Proposition. The lived experience of hope is the inventive renderings of dreams surfacing amid diverse engagements, while contentment arises in struggling with remote reflections of the joyful.

FINDINGS AND RELATED LITERATURE

The finding of the study for this group of children is the structure *the lived experience of hope is the envisioning of nurturing engagements while inventing possibilities.* The meaning of hope generated in this study is a synthesis of three core concepts, *envisioning, nurturing engagements,* and *inventing possibilities.* Each of these core concepts, written in the researcher's language, was derived from the participants' drawings and their descriptions of the drawings. The three core concepts are stated at incrementally higher levels of abstraction in the language of Parse's human becoming theory. This process is outlined in Table 1.

The first core concept, envisioning, suggests that hope for the participants involves visualizing their worlds as generally orderly and good, although not without challenges and struggles. Several participants depicted the peaceful coexistence of animals, plants, human beings, angels, and natural phenomena such as rainbows and oceans in their drawings and discussions about hope. The author was somewhat surprised by the participants' references to hope as peace and order between diverse groups of people, in nature and the universe.

The core concept of envisioning, depicted often as a multicolored rainbow, represents good fortune and an orderly, peaceful universe for most participants. The participants' cherished beliefs and desires for global peace define hope as

TABLE 1.
Progressive Abstraction of Core Concepts with Heuristic Interpretation

Core Concepts	Structural Transposition	Conceptual Integration
Envisioning	Inspiring conceptualization	Imaging
Nurturing engagements	Regardful involvements	Connecting-separating
Inventing possibilities	Ardent creating	Originating

Structure

The lived experience of hope is the envisioning of nurturing engagements while inventing possibilities.

Structural Transposition

Hope is inspiring conceptualizations with regardful involvements surfacing with ardent creating.

Conceptual Integration

Hope is imaging the connecting-separating of originating.

uplifting reflections of what could be, while contending with what is. Explicit reference to the divine by some participants reveals the presence of the super-natural in objects and natural phenomena. The participants conceptualize hope by seeing human (and some supernatural) beings in the natural order of things. A somewhat similar view of the universe was common in the eighteenth century, an example of which is Pope's (1733) poem:

> Hope springs eternal in the human breast. . . .
> See, thro' this air, this ocean, and this earth,
> All matter quick, and bursting into birth. . . .
> Vast chains of Being! which from God began,
> Natures ethereal, human, angel, man.
> Beast, bird, fish, insect, what no eye can see,
> No glass can reach; from Infinite to thee,
> from thee to Nothing. (pp. 100–105)

Downey (1998) quoted Emily Dickinson—"hope is the thing with feathers, that perches in the soul"—to support his theological reflection on hope as related to a belief in God's promise to be present in creation (p. 107).

Envisioning, as a core concept of hope, also was evident when participants drew and talked about themselves or close others as participating successfully in prized activities, such as basketball, or as achieving valued goals, like becoming a police officer. The ability to make linkages to desired ends and have strategies to reach these ends is similar to the definition of hope used by Hinton-Nelson, Roberts, and Snyder (1996) in their study about adolescents exposed to violence. Hinton-Nelson, et al. (1996), using a scale to measure hope (defined as believing in one's capabilities to produce pathways toward one's goals), found in their study that the eighty-nine seventh- and eighth-graders who had been exposed to violence were hopeful. The study reported here avoided a predetermined definition of hope, relying instead on the participants to define hope for themselves. There were references to violence, which reveal the complexity and paradoxical nature of hope for the participants. These findings did not arise as such in other studies on hope with children.

The comments and drawings about fighting and violence in some of the participants' drawings about hope seem at first to be contradictory to descriptions of hope related to peace and an orderly existence, but this shows the diverse, paradoxical meaning of hope. For some participants, hope is the ability to see beyond the violence to harmony. Fighting and violence are part of the everyday lives of the participants—in what they see on TV and around them, as they described in their drawings and discussions. The day after Anthony participated in this study, he and his brother went to stay with his father, and two days later his mother returned to his father's house also, even though, according to the shelter staff, there had been considerable violence in their parents' relationship in the past. Roy described hope as a protective ally, "a big mean dog." A few participants talked about hope as fighting. Michael said hope was about how the Black man on TV who was beat by the police was able to say "I love you" to those who beat him. His drawing and comments depict good and bad as polar opposites, which gives rise to conflict, which is also a process of separating and reuniting. Michael related hope as firm confidence that the good will win. Such confidence is not explained here by a sense of the invulnerability that some authors attribute to adolescents (Hinton-Nelson et al., 1996). The finding in the present study is interpreted as related to cherished beliefs and values. Violence and fighting within families also shows paradoxical aspects of the second core concept, nurturing engagements.

The mention of violence and fighting in the art and comments about hope suggests that conflict is a part of the participants' close and important relationships. *Nurturing engagements* represents for the participants in this study not only pleasant memories of helpful and loving connections, but also passionate struggles with and for close others. Freud (1952) considered such struggles and conflicts as central to human development: "Hatred of his father arises in a boy from rivalry for his mother" (p. 129). Girard (1977) rejected Freud's interpretation of such dynamics as essentially sexual drives and said that conflict and violence arise in triangles of desire that originate from the human inclination to imitate important others. In Girard's (1966) terms, mimesis is a source of conflict and violence in that disciples seek to be so like their models that they become intense rivals for the same object. In the perspective assumed in this study, Girard's (1966, 1977) theory, while more complex and less deterministic than psychoanalytic theory, continues to be somewhat reductionistic. Children in this study thought about hope as being like someone special, but at the same time they want to be different. Jose drew a boy in class picturing himself as a basketball player, but then said that boy wasn't him because he really wants to be an actor (see Figure 5).

According to the nursing perspective of this study, hope reflects evolving possibilities that arise from choices made in situations that involve being like and different from prized others. In other words, hope is choosing freely and cocreating patterns of relating that can be loving but that also can unfold in shifting patterns of violence. Girard (1977) also described the model of mimetic desire as an obstacle. In the terms of the human becoming theory, hope includes rhythmical patterns of relating that are diverse and paradoxical. Nurturing engagements is seen as cocreating patterns of relating, which always includes the limiting-enabling of connecting-separating with close others. Hope for the participants of this study represents nurturing engagements as the joyful helping and comforting of others, and as "fighting bad guys" and wanting to "do work so I can get a car like my dad's."

The third core concept is *inventing possibilities*, which unfolds in the articulation and depiction of artistic expressions of what hope is for each participant. This concept assumes that children, no less than adults, participate in the inventing of what will be by making it manifest in artistic expressions and words, a process of moving beyond with creative imagination. In other words, inventing possibilities is a process of making something present that wasn't there before. This core concept also relates to the wondrous hues and patterns that arise when contemplating hope. LaTania depicted hope as something with "lots of colors." She talked about rainbows with lots of colors that made her think of colorful sunsets, and she said, "I love sunsets." She also liked to draw people dressed in colorful clothing. Matthew said his drawing of colorful shapes was about hope, because they represented things he likes. His brother Danny drew a shape that he said was a star, and then he said Christmas was hopeful because things were so pretty.

The core concept of inventing possibilities arises from participants who took particular care in the drawings of human figures, which they said were themselves, or others, but which were of older persons, who were neat, well-dressed, cool, or athletic. The inventive aspect of these drawings and the participants' comments show the participants living the cocreational process. A few weeks prior to his participation in this study, Jose was hospitalized because he was overheard talking about suicide. Although he said he had trouble thinking about what to draw about hope, after a few minutes of silence with this researcher, he was able to create an artistic rendering of hope. Parse's (1981, 1992) human becoming theory guides the nurse, as it guided this researcher, to be present to persons in ways in which the hope hidden in hopelessness can be illuminated. Artistic rendering involves the creative use of symbols, hues, and patterns that move the artist beyond words and verbal dialogues. The participants' drawings also show that banal aspects of everyday life are contained in their meaning of hope.

Implications for further research and practice related to these findings will be discussed in the final chapter of this book with the findings from the other studies on hope reported here.

REFERENCES

Downey, M. (1998). *Hope begins where hope begins.* Maryknoll, NY: Orbis.

Freud, S. (1952). *Totem and taboo: Some points of agreement between mental lives of savages and neurotics* (J. Strachey, Trans.). New York: Norton.

Girard, R. (1966). *Deceit, desire and the novel: Self and others in literary structure* (Y. Freccero, Trans.). Baltimore: Johns Hopkins University Press. (Original work published 1961)

Girard, R. (1977). *Violence and the sacred* (P. Gregory, Trans.). Baltimore: Johns Hopkins University Press. (Original work published 1972)

Hinton-Nelson, M. D., Roberts, M. C., & Snyder, C. R. (1996). Early adolescents exposed to violence: Hope and vulnerability to victimization. *American Journal of Orthopsychiatry, 66,* 346–353.

Parse, R. R. (1981). *Man-living-health: A theory of nursing.* New York: Wiley.

Parse, R. R. (1992). Human becoming: Parse's theory of nursing. *Nursing Science Quarterly, 5,* 35–42.

Parse, R. R. (Ed.). (1995). *Illuminations: The human becoming theory in practice and research.* New York: NLN Press.

Parse, R. R. (1998). *The human becoming school of thought.* Thousand Oaks, CA: Sage

Pope, A. (1951). *Alexander Pope: Selected works* (L. Kronenberger, Ed.). New York: The Modern Library. (Original work published 1733)

Chapter 12

The Lived Experience of Hope for Women Residing in a Shelter

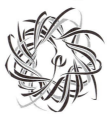

WILLIAM K. CODY
JAMES E. FILLER

The purpose of this study, guided by Parse's (1981, 1998) theory and using her research method (Parse, 1987, 1995, 1998), was to uncover the structure of the lived experience of hope for women residing in a shelter. Hope, cherishing a desire with anticipation of fulfillment (*Merriam Webster's Collegiate Dictionary*, 1995, is widely considered essential to human life, "a healing force," "a powerful coping mechanism," and "a significant personal resource" (Herth, 1996, p. 744). The findings of this study, however, reveal that the structure of the lived experience of hope is *attainment in persisting amid the arduous, while trusting in potentiality.*

LITERATURE RELATED TO HOMELESSNESS

According to the McKinney Act (1994), a person is considered homeless who "lacks a fixed, regular, and adequate nighttime residence and . . . has a primary night time residency that is: (a) a supervised publicly or privately operated shelter designed to provide temporary living accommodations . . . (b) an institution that provides a temporary residence for individuals intended to be institutionalized, or (c) a public or private place not designed for, or ordinarily used as, a regular sleeping accommodation for human beings." Link, Susser, Stueve, Phelan, Moore, and Struening (1994) reported that 4.6 percent of a random sample of the U.S. population ($N = 1507$) was homeless at some time between 1985 and 1990, and that 7.4 percent of their respondents reported being literally homeless at some point in their lives.

Homelessness is overwhelmingly associated with severe poverty. The number of poor people in the United States increased 41 percent between 1979 and 1990; families and children under 18 accounted for more than half of that increase (U.S. House of Representatives, 1992). Stagnating wages and changes in welfare programs are closely related to worsening poverty among families. In the median state, a woman making minimum wage would have to work eighty-three hours a week to afford a two-bedroom apartment at 30 percent of her income, which is the federal definition of affordable housing (Kaufman, 1997). Until its repeal in 1996, the largest cash assistance program for poor families was the Aid to Families with Dependent Children (AFDC) program. The Personal Responsibility and Work Opportunity Reconciliation Act of 1996 repealed the AFDC program and replaced it with a block grant program called Temporary Assistance to Needy Families (TANF). In most states, a person receiving TANF benefits would have an income of less than 75 percent of poverty level. In 49 states and 357 metropolitan areas, the maximum TANF grant level does not even cover the fair-market rent for a two-bedroom apartment (Kaufman, 1997).

Many of the women whose situation fits the definition of homelessness have had experiences with domestic violence, single parenthood, and/or substance abuse. It has been estimated that up to 50 percent of homeless women and children are fleeing abuse. Waxman and Hinderliter (1996) reported that 46 percent of cities surveyed by the U.S. Conference of Mayors identified domestic violence as a primary cause of homelessness. Of the millions of Americans whose situation may be defined as homeless, 40 percent are believed to be families with children (Shinn & Weitzman, 1996), and the vast majority of these are single women with children (Berne, Dato, Mason & Rafferty, 1990). Some sources have projected that in the near future a majority of the United States' overall homeless population will be single mothers with children (Berne et al., 1990).

Homelessness severely impacts the well-being of all family members. Compared with housed poor children, homeless children are reported to experience more developmental delays, anxiety, depression, behavioral problems, and lower educational achievement (Shinn & Weitzman, 1996). In addition, homeless children face barriers to attending school, such as transportation problems, residency requirements, inability to obtain previous school records, and lack of clothing and school supplies. A recent study of homeless and low-income families found that they experienced higher rates of depressive disorders than the overall female population, and that one-third of homeless mothers (and one-fourth of housed, low-income mothers) had made at least one suicide attempt (Bassuk, Weinreb, Buckner, Browne, Salomon & Bassuk, 1996). In both groups, over one-third of the sample had a chronic health condition.

Rates of alcohol and drug abuse are disproportionately high among the homeless population, but the increase in homelessness in the 1980s cannot be explained by substance abuse. During the 1980s, competition for low-income housing grew so intense that those with disabilities, such as chemical addiction and mental illness, were more likely to lose out and find themselves on the streets. Substance abuse increases the risk of displacement and diminishes one's chances of obtaining housing once on the streets. It is common for graduates of treatment programs to be discharged to the streets or shelters. One study of service providers found that 80 percent of the treatment programs surveyed could not meet demand and were forced to turn homeless clients away (Williams, 1992). The same study found that uninsured homeless persons seeking residential treatment for active substance abuse faced waits of fifteen to thirty days in California, thirty days in Massachusetts, fourteen days in North Carolina, and up to sixty days in New Jersey, Montana, and Washington.

There is a paucity of research describing hope qualitatively from the participants' perspectives (Kylmä & Vehviläinen-Julkunen, 1997). Further, there is a dearth of substantive literature interrelating women's experiences, homelessness, and hope. Kylmä and Vehviläinen-Julkunen (1997) report, in their meta-analysis of the nursing research on hope, that the majority of the research is quantitative and based on data gathered through questionnaires. From the existing literature, they concluded that hope may be regarded as an emotion, an experience, or a need. "There is a clear emphasis on the necessity and the dynamism of hope. As far as its dynamics are concerned, the most important dimension is the dialectic between hope and despair" (p. 364). They further concluded that "there is obvious need to carry out more qualitative longitudinal research" (p. 364). In a study of similarly broad scope, Morse and Doberneck (1995) found that the experience of hope included seven conceptual components.

These were "realistic initial assessment of threat or predicament," "the envisioning of alternatives and setting of goals," "bracing for negative outcomes," "a realistic assessment of personal resources and external conditions/resources," "the solicitation of mutually supportive relationships," "the continuous evaluation for signs that reinforce the selected goals," and "a determination to endure" (p. 281).

In writing of the experience of hope from the perspective of homeless families, Herth (1996) stated that the relative presence or absence of hope influenced homeless persons' perceptions of their situations. In concurrence with Wake and Miller (1992), Herth (1996) asserted that "counteracting hopelessness is critical in alleviating painful despair, mobilizing psychic energy needed for healing, creating a positive expectation for enjoying a positive future and preventing self-invitation to physical decline and death" (p. 744). In her study of hope among fifty-two homeless families, Herth identified six "hope-engendering strategies." These included "(a) interconnectedness with others," referring to human services staff as well as family and friends, "(b) personal attributes," predominantly patience and courage, and being "tough," "(c) cognitive strategies," such as envisioning hopeful images, "(d) attainable stepwise goals," emphasizing small successes, "(e) energizing moments," such as an inspiring sunset, and "(f) affirmation of worth," described as "having one's individuality accepted, honoured, valued, and acknowledged" (pp. 747–748).

PARTICIPANTS

This study was approved as a research project with human subjects by a university institutional review board in the usual manner. Women residing in a shelter in an urban area in North Carolina were invited through an intermediary on the staff of the shelter, or the staff of a nursing center within the shelter, to participate in the study. Volunteer participants were ensured confidentiality, given the names and numbers of the investigators, encouraged to call the investigators for any questions or problems, and asked to sign an informed consent. Ten women agreed to participate. Eight were African American; two were Caucasian American. Their ages ranged from mid-20s to early 50s. Although there was no intention in this study to focus on substance abuse, about half of the women were self-described as "in recovery" and were participating in a substance-abuse recovery program while residing in the shelter.

DIALOGICAL ENGAGEMENT

All dialogues were conducted in a private room in the shelter. Dialogues were audiorecorded. The participants were initially asked, "Please tell me about your lived experience of hope." Additional prompts by the investigator were limited to comments such as, "Go on," "Tell me more about that," and "Please tell me how what you've just said relates to your experience of hope." Participants were encouraged to speak about their experience of hope until they believed they had given a complete description and had nothing further to say.

EXTRACTION-SYNTHESIS

Betty's Story

Betty describes her struggles with alcohol and drug addiction. She is enrolled in the on-site substance abuse recovery program at the emergency shelter. She speaks tearfully about losses she suffered while using drugs, stating, "I had hope before my getting into alcohol and drugs, but then, after experiencing drugs and alcohol in my life, I lost hope, the hope of believing in who I am, the hope of spirituality, the hope of life itself." But she also states repeatedly that "hope is a beautiful thing," and describes the new hope for the future she is experiencing in the substance abuse recovery program and the hope of regaining a relationship with her family. She says that "hope is success; it's the hope of progress; it's the hope that things will get better. . . . Hope is wide-ranged, different things." She says, "My recovery is very important to me, and it does give me hope, and that's all I want to say."

Essences: Participant's Language

1. When the participant's life was all about drugs and alcohol she completely lost hope. But in recovery she believes that life is beautiful, and hope is believing in herself, her spirituality, and tomorrow.
2. The participant believes that taking suggestions and progressing toward something better will lead to regaining a relationship with family and having what she knows she can have.

Essences: Researcher's Language

1. Appreciation of persisting beyond desolation emerges with graceful trust in potentiality.
2. Venturing surfaces with dreams of communion with attainment.

Proposition. The lived experience of hope is persisting in venturing beyond desolation, as dreams of communion with attainment emerge with graceful trust in potentiality.

Joan's Story

Joan describes living with addiction and links her hopes to staying "clean and sober." She speaks of her memories of molestation at age 13, when she started drinking "to change my feelings about me," and she continues to hope for "feeling good about myself." She says that hope is "having my family close to me again . . . because I made everybody mad at me." She says she looks forward to "getting my kids back," having a big house, and "living with God on my side and hopefully being successful eventually."

Essences: Participant's Language

1. For the participant, hope means staying sober, getting an education and a job, being successful, getting her children back, having the family close again, and having those things that she and her children never had.

2. Living with God in her life and believing in prayer, the participant knows that God will help her.
3. Hope is feeling good about herself, getting to know herself better and not always having to hide who she is.

Essences: Researcher's Language

1. Persistent picturing amid the arduous arises with dreams of communion with attainment.
2. Trust in divine succor surfaces in abiding with the sacred.
3. Discovery with affirmation emerges with potentiality.

Proposition. The lived experience of hope is persistently picturing possibilities amid the arduous as trusting in divine succor arises with dreams of communion with attainment, while discovery with affirmation surfaces with potentiality.

Mary's Story

Mary speaks with great sadness about her husband's death, which robbed her of everything, even the desire to live. She describes hope as "a path, a destination, but you never get there; it is a happy light, a wish." She says, "I don't think you ever really get to the end of the road of hope; it's just something you always do throughout your life. . . . And the further you go, the more hopeful you get, but there's always something there gonna knock you down." She has attempted to kill herself three times, but she speaks about moving on with hope and recapturing life. She says, "I don't want to die any more. To me, now, that's hope right there, 'cause I don't want to kill myself anymore. I want to get on with my life." She describes a variety of specific hopes: "I hope to get another Corvette, a place to live . . . a hundred dollars. . . . But . . . my biggest hope is to restore my relationship with my husband's family." She says, "You can't have hope without faith," and, further, "My faith is in God. . . . He guides and directs me on this road where the little pitfalls are, and He's also the one who picks me up, you know, and I can continue on my road to hope."

Essences: Participant's Language

1. Hope is something the participant can see, a happy light—a wish, something that can be made to happen, a goal. She can point to it, but it remains just beyond reach.
2. Movement in a specific direction along a path with ruts and holes takes work; it doesn't just come. Sometimes you trip and fall, but each time you get up and keep moving toward that destination.
3. Holding in your hand what is longed for—a Corvette, a place to live, money, family relationships—would be a way of getting life back and being happy again.
4. God guides you along the road and picks you up when you fall. Like faith, hope lives inside your spirit; it nurtures your soul and helps you to grow.

Essences: Researcher's Language

1. A radiant anticipation of the feasible arises with inaccessibility.
2. Persisting amid the arduous arises with the inevitable.
3. Contemplating the cherished emerges with dreams of contentment in attaining communion.
4. Trust in divine succor in abiding with the sacred surfaces with potentiality.

Proposition. The lived experience of hope is anticipating the cherished while persisting amid the arduous, as trust in divine succor surfaces with dreams of attaining contentment.

Alice's Story

Alice speaks about her worries that recurrent aches and pains are forewarnings of some kind of disease. She also speaks about being very worried about cancer; she is waiting for the results of recent diagnostic tests. She describes the meaning of hope: "Hope for me is . . . having faith in myself and believing in and achieving things that I want and I need. . . . I want to stay sober and stay clean and all, hoping that my future to be with my children, be stable in a home." With regard to her worries about her medical problems, she says, "Hope is like a faith—something that makes me feel better, by knowing I have God on my side to help me overcome this illness."

Essences: Participant's Language

1. Knowing that God is on her side and that He will help makes the participant feel better. Hope is about having faith in self and having faith in God even though she is worried about cancer.
2. Hope is wanting and then accomplishing things—like getting married, paying bills, having food on the table, clean clothes, and baths for the children—living normally and having a stable home.

Essences: Researcher's Language

1. Comfort amid adversity emerges with abiding trust in divine succor.
2. Anticipating attainment of the longed-for surfaces with the everyday.

Proposition. The lived experience of hope is anticipating attainment of the longed-for with the everyday, as comfort amid adversity emerges with an abiding trust in divine succor.

Helen's Story

Helen tearfully remembers her losses—home, family, clothes, and jobs. She speaks of divorce, rape, and the toll alcohol has taken on her life. She says, "I was beat down, and lost a lot of things," and she isn't sure she can get them back. She describes hope as "seeing other people's accomplishments," and as "believing in God and trusting in God 'cause He will help you."

Essences: Participant's Language

1. Seeing others' accomplishments—homes, cars, good jobs, college, family—and knowing it can be done brings hope to the participant.
2. Believing that God will help her through the hard times gives the participant hope; you just have to surrender and admit that it can't be done alone.

Essences: Researcher's Language

1. Witnessing attainment emerges with dreams of potentialities.
2. Yielding with the limitations of solitude while trusting divine succor surfaces with persisting amid misfortune.

Proposition. The lived experience of hope is witnessing attainment with dreams of potentialities, as yielding with the limitations of solitude in trusting divine succor surfaces with persisting amid misfortune.

Audrey's Story

Audrey says that she came to the state with her husband in search of work. Neither has been successful in finding a job. She is awaiting news from a recent job interview. She says that hope is "a burning desire . . . a possibility that it just might will happen [*sic*]. It's something that deep down inside . . . you want so bad . . . but you aren't certain that this thing will come in place; you're just hoping and praying that it will." She says of the things that she is hoping for now—an apartment to share with her husband, an education, and a job—"I will just pray for it, and leave it in God's hands and hope that it will happen."

Essences: Participant's Language

1. Hope is a burning desire—something definitely wanted within one's lifetime; it is believing in the slightest chance that something will come to pass.
2. Getting a new apartment and an education, having a strong marriage, leaving the homeless shelter, leading a productive life, and establishing herself would make her feel very happy within.
3. Hope only works with the help of God; you've got to have some sort of power in front of you, and there's no greater power than the Lord.

Essences: Researcher's Language

1. Longing for a cherished potential emerges amid the improbable.
2. Dreams of attainment surface with anticipation of contentment.
3. Trust in divine succor arises in abiding with the potency of the sacred.

Proposition. The lived experience of hope is longing for a cherished potential amid the improbable, as dreams of attainment surface with anticipation of contentment, while trust in divine succor arises in abiding with the potency of the sacred.

Emily's Story

Emily states that she was fleeing an abusive relationship when she came to the shelter. Penniless, she describes how she fights to maintain her dignity. Faced with the prospect of a lengthy child custody battle, she says she is trying to "forget about the negative and look at the positive . . . that you have a roof over your head, and can get something accomplished." She goes on to say, "The hope comes in knowing what you have in mind and you can do it, that is your hope. . . . A person can do for themselves if they try. . . . So you really have to fight for your rights." She says that hope is believing that "God does come through for you, you just have to have patience . . . and have faith that if He closes one door He will open another."

Essences: Participant's Language

1. Hope is looking at the positive—trying to forget the bad, to let go of the past, not to give up, and to live for today and for the future.
2. Hope comes in knowing what you have in mind and that you can do it, but you have to work hard and fight for it.
3. Hope means having faith in God, knowing that He looks after us and will provide. Even though it's a hard struggle, you have to be thankful for each day that you're alive.

Essences: Researcher's Language

1. Anticipation of cherished potentialities in the now arises amid releasing prior misfortunes.
2. Longing for attainment surfaces in persisting with the arduous.
3. Trust in divine succor emerges with gratitude for the everyday.

Proposition. The lived experience of hope is anticipation of cherished potentialities in the now arising amid releasing prior misfortunes, as longing for attainment surfaces in persisting with the arduous, while trust in divine succor emerges with gratitude for the everyday.

Sally's Story

Sally says she traveled south in search of warmer weather. She speaks of run-down, overcrowded conditions in shelters in the North, and marvels at the cleanliness and comfort of the shelter. At the end of a long day wandering the rain-soaked streets, she speaks about the meaning of hope: "Hope for me is looking into the future. Future goals would be hope . . . where I'll be living, and after that, moving on from there to a new relationship." She continues, "I think if you're not optimistic when you're here . . . you're going to end up being stuck here for a long time."

Essences: Participant's Language

1. Hope is looking into the future with goals. You have to have that optimism or you'll get stuck.

2. Hope is moving on; moving away from the adverse—finding a new place to live, a new relationship, work—not just sitting back and letting people do things for her.

Essences: Researcher's Language

1. Anticipating the not-yet arises with trust in the potentiality of the cherished.
2. Persistently pursuing attainment amid the adverse emerges with independence.

Proposition. The lived experience of hope is anticipating the not-yet amid the adverse with trust in cherished potentiality while persistently pursuing attainment emerges with independence.

Edith's Story

Edith tells of "losing control" of her life to crack cocaine. She says when she is in control, she doesn't "have a clue as to what I need to do, you know, what's gonna be good for me." She reflects on her past behaviors, saying, "I didn't want to hear nothing nobody had to tell me." She says that hope is having faith in another person, "that they will give me advice or suggestions . . . as to what I need to do. . . . Hope is just believing in or having faith in something, that it will be okay." She states, "I had a mask on where I really didn't want people to see the real me. Now I'm able to let people see me as who I am." She also says that "if I turn my will over to God, He always sees me through. . . . As long as there is life, there is hope."

Essences: Participant's Language

1. For the participant, hope is life—as long as there is life, there is hope. If you can see, talk, walk, and sleep, there is hope. If you are open-minded, willing, and as honest as you can be, there is hope—even though she sometimes loses control and doesn't know what to do.
2. Hope is accepting advice and suggestions from others—believing they can help, letting them take control—and having faith that a higher power will see you through.

Essences: Researcher's Language

1. Persistently pursuing potentialities amid the adverse emerges with sincere contentment in attainment.
2. Abiding with sacred trust arises with affiliations.

Proposition. The lived experience of hope is pursuing potentiality amid the adverse with sincere persistence, as abiding with sacred trust arises in attaining contentment with affiliations.

Molly's Story

Molly recalls the agony of childhood and spousal abuse. She tells of being tied to a chair, beaten, and threatened with a loaded gun. Molly says, "Hope means never giving up. . . . It is a willpower, an inner strength that gets you through things that not everyone can get through." She says, "Hope is believing in yourself . . . [believing that] I could do anything I put my mind to . . . that I could overcome the obstacles." She goes on to say, "Hope is something that has to be nurtured, and built, and cared for. Everybody has it. Some people just don't know how to use it. You have to learn how to let it grow in you. And it gets stronger and stronger." She continues, "As long as you keep going, your hope can spread to other people, and there's plenty to go around. And I like to try to teach other people about the hope and faith, . . . [which] is all tied into love and charity, like a big circle, all interconnected."

Essences: Participant's Language

1. Hope is not giving in to self-pity but having faith in God; it is an inner strength that gets you through, but it has to be nurtured. It grows and grows until you believe you could fight this world one-on-one and come out a winner.
2. Hope is getting through abusive situations, not being afraid to reach out and touch others, and finding somebody to love her. Faith, hope, charity, and love form one big interconnected circle; when you have one, you can have the other.
3. Hope is building for the future, not looking back, but moving ahead, knowing it is going to get better. Hope is our dreams, our goals.

Essences: Researcher's Language

1. Trust in divine succor arises with the potency of yielding with attainment.
2. Courageously persisting amid the arduous emerges with fulfilling communion.
3. Anticipating contentment in the not-yet surfaces with the cherished.

Proposition. The lived experience of hope is anticipating cherished contentment in the not-yet while courageously persisting amid the arduous emerges with fulfilling communion, as trust in divine succor arises with the potency of yielding with attainment.

FINDINGS AND RELATED LITERATURE

The structure of the lived experience of hope generated through this study interrelated three core concepts: *picturing attainment, persisting amid the arduous,* and *trusting in potentiality.* The core concepts, structure, and heuristic interpretation in progressive levels of abstraction appear in Table 1.

Picturing attainment relates to envisioning success, dreaming of accomplishing one's goals, having that which is lacking—such as money, a job, a place to live, a car, and getting one's children back—and being happy. Picturing attainment is described by all ten participants as a constituent of hope. It is structurally transposed to the discourse of the theory as *envisioning triumphs.* This relates to the women's involvements in weaving the yearned-for not-yet while living in relative deprivation. Envisioning triumphs is integrated conceptually as

TABLE 1.
Core Concepts, Structure, and Heuristic Interpretation

Core Concepts	Structural Transposition	Conceptual Integration
Picturing attainment	Envisioning triumphs	Imaging transforming
Persisting amid the arduous	Pushing-resisting with the ups and downs	Powering enabling-limiting
Trusting in potentiality	Confirming possibilities	Valuing

Structure

The lived experience of hope is picturing attainment in persisting amid the arduous, while trusting in potentiality.

Structural Transposition

The lived experience of hope is envisioning triumphs while pushing-resisting with the ups and downs of confirming possibilities.

Conceptual Integration

The lived experience of hope is imaging transforming in powering enabling-limiting of valuing.

imaging transforming, linking the core concept directly with major concepts from Parse's theory. Imaging transforming is dreaming of a changed reality. All of the women in this study dreamed of a reality that was not yet present, a reality they longed for intently and for which they knew they would have to work. This connects the first core concept with the second, persisting amid the arduous.

Persisting amid the arduous relates to perseverance through difficult times, such as staying sober, getting an education, moving in a specific direction even though you trip and fall, paying the bills, surviving abusive situations, and generally making it through hard times. Persisting amid the arduous is described by all ten participants as a constituent of hope. It is structurally transposed to the discourse of the theory as *pushing-resisting with the ups and downs*. This relates to the women's resolute determination to overcome the numerous obstacles to progress in their paths, as, for example, many women spoke about getting knocked down and picking themselves up again. Common to all the participants was a volitional imperative to bend to adverse circumstances sufficiently to carry onward toward a brighter day. Pushing-resisting with the ups and downs was integrated conceptually as *powering enabling-limiting*. Powering enabling-limiting is affirming self as who one is in light of the possibility of non-being, while engaging with the opportunities and restrictions inherent in the challenges of everyday living. All of the women in the study expressed this strong sense of self in the face of overwhelming odds.

Trusting in potentiality relates to believing in tomorrow, having faith in God, nurturing the soul for personal growth, "knowing it can be done," believing even in the slightest chance that something will come to pass, and living for the future. Trusting in potentiality is described by all ten participants as a constituent of hope. It is structurally transposed to the discourse of the theory as *confirming possibilities*. This relates to the women's cherished beliefs in the possibility of a better tomorrow, specifically the *believing* itself, manifest with references variously to God, the self, family, and support networks. All of the women spoke in some way of the necessity of believing their dreams could come true. Confirming possibilities is conceptually integrated as *valuing*. Valuing is confirming–not-confirming cherished beliefs. In this case, the confirming was in the fore, as women spoke of hope in terms of a refusal to despair. Hope meant confirming precious beliefs and potential relationships and then believing in the possibility that these could be realized in one's life.

There are commonalities and differences among the findings of this research and the extant nursing literature on hope. The finding that *picturing attainment* is a core concept in the lived experience of hope for the women in this study relates to the identification by Morse and Doberneck (1995) of "envisioning alternatives and setting of goals" as a conceptual component of hope across four population groups (p. 291). Herth (1996) wrote of "cognitive strategies," such as envisioning hopeful images, and "attainable stepwise goals" (p. 747). The description of picturing attainment as a core concept in the lived experience of hope for ten sheltered women in this study is generally consistent with these particular components of earlier descriptions.

The finding that persisting amid the arduous is a core concept in the lived experience of hope appears to be similar to "a determination to endure," described by Morse and Doberneck (1995) as a component of hope in their conceptual analysis. Herth (1996) identified "patience and courage" and being "tough" in the category of "personal attributes," which she identified as one "hope-engendering strategy" (p. 747). Perhaps more pertinent to the concept that surfaced in this study, persisting amid the arduous, integrated with Parse's theory as powering enabling-limiting, was the finding of Kylmä and Vehviläinen-Julkunen (1997), in their meta-analysis, that "the most important dimension is the dialectic between hope and despair" (p. 364). In the present study, hope was described as energizing a refusal to despair, as the women persistently bounced back from even the most invidious trials.

The finding that trusting in potentiality was a core concept in the lived experience of hope appears distantly related to two conceptual components identified by Morse and Doberneck (1995), although not directly related to either one alone. These components were "envisioning of alternatives and setting of goals" and "a determination to endure" (p. 281). Between these two components, Morse and Doberneck's participants related experiences of anticipating possible outcomes, planning and working toward goals, and reinforcing beliefs on the basis of small gains. These experiences in general are not unlike those described by the women in this study in relation to hope. However, the women in the present study depicted trusting in potentiality with far richer descriptions of their faith in God, their belief in themselves, and their beliefs that their families, friends, and support networks would see them through. The belief itself, the volitional imperative, was stressed repeatedly throughout the study. One participant said:

> My hope will keep me focused, and I will overcome the obstacles, and I will reach that light at the end of that tunnel. It may take me forty years to do so, but the hope is reaching that light, because there is that light. It may be very dim right now, but it's there, and it is reachable. Hope gives you that chance to reach any goal you set in your life. Hope means that you are capable of doing anything you set your mind to. You could be anybody or anything you want to be. But you've got to have hope.

Implications for further research and practice are discussed along with the findings in other studies on hope in the final chapter of this book.

References

Bassuk, E., Weinreb, L. F., Buckner, J. C., Browne, A., Salomon, A., Bassuk, S. S. (1996). The characteristics and needs of homeless and low-income housed mothers. *Journal of the American Medical Association, 276,* 640–646.

Berne, A. S., Dato, C., Mason, D. J., & Rafferty, M. (1990). A nursing model for addressing the health needs of homeless families. *Image: Journal of Nursing Scholarship, 22,* 8–13.

Herth, K. (1996). Hope from the perspective of homeless families. *Journal of Advanced Nursing, 24,* 743–753.

Kaufman, T. L. (1997). *Out of reach: Rental housing at what cost?* Washington, DC: The National Low Income Housing Coalition.

Kylmä, J., & Vehviläinen-Julkunen, K. (1997). Hope in nursing research: A meta-analysis of the ontological and epistemological foundations of research on hope. *Journal of Advanced Nursing, 25,* 364–371.

Link, B. G., Susser, E., Stueve, A., Phelan, J., Moore, R.E., & Struening, E., (1994). Lifetime and five-year prevalence of homelessness in the United States. *American Journal of Public Health, 84,* 1907–1912.

McKinney Act of 1994, U.S.C. § 11301.

Merriam-Webster's Collegiate Dictionary (10th ed.). (1995). Springfield, MA: Merriam-Webster.

Morse, J. M., & Doberneck, B. (1995). Delineating the concept of hope. *Image: Journal of Nursing Scholarship, 27,* 277–285.

Parse, R. R. (1981). *Man-living-health: A theory of nursing.* New York: Wiley.

Parse, R. R. (1987). Parse's man-living-health theory of nursing. In R. R. Parse, *Nursing science: Major paradigms, theories, and critiques* (pp. 159–180). Philadelphia: Saunders.

Parse, R. R. (Ed.). (1995). *Illuminations: The human becoming theory in practice and research.* New York: NLN Press.

Parse, R. R. (1998). *The human becoming school of thought.* Thousand Oaks, CA: Sage.

Shinn, M., & Weitzman, B. C. (1996). Homeless families are different. In J. Baumohl (Ed.), *Homelessness in America* (pp. 109–122). Phoenix, AZ: Oryx Press.

U.S. House of Representatives Committee on Ways and Means. (1992). *Overview of entitlement programs: 1992 green book.* Washington, DC: U.S. Government Printing Office.

Wake, M., & Miller, J. (1992). Treating hopelessness: Nursing strategies from six countries. *Clinical Nursing Research, 1,* 347–365.

Waxman, L., & Hinderliter, S. (1996). *A status report on hunger and homelessness in America's cities: 1996.* Washington, DC: U.S. Conference of Mayors.

Williams, L. (1992). *Addictions on the streets: Substance abuse and homelessness in America.* Washington, DC: National Coalition for the Homeless.

Chapter 13

The Lived Experience of Hope for Those Working with Homeless Persons

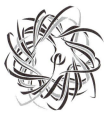

SANDRA SCHMIDT BUNKERS

> The Greeks told the story of the minotaur, the
> bull-headed flesh-eating man who lived in the
> center of the labyrinth.
> He was a threatening beast, and yet his name was
> Asterion-Star.
> I often think of this paradox as I sit with someone with
> tears in her eyes, searching for a way to deal with
> a death, a divorce, a depression.
> It is a beast, this thing that stirs in the core
> of her being, but it is also the star of
> her innermost nature.
> We have to care for this suffering with extreme reverence
> so that, in our fear and anger at the beast,
> we do not overlook the star.
>
> *T. Moore* (1992)

The illustrations of hope surfacing in the following study consist of paradoxes similar to what is described by Moore (1992). Hope is described by those working with homeless persons as a paradoxical life process of engaging-disengaging with others while discovering innovative ways of persisting with intense struggles of day-to-day living. The lived experience of hope emerged in this study as *envisioning possibilities amid disheartenment, as close alliances with isolating turmoil surface in inventive endeavoring.*

PARTICIPANTS

Participants in this study included ten persons (six women and four men) ranging from 25 to 50 years of age from South Dakota and Illinois, U.S. The participants were able to understand, read, and speak English and were able to focus on and describe the lived experience of hope. The discussions were audiorecorded and varied from 30 to 60 minutes in length, depending on how long the participant wished to discuss the experience.

DIALOGICAL ENGAGEMENT

The dialogical engagements took place in participants' places of employment. The discussion began with the researcher's statement as follows: "Tell me about the experience of hope in your life."

EXTRACTION-SYNTHESIS

Joe's Story

Joe, aged 45, has been working with homeless persons for over eight years. Joe talks intently about his lessons of hope in working with the poor, particularly underlining the lessons of hope learned while working with Mother Teresa on the streets of Calcutta. Joe states:

> Mother Teresa's work began in a culture where the Hindu philosophy and theology is very strong and the ethic is not for making change. Yet her presence in their midst created a new energy at work which was saying, "We can do something about these people who die on the streets." Her presence in the midst of much despair changed something. People don't die on the streets of Calcutta any more. I remember her describing how she began. She picked up her first person on the street and that person died in her arms. And she said, "Never again." She told me, "You pick up one person at a time." Basically, that is what she has done and that is a hopeful thing for me. It is hopeful in the sense that one person did something.

"When I think of hope," Joe continues, "I think of a quote from St. Augustine that goes something like this: 'Hope has two lovely daughters, Anger at the way things are and Courage to change them.' I think both of these [anger and courage] are part of the energy that drives me." Joe goes on to tell of painful life experiences of losing loved ones and needing to move to new places continuously and to try new things to keep feeling more alive. As he describes moving to different cities and new jobs he states with seriousness, "You know the world is not the way it ought to be. I get very angry about that." Joe shakes his head and continues, "I guess hope for me is having the ability to embrace the pain, brokenness, and darkness in life while being connected to a community of people."

Joe goes on:

> I really believe there is another presence at work even in the midst of the dark. And, maybe, ultimately, there is a sacred source in the brokenness . . . in the pain of life. So, going into the pain is not a scary thing for me because I believe it is going into the presence of God and discovering that Presence. God is a free Presence that can create something different out of what is. I just live in that freedom of knowing there can be newness, and that's enough to keep me going. That gives me hope.

Joe smiles and states:

> I've been talking and you have been listening, but I need to tell you one more thing. The one fear I have is that there may not be an ultimate tomorrow. I ask myself, "What if this is it? What if the difference we make here is for here, nowhere else?" I ask myself this existential question, "What is the use of all the things I do now if this is the end of it?" Yet I know there is a reason to go on. I have children. And this world is going to be a better place, a place with opportunity and freshness because of them. That's the hope for me.

Essences: Participant's Language

1. Hope is seeing and moving with courage to a new tomorrow that offers opportunity and freshness with the world being a better place; the fear is that there may not be an ultimate tomorrow.
2. Hope is the ability to embrace the painful life experiences, the brokenness, and the darkness in life with anger energy while being connected to a community of people; it involves a free God creating something different out of what is.

Essences: Researcher's Language

1. Envisioning novel achievements surfaces in endeavoring with ardent tenacity amid an ambiguous foreboding.
2. Contemplation of a solemn alliance emerges with honoring anguish in close affiliations.

Proposition. The lived experience of hope is envisioning novel achievements surfacing in endeavoring with ardent tenacity amid an ambiguous foreboding, as contemplation of a solemn alliance emerges with honoring anguish in close affiliations.

Emily's Story

"I think hope is a promise. . . . It is the beginning of the promise. I have a deep sense of hope and belief for a brighter life after death. . . . There is that promise." Thus begins Emily's description of hope in her life. Emily describes herself as a social activist. In her fifty years she has worked for over twelve years with people who are homeless. Emily continues her discussion of hope by sharing some of the losses in her life:

> I grew up in a small town where everyone helped everyone. I had a brother die of cancer. I remember when he died. A neighbor showed up with a can of coffee. Then someone came with a cake. I asked my mother, "Why are people bringing food? Can't we afford food?" My mother replied, "Emily, that is the way people try to help at a time like this." Then my sister died when I was 20. During her illness I went through a real tough time and got in trouble struggling with relationships. I remember walking alone in a city and looking up at a street light which seemed to have a halo around it. I thought, "God, if you'll just get me through this time, I know there's a better future out there." Faith in God and the power of God to help was a source of hope for me at that time.

When further discussing the meaning of hope, Emily cites her involvement in working with the poor and homeless:

> A gift that has been given to me is that I make a difference in other people's lives. Hope is a gift which you can give someone through

how you treat them, through how you are with them, through what you say to them. I think hope is a gift to be given away, if you've realized it yourself. Hope is something to be shared.

Emily tells a story about a man named Frank who frequents the soup kitchen where she works. Frank never talked until Emily started saying his name and greeting him. Emily states:

So each day I say, "Hello Frank. I hope you have a good day." Now he has started answering me. And instead of just one sentence he is up to about three or four sentences. This is great progress. And so how do you measure hope? I don't know. If I can just choose one person at a time and call them by name, that is something very special . . . to call another by name. I always refer back to the scriptures: "I have called you by name; you are mine."

Emily shakes her head slowly, pausing briefly.

I think of a lack of hope when I talk with young college people who volunteer here in the soup kitchen. I request that when they work here they ask the young people what their dreams for the future are. I want the children to share their dreams because it will encourage them in thinking about a future. Well, at closing time one day one of the young helpers said to me, "You know that question you wanted us to ask the kids. Well, I was sitting at a table with a family and I asked the kids what they wanted to be when they grew up. And the father said, 'Don't ask my kids that because they can't go to college like you can. I don't want you putting thoughts like that in their minds because they can't do that.'" The college youth was embarrassed. I said, "That's okay that you asked the question. Those kids will remember that somebody said they can have a future. Far too many kids are being told 'Don't think about that; you can't do that.' Be glad that you asked the question!"

"I put the word of God into action. . . . I have a strong faith. . . . I put hope into action," Emily says with a smile. "So hope for me is a yearning and an aching. It takes courage to have hope and to follow dreams. You put all your energy, all your being into it."

Essences: Participant's Language

1. Hope is a belief in a God that loves and a faith in His promise of an end to struggling alone and in need of help in relationships; it is a belief in a better life after death.
2. Hope is being able to make a difference in people's lives; it involves choosing to be with another and calling that person by name.

3. Hope is a promise, a yearning you put all your energy into; it involves having goals and dreams and the courage to follow the dreams.

Essences: Researcher's Language

1. Disheartenment with isolating turmoil surfaces amid a covenant with a solemn alliance in contemplating a hereafter.
2. Compassion emerges with an intimate regard for others.
3. Envisioning possibilities arises with enduring resolve for pushing on with novel endeavors.

Proposition. The lived experience of hope is envisioning possibilities arising with enduring resolve for pushing on with novel endeavors, as compassion emerges with an intimate regard for others, while disheartenment with isolating turmoil surfaces amid a covenant with a solemn alliance in contemplating a hereafter.

Tanya's Story

"There are three particular experiences which come to mind when I think about hope. The first experience concerns a patient I have known for many years, but I found out recently I didn't really know her." This first story begins Tanya's tales of how an understanding of hope has emerged in her life. Tanya, 40 years old, has held a supervisory position in a clinic working with the indigent and homeless for fourteen years. Tanya begins:

> Carol, the patient I will now tell you about, has been coming to the clinic for several years. She usually comes when she is intoxicated and needs help getting medications or hospitalized. One day she comes in complaining of pain in her stomach. Carol was quite intoxicated, so I placed her in a room to wait for the lab results. We were very busy in the clinic so she was inadvertently passed by. So, a couple hours later I hurried to the room where she was waiting. Carol was sound asleep. I awoke her and apologized for the inconvenience. She seemed quite comfortable with the unexpected wait. Feeling very apologetic, I sat down to talk with her until she could be seen by one of the physicians. Carol started talking about herself. She wanted to talk about her losses in the past couple years. We talked about her mom who had died a year ago and how she missed her. Carol stated there was no longer a sense of togetherness in her life nor closeness with the rest of her family. We discussed a friend who had died and how she mourns him terribly. He had been a companion for her. Then she broke down and started to cry and explained to me that she didn't want to live her life the way it was going. So we talked about her drinking and she explained that she really didn't want to drink. She said, "Do you think I want to have my life go like this? I wish I could have a happy life. My life is not happy. I don't want to drink." I asked her what would make

her life happy and she said, "I would be happy if I could have a normal life." And I said, "Well, what is normal?" To her a normal life was to have a roof to go home to every night, to be sober, and to have children around her. It doesn't sound like she has any of that right now.

Tanya smiles and states:

Until I sat down and listened to her story, I really didn't understand this woman. So the real hope I have coming out of this story is that Carol has agreed to go into treatment in December. She wants to find satisfaction in life, warmth, and family support. She looks forward to finding peace and sobriety. My hope for her is that she finds a meaning for her life.

Tanya goes on to her second story:

I can think of an experience of hope I had when my father was dying of cancer. We knew that he was terminal, but the hope came from watching a family of seven kids and my mom pull together and make his last days what he wanted them to be. I knew I couldn't prolong his life, but I was there for him. I watched my mother and father become closer as she cared for him. That is a big picture of hope in my life.

The third story is told with a voice filled with concern:

World peace is something that I have not been very hopeful for. However, we here at the clinic have just helped resettle 190 refugees in this city who have experienced terrible abuse and beatings in their home countries. As I watch them make something out of their lives, work on their English, and get their kids in school, I get hopeful that they will have a better life. These are such things in which I see hope.

Essences: Participant's Language

1. Hope is watching people make something out of their lives as they move toward feeling whole and finding peace and meaning in life.
2. Hope is about pulling together as a family during a time of terminal illness; it is finding many ways of being there and becoming closer to each other.
3. Hope is seeing community caregivers make an effort to help refugees who share terrible stories of abuse and beatings in home countries; less hope exists for world peace.

Essences: Researcher's Language

1. Reflecting on possibilities for creating anew emerges in dwelling with purposeful serenity.
2. Genuine closeness surfaces with witnessing agony.
3. Sustaining endeavors arise amid anguishing apprehensions.

Proposition. The lived experience of hope is reflecting on possibilities for creating anew in dwelling with purposeful serenity, as genuine closeness surfaces with witnessing agony, while sustaining endeavors arise amid anguishing apprehensions.

Ellen's Story

"I live my experience of hope by what I do for a living." This is the essence of hope in Ellen's life. Ellen, aged 25, has worked with indigent and homeless persons for over two years. Ellen continues:

> I do a lot of listening and I try to meet people where they are. I am the sort of person who carries the weight of the world on my shoulders. I can't walk down the street and ignore all the sad problems that I see. So I'm pretty much dedicated to service. I have a lot of hope.

Ellen's face looks solemn as she continues talking about the discord in the world:

> Everything is getting worse, such as the violence in this country and the way resources are being stripped away from those who need help. It is discouraging and scary. It's hard to act on the individual level when all these things are going on in politics and government. Sometimes I wish I could instill in the leaders of this country the hope that I and the people that work with me feel. There just aren't enough people that care about each other. It's like you take little baby steps.

Then she smiles and adds, "Although I know a lot of people who were homeless that are definitely success stories, whose lives have changed, and those are the people that keep me going.

Ellen describes with detail the involvement she has with homeless people:

> You know, I get emotionally involved and I have been driven to tears. It's impossible to work with people whose lives are this sad and not feel involved. I share their tears. I live my experience of hope by trying to make a difference in people's lives. That is the hope that drives me.

Essences: Participant's Language

1. Hope is success stories for the homeless as their lives change; it's getting emotionally involved with people and sharing in their tears.
2. Hope is a driving force to make things better for people even when resources are being stripped away from people and violence in the country is discouraging and scary.

Essences: Researcher's Language

1. Acknowledging possibilities amid turmoil surfaces with close affiliations.
2. Isolating disheartenment arises with launching inventive endeavors.

Proposition. The lived experience of hope is acknowledging possibilities amid turmoil surfacing with close affiliations, as isolating disheartenment arises with launching inventive endeavors.

Jeffrey's Story

> I'm living with a fatal disease. I've been HIV positive for sixteen years and have had AIDS for over six years. I'm going to die eventually, but we all do. Right now I'm going through a major change in my life because I'm applying for disability retirement. My whole life has been identified with being a professional. I'm giving up the profession I really love. I have to. I'm just too worn out. But I think hope is what gets me out of bed in the morning, along with a sense of accomplishment or a sense of trying to accomplish something and live certain dreams that I haven't fulfilled yet. I'm still hoping to get them. When I retire I think I might even sit down and write my hope list.

Jeffrey, 47 years old, has established his career as a public health service professional. He has worked with the underprivileged his entire career. Hope, for Jeffrey, resides with people, places, and accomplishments. Jeffrey states:

> I'm hoping retirement will allow me to investigate a lot of areas in my life that I haven't been able to because I've been so tied into work. A lot of people I know work, go home, and die. I'm determined not to let that happen to me. So that's a big definition of what I'm hoping for.

Jeffrey talks about the losses and challenges he has faced related to living with AIDS.

> This morning I attended the funeral of a friend who died of AIDS. And I'm going out to California shortly to make my last visit to a friend who is on his way out. . . . I'm working with young people who are looking death in the face at an early age. It's a real challenge. All my friends are HIV positive and we have all lost so much. It's a never-ending nightmare. It's real difficult to maintain hope sometimes. One by one dreams and hopes have to be eliminated. You have to concentrate on those that are obtainable and not give in to the hopelessness.

Jeffrey shifts in his chair and states:

> I'm not used to going on like this, but I am a Christian and I think religion instills hope. I also volunteer for an agency that distributes hot

meals and lunches to people with AIDS and to homebound people. There is a real sense of joy for me in doing that. You bring the very basics: food to people who can't afford it or are unable to fix it. The people are so grateful. So, if there is such a thing as a hope quotient, this raises it.

Jeffrey begins talking about his mother:

I think my mother is a pretty good example of living with a perspective of hope. She's having a real hard time now. She's a recent widow with financial problems, but she won't let it show. Another side of hope is that constant forging ahead and not letting things get you down.

Jeffrey then begins talking about his work with the homeless and people who are HIV positive:

I think I'm setting an example, too, for other people so that they can have hope. I spoke at church last night, and people who may not even be involved with the homeless or those with terminal disease can appreciate what other people are going through. The whole mission at this agency about healthcare for the homeless is certainly doing more than medical care. I think we are giving the clients a lot of hope. Coming here is a big deal for them. They are treated like human beings; they are welcomed here and I think that instills hope. I try to work with the whole person and help clients solve problems.

Jeffrey concludes his dialogue concerning hope with an example of being treated with respect:

I have had wonderful acceptance here. The staff accepts me, my diagnosis, my lifestyle. In this place you don't hear people judged. Treating people with respect is part of hope. Maybe I have a lot of hope because I have a lot of self-respect.

Essences: Participant's Language

1. Hope is a sense of joy in having set an example for other people while living with the fatal disease of AIDS; it involves looking forward to living certain dreams that aren't fulfilled yet.
2. Hope is not giving in even while living the hopeless nightmare of friends dying and working with young people who are looking death in the face; it involves religion and a mother who in difficult times keeps forging ahead.
3. Hope is working with people and helping them problem-solve situations; it includes acceptance, respect, and being treated as a whole human being.

Essences: Researcher's Language

1. Envisioning possibilities emerges with delighting in achievements amid the recognition of mortality.

2. Inspiring alliances surface in struggling with the agony of futility.
3. Honoring uniqueness arises with undertaking innovative endeavors.

Proposition. The lived experience of hope is envisioning possibilities while delighting in achievements amid the recognition of mortality, as inspiring alliances surface in struggling with the agony of futility, while honoring uniqueness arises with undertaking innovative endeavors.

Alan's Story

Alan, 49 years old, has been a case manager and street outreach worker with homeless persons for over two years. He begins describing hope in his life by focusing on his past:

> I will have to describe the experience of hope in my life in a couple of ways, including a look at my past life. It is impossible for me to discuss this subject without talking about myself as a recovering alcoholic and drug addict. I was so beat down from the disease and so hopeless. Then I saw that help was all around me; I just needed to reach out to others. I've come to think of it as divine intervention. I have nine years in recovery at this point. Recovery helped me value myself. So that kind of very personal experience is one way that I look at hope in my life.

Alan begins talking about his work with homeless persons:

> I really can't identify a hopeless situation. However, the work can be very difficult, very challenging. Clients' issues are often complex. There are times when you can't see any movement with clients. As a case worker, that can make it very difficult to maintain your commitment. But, when I sit down with an individual, I'm always maintaining hope that there is something we can do together. If a client is willing to work on their situation and put one foot in front of another and follow through, then we can do something.

Alan continues:

> I do know there are many staff involved in this struggle who genuinely care and are trying to make a difference in the world. Recently I attended a homeless coalition meeting. The fact that a number of us were working together was energizing. There is a lot of good work being done by people and that gives me hope.

Essences: Participant's Language

1. Hope is genuinely caring about making a difference in the world; it is energizing working with others.

2. Hope is continuing in relationships when complex problems are a challenge and it is hard to see progress; it consists of putting one foot in front of the other and following through.
3. Hope is reaching out and receiving help from others when feeling hopeless and beaten down; it involves divine intervention.

Essences: Researcher's Language

1. Committing to envisioned possibilities arises with engaging alliances.
2. Disheartenment surfaces with ingenious endeavors for pushing on.
3. Solemn, attentive closeness emerges amid anguishing estrangement.

Proposition. The lived experience of hope is committing to envisioned possibilities arising with engaging alliances, as disheartenment surfaces with ingenious endeavors for pushing on, while solemn, attentive closeness emerges amid anguishing estrangement.

Ida's Story

"I can't imagine a life without hope," Ida, a 32-year-old woman who has worked with homeless persons for over three years, states emphatically.

> I think there is always hope in someone's life. I don't know if I would want to live if I couldn't hope for something. Even if people say they are hopeless, then I think they are hoping to have hope about something! I know that sometimes I go through a couple weeks where I'm hopeful and have a lot of energy and am happier. Then I can become sadder and am less hopeful. It's obviously a cyclical thing for me, a cycle of high hope and then low hope. I hope for a lot of things at the same time, like things for my family, being happy in my marriage, creating new accomplishments and being healthy.

Ida then talks about hope in relation to her community:

> When I think about hope, it is frustrating to me that homeless people hope for things I think they should already have. There are tons of homeless people that don't have access to healthcare or can't get into the system . . . or can't have a place to live. I get mad that this is what they have to hope for. I go home sometimes and wonder if there is hope for the homeless population. Can we hope that there won't be homeless people?

Ida slowly shakes her head and states:

> One of the things that I was very unhopeful about lately was that we had a celebration because our agency had been in existence ten years. I didn't like the idea of celebrating at all. I think it's sad that we have been needed for that long. Can we hope that we will not be needed any more

to provide these services? Realistically I know we won't go away because we're not needed, but that is something that I hope for. It is sad, but this agency is the last resort for a lot of homeless people. We provide them with healthcare, we may be able to have someone here that speaks their language, and we refer them to other sources of assistance. For many people, there's no place for them to go but here. We are their hope.

Ida shifts the conversation and begins talking about God:

I think people who believe in God have stronger hopes, although right now I feel God is missing from my life. I wasn't brought up in a religious household and right now don't go to church. But I want to join a church for two reasons: for a sense of community and, as I get older, the divine becomes more important. I'm sure the divine and hope interact. You see, I hope for many things. It's especially fun to hope for something that you think you're really going to get or achieve. I hope to always be challenged. It is important to be doing something in my life that makes me think and grow and question things I've believed. My belief in God makes me hopeful that things can happen.

Essences: Participant's Language

1. Hope is wanting all sorts of things and having desires; it involves a cycle of high hope and then low hope.
2. Hope is believing in a God even when God seems to be missing; it includes growing with many opportunities that give energy and happiness.
3. Hope is community with others; it involves providing services to the homeless while experiencing sadness and frustration in seeing their lack of access to care.

Essences: Researcher's Language

1. Envisioning possibilities arises with the ebb and flow of anticipation.
2. Inspiration amid solemn estrangement emerges with the spirited engagement of the novel.
3. Close alliances amid disheartenment surface with inventive endeavors.

Proposition. The lived experience of hope is envisioning possibilities arising with the ebb and flow of anticipation, as inspiration amid solemn estrangement emerges with the spirited engagement of the novel, while close alliances amid disheartenment surface with inventive endeavors.

Pamela's Story

Pamela is a 32-year-old community health nurse who has been working with homeless persons for over two years. She describes her experience of hope while sharing certain struggles in her life.

I think as a child I didn't know what tomorrow was or what hope was. I knew more about the uncomfortableness and the pain associated with growing up with an alcoholic father, abuse, and a separation and divorce. I was an only child so I didn't have siblings or friends to share my experience with. I didn't share with friends because I thought they were different than me. My childhood was pretty painful and I didn't have any hope that it would be different. I just thought that this was how life was. However, as I've gotten older I feel extremely hopeful. Now I feel as if I have hope every day that there is a tomorrow and that tomorrow is going to be better than today. I feel that hope is an essence of myself. I think those significant experiences of my childhood influenced who I am today and the fact that I have compassion and empathy for people.

Pamela smiled faintly and added, "I think it's been in the last five years that I have realized there is so much more beyond the pain, beyond that feeling of being betrayed and victimized."

The discussion changes to Pamela's experience with her spiritual path:

In the last five years I have been on a spiritual path and that has created hopefulness and a zest for life and a yearning for more. I thank my higher power for today. I've found that spirituality is a core part of me. I still don't have an identifiable religion, but spirituality has become an inner thing, an inner presence and peacefulness that gives me hope. Sometimes the energy or the force of negativism pushes me down. I think then, "Oh my God, it will never get better because this happens and war here and famine there." So I go from the feeling of being hopeless with fear to feeling a sense of hope. I think doing good is the same as wanting or having hope. Doing good in anything in my life whether it be relationships or in my work is hopeful. I can create hope; it is very internal. So creating is related to hope.

Pamela continues to talk about creating and hope:

I wonder if you have to have hope to have creativity. They just seem to go together. I'm in a transition period in that I'm living in one place but plan on moving out of state. I'm looking for opportunities. I'm moving on. That's hopeful. I yearn to be elsewhere within a year's time, and I am creating that real desire. I don't know exactly where I will be and what I will be doing, and the unknowing and not familiar is hard.

The discussion turns to Pamela's desire to write:

My writing is a vehicle to get to hope. I tend to ask questions that require introspection so I write. I write and then I just know by writing.

Usually when I'm writing it is about some decision, some situation, be it negative or positive. I use writing to get through whatever it is I'm trying to get through. Sometimes the answer I find isn't always what I want it to be or would like it to be. But I find hope in knowing that there is an answer.

Essences: Participant's Language

1. Hope is knowing there will be a tomorrow; it involves moving between feelings of being abused, hopeless, and different from others to feeling tomorrow will be a better day.
2. Hope is creating opportunities for moving on with the unknown and doing good in relationships and work; it consists of having compassion and empathy.
3. Hope is finding answers through introspection; it includes a spiritual path with a higher power providing a zest for life and a yearning for more.

Essences: Researcher's Language

1. Optimistic expectations arise amid the uncertain trepidation of agonizing alienation.
2. Formulating ingenious endeavors surfaces with close affiliations.
3. Vitality emerges with contemplation amid recognition of a solemn alliance.

Proposition. The lived experience of hope is optimistic expectations arising amid the uncertain trepidation of agonizing alienation as vitality emerges with contemplation amid recognition of a solemn alliance, while formulating ingenious endeavors surfaces with close affiliations.

Gary's Story

Gary, a 28-year-old man who has been an outreach worker and driver for homeless people for over four years, is excited about all the hope he has for his life. He states:

> I want to do so much, but I got to work with what I have. I hope to become a better person as I accomplish my goals. I hope I can help my clients. I really want to buy my own building so my clients, maybe thirty of them, would have their own shelter. I hope to help as many people as I can and to maintain and keep my wife and children happy. My hope when I was 20 years old was to be married when I was 21. I accomplished that.

Gary continues to talk about his work with homeless people:

> I love coming to work. You know there are people who turn their back on everybody. Well, I'm not that kind of person. I treat everybody like

they are supposed to be treated. I go out of my way for my clients no matter what. I feel like I am on the same level they are, only I have a place to go stay at night and they don't. I'm giving people a chance to help themselves, and many tell me they hope they can be somebody. They come in here to talk with me. I'm somebody they can trust. I'm their hope for something.

Gary begins to talk about how he deals with his work:

I really keep everything inside of me. I hold it in. I may tell my wife a little bit about what I've done, but other than that I really don't talk to anybody. As I drive home at night I just sit there and say to myself, "I did it; I did it again. I helped somebody again. I'm that hope." And I hope I can be here another ten years. However long it takes.

Essences: Participant's Language

1. Hope is about setting goals and reaching them; it involves becoming a better person as goals are accomplished.
2. Hope is being there for people, to listen to them, and treat them right; it entails holding things inside and not sharing experiences of helping others, but saying to yourself, "I did it; I did it again; I helped somebody again. I'm that hope."
3. Hope is about giving people a chance to help themselves even though there are people who turn their back on everybody; it is about going out of the way for people no matter what.

Essences: Researcher's Language

1. Envisioning possibilities arises amid acknowledging achievements.
2. Disquieting aloneness emerges with a regard for close affiliations.
3. Disheartenment with alienation surfaces while launching diverse endeavors.

Proposition. The lived experience of hope is envisioning possibilities amid acknowledging achievements, as disquieting aloneness emerges with a regard for close affiliations, while disheartenment with alienation surfaces while launching diverse endeavors.

Janet's Story

"This is the best job I've ever had in nursing." Janet, a 48-year-old community health nurse who has worked with homeless people for over three years, makes this statement boldly as she discusses her experience of hope:

The people that I am working with have inspired me. They are wonderful people who have managed under all sorts of terrible situations to maintain their humanity and to maintain their thoughtfulness. The people we see here at this clinic are warm and grateful for the care they receive. They make it very easy for me to take care of them and work with them. Some people say to me, "Isn't your work depressing?" I say, "No, in fact it is just the opposite. It is not depressing at all; it is joyful because we interact and have a good time."

Janet talks about her hope for nursing in the community:

This is such a good place for nursing. Nursing can have influence as to what is going on in this field. I am writing a grant right now. I can't just sit here and think someone else is going to do it for me. I need to start making positive moves on my own. If I get my grant it would provide substance abuse treatment for women who are homeless. So . . . you have to put action to what you feel. I hope for my clients; I want them to get something.

Janet sighs and continues, "You know, I get angry because sometimes it looks so bleak and overwhelming when I see someone that has absolutely nothing and no opportunity. Then I just hope for what that person needs right now and hope I can make a difference in their experience."

Janet focuses on her faith. "I think hope goes hand in hand with my faith. I'm not a religious person but I'd like to consider myself a spiritual person. I have a strong faith in God. I feel like I can have hope because I have faith."

Essences: Participant's Language

1. Hope is having influence in working with the homeless in the community; it involves dealing with anger when observing the lack of opportunity, the homeless experience.
2. Hope is faith in God and joy in working with people who are warm and grateful.
3. Hope is making positive moves and putting action into what you feel even though it seems bleak for those who have nothing and their situations seem overwhelming.

Essences: Researcher's Language

1. Anticipating possibilities arises amid disturbing turmoil.
2. A solemn alliance surfaces with the delight of close affiliations.
3. Disheartenment with estrangement emerges in launching inventive endeavors.

Proposition. The lived experience of hope is anticipating possibilities arising amid disturbing turmoil, as a solemn alliance surfaces with the delight of close affiliations, while disheartenment with estrangement emerges in launching inventive endeavors.

FINDINGS AND RELATED LITERATURE

The central finding of this study is that the lived experience of hope is *envisioning possibilities amid disheartenment, as close alliances with isolating turmoil surface in inventive endeavoring.* Propositions derived from the ten participant descriptions revealed three core concepts: *envisioning possibilities amid disheartenment, close alliances with isolating turmoil,* and *inventive endeavoring.* (See Tables 1–3.) The meaning of hope is explained in the process of heuristic interpretation where the core concepts are linked with the human becoming theory. (See Table 4.) At the level of structural transposition, hope is *pondering the will-be amid tribulation, as communion-aloneness surfaces in pressing with the not-yet.* At the conceptual integration level of the human becoming theory, hope is *imaging the connecting-separating of powering originating.*

The first core concept, *envisioning possibilities amid disheartenment,* was described by participants as a considering of opportunities for tomorrow while at the same time realizing the discouragement that the world is not what they want it to be. The words of the participants portray the imaginings of what could be while at the same time struggling with the challenges of day-to-day evolving. Examples of participant statements follow: "Even when I get depressed I know

TABLE 1.
Concept Evident in Propositions of Participants:
Envisioning Possibilities Amid Disheartenment

Concept:	**Envisioning possibilities amid disheartenment**
Structural Transposition:	**Pondering the will-be amid tribulation**
Conceptual Integration:	**Imaging**

1. envisioning novel achievements . . . amid ambiguous foreboding
2. envisioning possibilities . . . disheartenment
3. reflecting on possibilities . . . anguishing apprehensions
4. acknowledging possibilities . . . isolating disheartenment
5. envisioning possibilities . . . struggling with . . . futility
6. committing to envisioned possibilities . . . disheartenment surfaces
7. envisioning possibilities . . . with the ebb and flow of anticipation . . . disheartenment
8. optimistic expectations . . . uncertain trepidation
9. envisioning possibilities . . . disheartenment with alienation
10. anticipating possibilities . . . disheartenment

TABLE 2.
Concept Evident in Propositions of Participants:
Close Alliances with Isolating Turmoil

Concept:	Close alliances with isolating turmoil
Structural Transposition:	Communion-aloneness
Conceptual Integration:	Connecting-separating

1. a solemn alliance . . . honoring anguish . . . close affiliations

2. intimate regard for others . . . isolating turmoil . . . a covenant with a solemn alliance

3. genuine closeness surfaces with witnessing agony

4. turmoil . . . close affiliations

5. inspiring alliances . . . recognition of mortality . . . struggling with the agony of futility

6. engaging alliances . . . solemn, attentive closeness emerges amid anguishing estrangement

7. close alliances . . . solemn estrangement

8. a solemn alliance . . . close affiliations . . . agonizing alienation

9. regard for close affiliations . . . disquieting aloneness

10. solemn alliance . . . delight of close affiliations . . . disturbing turmoil . . . estrangement

that I'm not the only resource at work here. There is a God free to do something new." "Whatever I learned from today, felt from today . . . those things give me hope for a better tomorrow."

Envisioning possibilities amid disheartenment was integrated with the theory of human becoming as *pondering the will-be amid tribulation.* Parse (1990) writes, "Envisioning the not-yet is the persistent picturing of possibles" (p. 15). Bunkers (1996) describes "pondering the possibles" as moving a person beyond the moment and thus "diversifying one's way of becoming" (p. 146). Pondering the will-be amid tribulation is *imaging* a way of structuring meaning and cocreating reality, and is connected with the first principle of Parse's theory (1995): "Structuring meaning multidimensionally is cocreating reality through the languaging of valuing and imaging" (p. 6). Imaging involves explicit-tacit knowing. As the philosopher Fisher (1985) suggests, imagining is a fundamental way of knowing and is central to human becoming. Thus, hope can be understood as an explicit-tacit knowing. As images arise of what will be, new understandings evolve for moving on. Parse (1990) describes this imaging process as "anticipating possibilities through envisioning the not-yet" and in a

TABLE 3.
Concept Evident in Propositions of Participants: Inventive Endeavoring

Concept:	Inventive endeavoring
Structural Transposition:	**Pressing with the not-yet**
Conceptual Integration:	**Powering originating**

1. endeavoring with ardent tenacity
2. enduring resolve for pushing on with novel endeavors
3. sustaining endeavors arise
4. launching inventive endeavors
5. undertaking innovative endeavors
6. ingenious endeavors for pushing on
7. inventive endeavors
8. formulating ingenious endeavors
9. launching diverse endeavors
10. launching inventive endeavors

study on the experience of laughter as "contemplative envisioning" (Parse, 1993, p. 41). It is also similar to what Bunkers (1998) described in a study of considering tomorrow as "contemplating desired endeavors" (p. 59).

Related literature that is consistent with the notion of envisioning possibilities amid disheartenment includes writings of philosophers Marcel, Fromm, and Frankl. Marcel (1962) sees hope situated within the framework of a trial. He writes, "The truth is that there can strictly speaking be no hope except when the temptation to despair exists. Hope is the act by which this temptation is actively or victoriously overcome" (p. 36). Fromm (1968) says, "Hope is paradoxical. It is neither passive waiting nor is it unrealistic forcing of circumstances that cannot occur. It is like a crouched tiger, which will jump only when the moment for jumping has come" (p. 9). Frankl (1984) indicates that finding meaning in suffering holds the possibility of surfacing hope and optimism in the face of no-hope and tragedy.

Envisioning possibilities amid disheartenment is creating new images of what can be while encountering what was, what is, and what is not yet all-at-once. The philosopher Wu (1972) writes, "Hope is that creative pull between the now and the future, originating from the contrast of the actual with the ideal. Hope is our life-nisus to a better tomorrow, spurred on by the disillusionment of today" (p. 135). The participants in this study lived hope by envisioning new ways of living health.

Close alliances with isolating turmoil, the second core concept, reflects the paradoxical rhythm of being close to others while at the same time experiencing

TABLE 4.
Heuristic Interpretation: Progressive Abstraction of Core Concepts of Hope

Core Concepts	Structural Transposition	Conceptual Integration
Envisioning possibilities amid disheartenment	Pondering the will-be amid tribulation	Imaging
Close alliances with isolating turmoil	Communion-aloneness	Connecting-separating
Inventive endeavoring	Pressing with the not-yet	Powering originating

Structure

The lived experience of hope is envisioning possibilities amid disheartenment, as close alliances with isolating turmoil surface in inventive endeavoring.

Structural Transposition

The lived experience of hope is pondering the will-be amid tribulation as communion-aloneness surfaces in pressing with the not-yet.

Conceptual Integration

The lived experience of hope is imaging the connecting-separating of powering originating.

distancing unrest in close relational activities. Such isolating unrest surfaces with an individual's freedom to react to the adversity and unpredictability in the world. Sartre (1956) suggests that "every free project in projecting itself anticipates a margin of unpredictability due to the independence of things precisely because this independence is that in terms of which a freedom is constituted" (p. 650). Participants expressed feeling close to others while at the same time sensing an aloneness in such statements as these: "Sometimes it looks pretty bleak when you see someone who has absolutely nothing. . . . But these people I'm working with are warm, wonderful people." "Sometimes you might sit across from someone who won't even speak to you. That's okay; they still feel good that you with the yellow name tag have come to sit with them. You chose them to sit with in this dining hall."

At the level of structural transposition, close alliances with isolating turmoil is *communion-aloneness*. Communion-aloneness portrays the participants' involvement with others while having a separateness of personal experiences and meanings. This involvement-with-separateness is similar to Parse's (1996) concept of "close-to–apart-from" in her quality of life study. Also, Cody (1995), in a study on grieving, identified a similar concept of "bearing witness to aloneness with togetherness," and Bunkers (1998), in a study on considering tomorrow, identified the concept of "intimate alliances with isolating distance" as a rhythmical paradoxical pattern of engaging-disengaging with persons and events. The concept of communion-aloneness is consistent with Marcel's (1962) notion that hope is experienced in communion with a situation and those in the situation. Marcel's thesis concerning hope for liberation and salvation is "I hope in thee for us" (p. 60). Communion-aloneness is *connecting-separating* with persons, events, and meanings as one immerses one's self in new involvements. Connecting-separating is a coming together with others and various phenomena while simultaneously separating from other possibilities (Parse, 1981) and is related to the second principle of the human becoming theory: "Cocreating rhythmical patterns of relating is living the paradoxical unity of revealing-concealing and enabling-limiting while connecting-separating" (Parse 1995, p. 7).

Connecting-separating involves choosing at multidimensional levels to participate in engaging and disengaging with others and the universe. This interrelational rhythm of being with and apart from others in living hope is similar to what Steindl-Rast (1984) describes concerning the dance of hope: "In the youthfulness of hope the stillness of waiting is one with the dancing" (p. 138). Connecting-separating is described by Parse (1981) as people coming "together in an intersubjective relationship; that is, they are truly present to each other, simultaneously unifying and separating as their togetherness evolves" (p. 54). Close alliances with isolating turmoil is unifying with others in intentional activity while separating in the process of ascribing personal meaning and purpose to the connectedness-separateness. The participants in this study lived hope as a rhythmical interconnectedness which involved a moving toward and away from and a being with and apart from others and situations all-at-once.

The third core concept of hope, *inventive endeavoring*, reflects a process of constructive inventiveness in the pushing-resisting encounters of human existence. Inventive endeavoring is described by participants in the stories of how they lived out their hope in creative works by statements such as the following: "I see people pulling together more and making an effort to help, and I'm hopeful about that." "I'm using my skills to help other people as much as I can." "I'm setting an example for other people. . . . When you work with populations like I do you just don't pull teeth . . . you try to work with the whole person. . . . Many times you get involved in family situations."

Inventive endeavoring is interpreted at the structural transposition level of theory as *pressing with the not-yet*. Pressing with the not-yet depicts the participants' pushing forward with others toward new opportunities. This pushing forward with the new is similar to Rendon, Sales, Leal, and Pique's (1995) concept of "forceful enlivening," emerging in a study on aging; Smith's (1990) concept of "mobilizing the possibles in the rhythms of becoming through asserting being," identified in a study on struggling through a difficult time; and Bunkers' (1996) considering tomorrow concept of "resilient endurance amid disturbing unsureness," depicting the process of "struggling with the paradoxical nature of being sure and not-sure while moving beyond the now with resoluteness to the not-yet" (p. 167). Pressing with the not-yet entails cocreating possibilities for human well-being and quality of life while confronting the actualities of the moment. Kierkegaard (1980) suggests that a human being is a synthesis of the limited (actuality) and the unlimited (potentiality) and exists in movement. Bishop and Scudder (1996) write, "A possible future project that seems destined to foster human well-being calls us into action" (p. 70). Pressing with the not-yet is *powering originating* and is connected with the third principle of the human becoming theory (Parse, 1995): "Cotranscending with the possibles is powering unique ways of originating in the process of transforming" (p. 7). Parse (1981) denotes, "Powering is a continuous rhythmical process incarnating one's intentions and actions in moving toward possibilities" (p. 57). Powering is fundamental to being and "is the force of human existence and underpins the courage to be" (Parse, 1981, p. 57). Originating is "inventing new ways of conforming-not conforming in the certainty-uncertainty of living" (Parse, 1998, p. 49). Powering originating in hope involves forging ahead and holding back while inventing novel ways of becoming in challenging life situations. Inventive endeavoring is cocreating opportunities for human well-being and quality of life. It is a compelling individual-communal endeavor inherent in human becoming. The core concept of inventive endeavoring can be further understood through the following:

> A knight in full armor is riding through a valley, accompanied by the figure of death on one side, the devil on the other. Fearlessly, concentrated, confident the knight looks ahead. The knight is alone but not lonely. In solitude the knight participates in the power which gives courage to affirm self in spite of the presence of the negativities of existence. (Tillich, 1952, p. 161)

Inventive endeavoring is creating new paths in the struggle of being with nonbeing. The inventive endeavoring of hope involves a synthesis of human actuality and potentiality all-at-once.

Implications for practice and research will be discussed in the final chapter of this book along with findings from the other studies.

REFERENCES

Bishop, A., & Scudder, J. (1996). *Nursing ethics: Therapeutic caring presence.* Boston: Jones and Bartlett Publishers.

Bunkers, S. S. (1996). *Considering tomorrow: Parse's theory-guided research.* Unpublished doctoral dissertation, Loyola University Chicago, Chicago, Illinois.

Bunkers, S. S. (1998). Considering tomorrow: Parse's theory-guided research. *Nursing Science Quarterly, 11,* 56–61.

Cody, W. (1995). The lived experience of grieving, for families living with AIDS. In R. R. Parse (Ed.), *Illuminations: The human becoming theory in practice and research* (pp. 197–237). New York: National League for Nursing.

Fisher, K. (1985). The imagination, justice, peace. *Studies In Formative Spirituality, VI* (1), 29–37.

Frankl, V. (1984). *Man's search for meaning.* New York: Simon & Schuster.

Fromm, E. (1968). *The revolution of hope.* New York: Harper & Row.

Kierkegaard, S. (1980). *The sickness unto death.* Princeton, NJ: Princeton University Press.

Marcel, G. (1962). *Homo viator : A metaphysics of hope.* New York: Harper & Row.

Moore, T. (1992). *Care of the soul.* New York: HarperCollins.

Parse, R. R. (1981). *Man-living-health: A theory of nursing.* New York: Wiley.

Parse, R. R. (1990). Parse's research methodology with an illustration of the lived experience of hope. *Nursing Science Quarterly, 3,* 9–17.

Parse, R. R. (1993). The experience of laughter: A phenomenological study. *Nursing Science Quarterly, 6,* 39–43.

Parse, R. R. (1995). The human becoming theory. In R. R. Parse (Ed.), *Illuminations: The human becoming theory in practice and research* (pp. 5–8). New York: National League for Nursing.

Parse, R. R. (1996). Quality of life for persons living with Alzheimer's disease: The human becoming perspective. *Nursing Science Quarterly, 9,* 126–133.

Parse, R. R. (1998). *The human becoming school of thought: A perspective for nurses and other health professionals.* Thousand Oaks, CA: Sage.

Rendon, D., Sales, R., Leal, I., & Pique, J. (1995). The lived experience of aging in community-dwelling elders in Valencia, Spain: A phenomenological study. *Nursing Science Quarterly, 8,* 152–157.

Sartre, J.-P. (1956). *Being and nothingness.* New York: Simon & Schuster.

Smith, M. C. (1990). Struggling through a difficult time for unemployed persons. *Nursing Science Quarterly, 1,* 60–67.

Steindl-Rast, D. (1984). *Gratefulness, the heart of prayer.* New York: Paulist Press.

Tillich, P. (1952). *The courage to be.* London: Yale University Press.

Wu, K.-M. (1972). Hope and world survival. *Philosophy Forum, 12,* 131–148.

Chapter 14

Hope as Lived by Native Americans

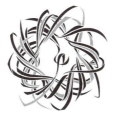

LOIS S. KELLEY

I Watched an Eagle Soar

Grandmother,
I watched an eagle soar
high in the sky
Until a cloud covered him up.
Grandmother,
I still saw the eagle
Behind my eyes.

Virginia Driving Hawk Sneve (1989)

Something beautiful, multidimensional, and "close to the Earth" is found in the Native American participants' perspectives on hope shared in this chapter. A Native American perspective according to Bray (1997) "protects people and cultures that are beautiful and unique and timeless" (p. 42). Doll (1994) describes the people of the Sioux Indian Nation as having survived broken treaties and broken promises of the past even as they seek to make a difference by continuing to carry the traditions and culture of their people to future generations. However, many Native Americans have lost their connection to their own indigenous roots, and as Gustafson (1997) notes, there exists a profound sadness and longing for its return.

PARTICIPANTS

The ten participants are Native Americans from South Dakota, from the Sioux Indian Nation, and among those featured in Doll's *Vision Quest* (1994). The five men and five women between the ages of 46 and 78 were either Lakotas, Dakotas, or Nakotas.

DIALOGICAL ENGAGEMENT

Researcher-participant discussions proceeded through dialogical engagement, which is an intersubjective "being with" (the researcher in true presence moves with the participants through an unstructured discussion of the lived experience of hope). The dialogical engagements occurred on and off reservations, in homes, schools, offices, and restaurants. All that was recounted by participants at the moment of telling to the researcher told of the essences of the meaning of hope.

EXTRACTION-SYNTHESIS

Hope, from the qualitative research findings of ten dialogical engagements with Native Americans, was revealed as *transfiguring enlightenment arising with engaging affiliations, as encircling the legendary surfaces with fortification.* The three core concepts comprising the structure were (a) transfiguring enlightenment, (b) engaging affiliations, and (c) encircling the legendary with fortification. The ten participants, in telling their stories, brought to light the meaning of hope. At the human becoming theoretical level (Parse, 1981, 1992), the lived experience of hope is *transforming the connecting-separating in languaging powering.* See Tables 1 through 4 for evidence of the core concepts leading to the structure of the lived experience of hope; the tables also show the ascending levels of discourse from structure to theory.

The following life stories depict the core concepts in the very words of the participants. Words are chosen carefully by Native Americans and rarely are wasted. Furthermore, the Native American needs no writings; words that are true sink deep into the heart where they remain, never forgotten (Sneve, 1989). It has long been recognized that the qualities of wonder, hope, and awe return to the Native American people when the healing salves of storytelling, singing, dancing, and silence are maintained and retrieved (Arrien, 1993). The intent is that the "truth of it" sink deeply into the heart of the reader and inspire hope for both Native American and non-Native American.

Fancy Dancer's Story

Fancy Dancer is a 58-year-old man who has been active with the American Indian Movement since its early days in the 1960s. He continues to work to reduce institutional racism in sports, movies, and everyday life. For Fancy Dancer, the closest thing to hope happens during sundancing when he is pierced. Hope is "a transcendence into another plane of spirituality, of spiritual consciousness, if you will.

TABLE 1.
First Core Concept as Evident in Propositions

Core Concept:	Transfiguring enlightenment
Structural Transposition:	Numinous vivification
Conceptual Integration:	Transforming

1. transfiguring enlightenment
2. transfiguring
3. shifting with the new
4. metaphysical shifting
5. uncovering the beauteous
6. transfiguring affirmation
7. transfiguring oneness . . . shifting anticipation
8. shifting anticipation
9. shifting ultimate rhythms
10. shifting arduous positionings

TABLE 2.
Second Core Concept as Evident in Propositions

Core Concept:	Engaging affiliations
Structural Transposition:	**Coming together and moving apart**
Conceptual Integration:	**Connecting-separating**

1. meditative communion
2. intermingling . . . unconditional engaging . . . procreatory affiliations
3. emerging affiliations
4. engaging
5. expressions with affiliations
6. enlivened affiliations . . . embracing
7. exposing treasured affiliation
8. engagements
9. nurturing affiliations
10. essential mutuality

When you break through to just communicating with the Great Spirit, everything is spirit; and you have a knowing in a way that you begin to understand the meaning of life." Hope is something more than a moment in which you experience something extraordinary. It is mingled with participating in an imperfect world with "tricksters, worries, temptations, and real dangers to your very life." It is listening above the jungle with expansive sight for a beginning understanding of the meaning of life while letting go of stupid worries in order to be truly free. Fancy Dancer says that hope changes you so that you are free even as you experience the worst. Hope is "a prayerful communication of root teachings and the wisdom that comes from a life of learning from the spirits which brings happiness in knowing that life takes care of itself, that everything will be okay."

Essences: Participant's Language

1. Hope is an experience within sundancing between "transcendental praying while barely feeling the piercing pain" and "breaking free to an even higher level where everything is spirit."
2. Hope is listening above the jungle with expansive sight for a beginning understanding of the meaning of life while letting go of stupid worry in order to be truly free.
3. Hope is prayerful communication of root teachings and the wisdom that comes from a life of learning from the spirits, which brings happiness in knowing that life takes care of itself.

TABLE 3.
Third Core Concept as Evident in Propositions

Core Concept:	Encircling the legendary with fortification
Structural Transposition:	Mythologems unfold unequivocal potency
Conceptual Integration:	Languaging powering

1. rhythms . . . ethereal . . . contented certitude
2. certitude . . . coalescing the cherished . . . näiveté with sagacity
3. steadfast certitude . . . prevailing venerated symbols awaken the beneficent
4. venerated symbols . . . fortitude
5. legendary wisdom . . . fortifying treasured
6. propelling certitude . . . enduring . . . covenant . . . nurturing legendary wisdom
7. enduring . . . perpetuating the venerated
8. buoyancy . . . revelation . . . encircling patterns
9. enduring . . . poignant recollections . . . reviving legendary wisdom
10. elevating . . . polestars . . . prized legendary wisdom

Essences: Researcher's Language

1. Transfiguring with distinct sensations emerges at one with celebratory rhythms.
2. Rising to the ethereal surfaces with relieving the commonplace amid liberating enlightenment.
3. Contented certitude arises in meditative communion.

Proposition. The lived experience of hope is transfiguring with distinct sensations emerging at one with celebratory rhythms, while rising to the ethereal surfaces with relieving the commonplace amid liberating enlightenment, as contented certitude arises in meditative communion.

Stone Healer's Story

Stone Healer is a 45-year-old man who originated an alcohol treatment program that incorporates native spirituality, ceremonies, and songs. He prays to his Creator for the right words to bring to his people and all peoples. For Stone Healer, hope involves bringing the spirit world into the physical world, and the knowingness that comes with this emerging. Elders have visions based on such knowingness and the potentials of such knowing. Hope is an option of the young to be able to dream and to exercise their talents and test themselves,

TABLE 4.
Progressive Abstraction of the Core Concepts with Heuristic Interpretation

Core Concept	Structural Transposition	Conceptual Integration
Transfiguring enlightenment	Numinous vivification	Transforming
Engaging affiliations	Coming together and moving apart	Connecting-separating
Encircling the legendary with fortification	Mythologems unfold unequivocal potency	Languaging powering

Structure

The lived experience of hope is transfiguring enlightenment arising with engaging affiliations, as encircling the legendary surfaces with fortification.

Structural Transposition

The lived experience of hope is numinous vivification in coming together and moving apart as mythologems unfold unequivocal potency.

Conceptual Integration

The lived experience of hope is transforming the connecting-separating in languaging powering.

---

face themselves, and take what they learn and be examples as they mature. Hope involves exercising one's talents and learning, trying, and trying again, not for the benefit of personal gain, but for those who are following and to see how that fits in with those who have gone before. Stone Healer states:

> [H]ope is an opportunity to be a player in the game. Once we have mastered the game, then we move into another level, exactly the same game, but it is something different now. It is almost like parents looking at a leaf through the child's eyes, the first time in a small child. Even though the parents have seen thousands of leaves, have experience in touching many leaves, when that child picks up that leaf and turns it, you, the parents are looking at it in a different way for the first time. Even though you don't physically touch the leaf, you touch it more intensely than when you did physically touch it. Because you touch it with the love of not only experiencing that yourself but with the love of the child.

For each successive generation the experience becomes more intense. There is this knowledge that everything is going to work out. "Hope is reflected in the blossoming child and in the wisdom of the elder; the circle is complete when both experience hope in the other," according to Stone Healer.

Essences: Participant's Language

1. Hope is maturing experiences that lack something; between dreaming dreams and having visions, you bring the spiritual world into the physical world and know that things will work out.
2. Hope is reflected in a blossoming child and in the wisdom of an elder; the circle is tested and complete when both experience hope in the other.
3. Hope is touching with love; it is important channeling and sharing of personal gifts and talents with those who follow and seeing how that fits with those who have gone before.

Essences: Researcher's Language

1. Transfiguring certitude emerges with coalescing the cherished.
2. All-encompassing mutuality arises with the intermingling of näiveté with sagacity.
3. Unconditional engaging with endowments surfaces with recollecting pro-creatory affiliations.

Proposition. The lived experience of hope is transfiguring certitude emerging with coalescing the cherished, as all-encompassing mutuality arises with the intermingling of näiveté with sagacity, while unconditional engaging with endowments surfaces with recollecting procreatory affiliations.

Buffalo Hunter's Story

Buffalo Hunter, 54 years of age, serves as Commissioner for Indian Affairs for the state of South Dakota and oversees the official reconciliation program with the Lakota. He believes that Indians who know the language of the culture can best be in tune with traditional cultural ways of living. For Buffalo Hunter, hope means seeking "a peaceful way of living" that combines all other Native American values, including being broad-minded, having patience and discipline, and accepting things. If you strike out or engage in public debate, the other person has already taken your mind. The closest thing to hope is:

> . . . giving a person life rules to work with and then letting him go out and be expected to make the right decision. You recognize that life situations may make some accomplishments almost impossible, so you experience arrivals along the way with surprise and celebration; you experience the surprise of living on when you thought you were dead.

Hope, for Buffalo Hunter, is "like 'waiting' as relationships move from narrow to broad, where true expectations of finality of decisions and 'what happens happens' are honored, and where you accept responsibility for the good way and its consequences."

Buffalo Hunter speaks further of acceptance as a Lakota way.

I remember my brother. He died of a cerebral hemorrhage. He did not want to go to the hospital. So we just accepted it. Whatever happens happens. He does not want to do it, so that is it. And we waited. It was not like, "Well I hope he makes it, that he lives, I hope." . . . It was just that he had made a decision and whatever decision he made was okay. We will abide by it. There really is a finality in decisions. If you go to the English side and say "Unless he goes to the hospital, he won't have the best chance of living," then this creates kind of false things in you.

Essences: Participant's Language

1. Hope means knowing that no one has taken your cultural mind while you persist in making right decisions that are good and peaceful in starting again surprisingly differently.
2. Hope means waiting without shame as relationships move from narrow to broad, where true expectations of the finality of decisions and "what happens happens" are honored.
3. Hope means giving the person rules to work with and the freedom to make the right decision; it is accepting one's responsibilities and consequences and expecting to do the right thing.

Essences: Researcher's Language

1. Shifting with the new amid steadfast certitude surfaces with a wondering quiet.
2. Anticipation with emerging affiliations expands at one with impudent possibilities.
3. Prevailing venerated symbols awaken the beneficent.

Proposition. The lived experience of hope is shifting with the new amid steadfast certitude that surfaces with a wondering quiet, as anticipation with emerging affiliations expands at one with impudent possibilities, while prevailing venerated symbols awaken the beneficent.

Chaske's Story

Chaske is a 57-year-old man who has been a tribal chairman for a long time. He continues to work on legislation protecting human rights in repatriation, religious freedom, and protection of sacred sites. Chaske speaks of hope as a spiritual oneness where your "heart and mind function simultaneously and it gives you awesome power." Persons with this power can physically change their beings, for example, into animals; in some cases they would use this power in life-giving sacred healing to others, and on rare occasions to "hex" others. Based on the many traumas that the Native Americans have experienced, many have lost the ability to put their mind and heart together, and to be strengthened by spirit helpers. When they can do this again, the power to "shape shift" would be there again and with it the awesome power to do good for others.

As an example, Chaske tells about sundancing and healing. A young girl had gone through chemotherapy, radiation, gone through everything, and the cancer was still there. They had told the girl and the parents that she had ninety days at the most. So the woman brought her daughter to the Sundance on the third day for prayers. She was healed and is now married and has two children. According to Chaske, she was healed because "her heart and mind were functioning simultaneously."

Chaske went on to say:

> Of course, some who came there for prayers died. But the teaching that we listen to from the elders is never to be concerned about whether the prayer or medicine heals or does not heal. It is more important to have the people there for the purpose of prayer than whether the person who is there for the prayers is healed.

As Chaske sums it up, "Hope is a spiritual essence, a spiritual invocation of the heart, and if that is not working, then hope does not exist. Hope is a spiritual concoction that has the help of spirits from many directions; you are made stronger, free of clutter, to live the good way."

Essences: Participant's Language

1. Hope is life-giving sacred energy that comes from spirituality in the heart working with many spirit helpers to strengthen self and others for miraculous healings and form changes.
2. Hope is colors of many directions that helps one stay uncluttered and unscrambled by the mind or mental consternation.
3. Hope is a spiritual invocation of the heart, a spiritual essence, that is alive in a good way and with you all the time, made stronger by sundancing, pipe, and other ceremonies.

Essences: Researcher's Language

1. Metaphysical shifting arises with the vigor of ineffable reverence.
2. Diverse meditative rhythms emerge with a rigorous chosen stance.
3. Engaging venerated symbols surfaces with fortitude amid quietude.

Proposition. The lived experience of hope is a metaphysical shifting that arises with the vigor of ineffable reverence, while diverse meditative rhythms emerge with a chosen stance, as engaging venerated symbols surface with fortitude amid quietude.

Winyan's Story

Winyan is a 77-year-old woman. Now retired, she had been active in numerous capacities in the Indian Health Service and has held key leadership roles within a national Indian women's group. She continues to devote her energies to improving the image of the Indian. For Winyan, hope means being strong enough to set a good example, having surprising successes in jobs, and meeting beautiful people. Life was hard, such as the pain of doctoring a wound with tobacco, but it was also beautiful with respected love for each other in the home. Achieving success involves being good examples as human beings, letting the beauty come forth. Hope means not letting habits keep people from succeeding. They must be on time, complying to the rules and regulations if they are to stay in the workplace. Winyan recalls that "it was a matter of talking all the time to get them there. I was able to help them assimilate, to help them succeed in the predominant culture where the work was."

However, within this struggle, there was and is beauty. The beautiful comes through in their language and the customs and traditions. The hope is in teaching the little ones what traditions are all about, such as give-aways, a ceremony that occurs a year after a loved one dies. The Native Americans teach the children that you can show love and respect by doing this and also that there is a special meaning to it.

Winyan also said that hope comes in surprising ways. For example, a young woman who had cancer was being honored. As Winyan remembers:

> I had been drawn to her because of her cancer, since I had a history of cancer. I had visited her during her last days in the hospital. At the time, I had been feeling badly because she had lost her hair; she had on a stocking cap. However she was so cheerful. And I was going there to cheer her up and it was just turned around. She was the one who cheered me. She was saying that she had a good life and she was not afraid to die. She knew she was not going to get well, and she was eager to meet her Maker. There was a beauty in how she was with her situation. She gave me hope for a better life for all of us . . . and the ability to do the work God has planned for me to continue, to make the beautiful visible.

Essences: Participant's Language

1. Hope is having surprising successes in the job while living with what is rough but what gets healed.
2. Hope means learning the rules and regulations of dominant society and knowing when choices cannot be made according to habits of one's own for the good life.
3. Hope is being strong enough to set a good example while all are living together within customs to make the beautiful visible.

Essences: Researcher's Language

1. Astonishing realization emerges with the arduous.
2. Discerning judgments arise with the disjoining of legendary wisdom.
3. Fortifying treasured expressions with affiliations surface with uncovering the beauteous.

Proposition. The lived experience of hope is an astonishing realization emerging with the arduous, as discerning judgments arise with the disjoining of legendary wisdom, while fortifying treasured expressions with affiliations surface with uncovering the beauteous.

High Eagle's Story

High Eagle, a 65-year-old nun and educator, returned to the reservation after thirty years to found a home for children "whom no one else wants." She continues to grapple with reconciling her Christian religion and her Indian spirituality and is happy in what she is doing. Hope for High Eagle means willingness to give up ever coming home again with a faith in God's promise. If you leave everything, you will have many brothers and sisters, but there will be crosses with it. There will be suffering. She said:

> The most difficult thing was giving up living in a wonderful Christian family. My hope comes from that and in the changes that occurred over the thirty years in the religious order that did permit me to return home. My hope always is that God is present in all of this. . . . My hope is the spirit of family and community where the center of my being is never left without help, rooted in culture and sacred order. There is a resiliency where underlying terrible tragedies happen to people over and over again, but they can come out of it. If given a little bit of help, they can live a happy life.

> Hope is reflected in the image of an eagle soaring. As High Eagle says:

> Sometimes we have forgotten how we have been put into cages with repeated tragedy, raised with chickens, and we do not realize our power, our potential. But once we realize our power and potential, like the spirit of an eagle, we find out that we can fly and know who we really are. When I forget who I really am, who my people are, then the hopeless image that I have is a chicken pecking on the ground. Within the image of soaring is the belief that in the center of who I am and every one of who these children are and in all peoples, God dwells there. Hope is in having the spirit so we can soar; it is God's promise about who we are—that we claim who we are . . . that is the hope that I have. I remember that my grandma was a whole woman. She became a Christian but she still practiced her cultural traditions. Many people like my parents believed that to practice traditions was devil worship. My grandma never did. She knew she met God before she ever became a Christian. I remembered that. There is hope in that, as it shows me that God was always with my people, and that who we are is wonderful. There is hope in reclaiming that; it gives me strength and courage.

Essences: Participant's Language

1. Hope is the resiliency of repeated tragedy and coming out of it to fly and soar like the eagle and know who I really am anew.
2. Hope means bearing the cross of giving up family on God's promise that in doing so one will have many brothers and sisters.
3. Hope is the spirit of community where the center of my being is never left without help rooted in culture and sacred order.

Essences: Researcher's Language

1. Propelling certitude with transfiguring affirmation surfaces amid enduring adversity.
2. Embracing the ponderous covenant arises in yielding with the cherished.
3. Enlivened affiliations emerge with nurturing legendary wisdom.

Proposition. The lived experience of hope is propelling certitude with transfiguring affirmation surfacing amid enduring adversity, while embracing the ponderous covenant arises in yielding with the cherished, as enlivened affiliations emerge with nurturing legendary wisdom.

Charlotte Black Elk's Story

Charlotte, a 45-year-old woman, is the daughter of a renowned Indian of a historic family. Active in environmental issues and an authority in Lakota oral tradition, Charlotte works for the return of the Black Hills to the Sioux Nation. For Charlotte, hope means surviving the pervasive incorporated persecution of a people embodied in the cosmology of the Black Hills.

> The cosmology is "stars with earth sites" that show us all of the sacred sites and ceremonies associated with those sites. There is a connectedness, a continuum, the past, present and the future. It probably is difficult for the average European American or even Afro American to comprehend this continuity, as they have someone in the homeland that is preserving their language so they can be what they choose here. They don't have to know their culture, because someone back home is maintaining it. That is not true for Native Americans. This is our home. If you do not maintain it, endure the persecution, then it does not exist.

Charlotte continues:

> With the young people, there is now an openness, a possessiveness, I guess, of that culture . . . and it is embodied in the cosmology. There is hope for me when I witness the return of children participating in religious ceremonies, both the sacred and teaching ceremonies, at many, many levels. There is hope when there is a complete culture that maintains a relationship where there is the blending of land, experience, and practice. Your culture is tied to the land you are from. You

have people that are complete, who can dream backward as well as dream forward. Hope requires active generational interaction, responsibility, and action from people.

Charlotte relates a story that represents hope for her family:

When Sitting Bull was killed by the Indian police, my great-grand-mother was among his followers. His followers headed out toward the Cheyenne River to where Big Foot's people were. And they walked through snow, on the 15th of December, and the blizzard came through, and they did not have many horses, so the few horses they had, they put the children on them. My great-grandmother was a young woman, and she often told her son how she cried with her tears froze to her face. She cried not just for Sitting Bull having been killed, not just for herself or the harsh winter, but because she wondered if she would ever have children and if she did have children, would her children be able to survive. But more importantly, would the great-grandchildren of her grandchildren ever be Lakota. . . . Then, in 1990 my son made that ride along Big Foot's final journey, and that was one of the stories told when he made that journey. He rode from the 23rd of December and arrived at Wounded Knee on the 28th and then went through the whole "wiping of the tears" ceremony. For our fam-ily, that has been one of our stories of hope. It also is a story that has connected us with the past. The hope that my grandmother and great-grandmother had that her great grandchildren would be Lakota. It required that my father be raised a certain way, that he be told the story, and that my father raise me a certain way, and that I raise my son with those stories. Hope is in this active generational interaction.

Essences: Participant's Language

1. Hope means surviving pervasive incorporated persecution with embodi-ment in the cosmology.
2. Hope is dreaming forward and backward to maintain the possessive con-necting relationship of land, experience, and practice.
3. Hope is showing the responsible continuum of active generational inter-action through culturally sacred and teaching ceremonies.

Essences: Researcher's Language

1. Transfiguring oneness arises with enduring immersion.
2. Shifting anticipations of the was and will-be emerges amid incumbencies.
3. Exposing treasured affiliations arises in perpetuating the venerated.

Proposition. The lived experience of hope is transfiguring oneness arising with enduring immersion, while shifting anticipation of the was and will-be emerges amid incumbencies, as exposing treasured affiliations arises in perpet-uating the venerated.

Ena's Story

Ena, a 47-year-old specialist in pediatrics and internal medicine, has four birth children and one adopted child with fetal alcohol syndrome. She values her strong sense of family, not only parents, sisters, and brothers but also grandparents, uncles, aunts, and cousins. Ena says about hope:

> Hope helps you to think of the future with the positive thoughts from "behind." You are led by the positive thoughts, by what you would wish for "that is good," not in tangible things, but in intangibles. But with children, you help them to understand a wish as something tangible in the future and color it with bright or morning colors. You would describe hope as something tangible that leads you to have an uplifting feeling. Hope is knowing what you are unable to do, do what you can, and don't worry what you cannot do, and then just carrying on, even without the highest degree of elation. Hope involves going from the tangible to the intangible, from developing their own sense of being well enough to think of other senses of being.

Ena tells this story about her family:

> And when I think of my adopted son, I am reminded of other people who have adopted children, and the adoption turned out to be not as they expected. They might have had a child that they thought would be okay and perhaps have some problems, and when the child got older, they were not able to handle the behavior problems that arise and they gave the kid back. I cannot for the life of me understand that. When you adopt someone, you adopt them; if they have problems, you cope with it. If they have to be institutionalized because you could not handle it, fine, you did not fail. It is a problem you could not handle. But you do not give them back. So I teach this emotional type feeling of a familial bond that goes on and on, no matter what. There is hope in that.

There is hope in trying to keep daily life centered around handling everything as it comes along and dealing with it right or wrong. If one makes a mistake, a lesson is learned from it and then the person goes on. And, by having a positive attitude about it, people may be pulled forward by the wishes and dreams. One should never say that anything is totally impossible. According to Ena, hope is "reaching for it with a confidence in yourself, that no matter what happens, you can always keep striving and keep going on. In the end you go with what happens but are uplifted spiritually as you face what happens all along the way."

Essences: Participant's Language

1. Hope is accepting a series of tangible experiences in which you can fail but not be a failure while it gives you an intangible lift.

2. Hope is not worrying about what you cannot do and remembering what you can use for the future, trying to keep life centered around handling what comes.
3. Hope is having positive thoughts from behind as you are being pulled forward by the familial bond of repeating ways.

Essences: Researcher's Language

1. Buoyancy arises in yielding with essentials despite possible futility.
2. Commitment emerges with shifting anticipation of new possibilities.
3. Revelation surfaces with engagements amid the tensions of encircling patterns.

Proposition. The lived experience of hope is a buoyancy in yielding with essentials despite possible futility, as commitment emerges with shifting anticipation of new possibilities, while revelation surfaces with engagements amid the tensions of encircling patterns.

Lakota Man's Story

Lakota Man is a 62-year-old who founded the only Indian-owned weekly newspaper in the United States and provides his syndicated weekly column to more than 300 newspapers nationwide. For Lakota Man, hope is in the surprise of being able to return to his own community and do something to change things that he never dreamed he could do in his entire lifetime. He had always been told that to be successful you had to leave the reservation, leave being an Indian. He explains:

> So to me I can sit here today and wonder how I did it or why I did it, or what pushed me to do it, to allow the turmoil that became part of trying to build the paper, the animosity, the hatred, the violence, that was directed at us as a newspaper at the beginning. And I think that I have reached that point now where the paper is as I had hoped, a paper that can go on without me and continue to serve all the peoples of Indian country nationwide now, and eventually Canada. All my life I wanted to be a writer. I have always believed that the pen was mightier than the sword. So that's been the point of all my hopes in life—to be doing exactly what I am doing right now. . . . I draw hope every week when I write. I use my writing to inspire, to encourage, and I am called to speak at many functions, such as high school graduations and tribal functions. And my message is always one of hope. We cannot do anything about where we have been, we only do something about where we are and where we are going.

Lakota Man believes it is extremely important that the young people know that there are Indians who are doctors, lawyers, journalists, authors, and artists that they can look at and say, "Yes, I would like to do something like that with my life. I would like to become something like these folks are, these people who are also Indian." Lakota Man sees hope as having something to look forward to by having a role model to emulate in making a difference to the community.

One major issue that Lakota Man cites is to help lessen the use of alcohol on the reservations. Lakota Man says:

> Many real strong stories on this issue have been written. And the fact now is that, after all these years, I see people running for elective office on the reservations and running on what they call a sobriety ticket. This is something that I have never seen in my entire life. The young people in the schools on the reservation are marching in protest against alcoholism. This is an example of lessening a major destroyer of our culture and our people, and I think that through our writings and our efforts to inform and educate, we helped bring about this attack against alcoholism, and I guess that we will eventually win. Hope is to return to the culture, to the traditions and spirituality where we were at one time in our history.

Essences: Participant's Language

1. Hope is the surprise of overcoming major destroyers of the culture as astounding facts happen that the participant says he never dreamed could happen in his lifetime.
2. Hope is found in communications that give young people new mentors to emulate and the possibility of eventually winning by getting jobs.
3. Hope is progress toward the goal of returning to the culture, with its original strength and spirituality. It is something to look forward to.

Essences: Researcher's Language

1. Astonishing, unanticipated occurrences arise amid enduring ruin.
2. Shifting ultimate rhythms emerge with nurturing affiliations.
3. Poignant recollections with anticipation surface in reviving legendary wisdom.

Proposition. The lived experience of hope is astonishing, unanticipated occurrences arising amid enduring ruin, as shifting ultimate rhythms emerge with nurturing affiliations, while poignant recollections with anticipation surface in reviving legendary wisdom.

Wacantekiye Win's Story

Wacantekiye Win is a 70-year-old woman who is a school principal on the reservation. She has received honors as an educator and continues to implement creative curricula to incorporate the Lakota culture and a positive self-concept. Hope for Wacantekiye Win is the community finding a way to release the human energy so that talents are tapped and not wasted and so that potential is fulfilled. "It involves a process of raising our standards or 'stand points' in every entity and institution in our little reservation."

Wacantekiye Win notes within the reservation that families are breaking up because of the lack of spiritual teachings. "In homes, you need to be taught to respect other people, no matter what. Then when they come to school, they bring that respect and are not continuously causing a disturbance."

She notes that interdependence in regard to businesses is not developed:

> There is no need for us to go twenty miles to wash or ten miles to buy milk. We could do it here. Instead we have an environment where there is much jealousy that we do not let each other succeed. We tear down more than we build. When children live in this environment, they see this, and they will do this. Schools can help students with positive actions, but it takes a return to the value of cooperation by the community and to electing talented leaders who are visionary and live a life of full respect to all living and nonliving things.

Wacantekiye Win sees hope for the children to change and to become truly successful, first-class citizens, and not being prone to saying "Okay, lower the standards; somebody wants the job."

She points to a problem in their limited English proficiency:

> Many families do not use Lakota language in the home, and they are not so good at English either. So we do a lot of discussions to increase vocabulary and increase their utilization of English. Since we have to go into the dominant culture, our schools have a role to play in releasing the talents that so many of our children have. We send some good students to our neighboring public schools, but somehow or someway they never get on the honor roll no matter how they try. When I talk to them, they say, "It is English; it is English." So I say, "Okay, you need to study a bit more of English. You need to read more and increase your vocabulary." This year we had two students that got on the honor roll. I was extremely happy. That was a desired feeling that I had. It continues to be my hope and dream that the children's talents can be released and they can find themselves successful among their counterparts, feeling that their Lakota stuff is just as good as the white person's.

Essences: Participant's Language

1. Hope is struggling with stand points to success, from being second-class citizens to releasing the energy to become first-class citizens.
2. Hope is the interdependence of family, school, and businesses while taking positive action to let go of bickering with community.
3. Hope is bringing back a selection of leaders with right attitudes, religious entities, and spiritual teachings.

Essences: Researcher's Language

1. Spirited fruition emerges in shifting arduous positionings.
2. Essential mutuality arises with the yielding of acrimony.
3. Elevating preferred polestars surfaces with prized legendary wisdom.

Proposition. The lived experience of hope is a spirited fruition emerging with shifting arduous positionings, as essential mutuality arises with the yielding of acrimony, while elevating preferred polestars surfaces with prized legendary wisdom.

FINDINGS AND RELATED LITERATURE

The stories and findings in this study speak to the human condition. As Arendt (1958) notes, the human condition is where a life of action has humanness in relationships as the highest good, and gives the most mortal thing, human life, a position with the cosmos, of immortality. Native Americans seek the good life, value relationships, and relate the connection of all life to the universe.

For the Native Americans in this study, hope is a *transfiguring enlightenment arising with engaging affiliations as encircling the legendary surfaces with fortification.* A discussion of each of the three core concepts follows.

Transfiguring Enlightenment

In this study, the *transfiguring enlightenment* is *numinous vivification*, which is *transforming.* (See Table 1.) There is a oneness with human-cosmic connections. According to Parse (1981), transforming is the changing of change, with a person increasing in diversity while integrating new discoveries and continuously becoming the not-yet. It is a shift to a different vantage point; it is self-initiated and creative.

In this study it was found that participants made choices to be in "readiness" for change, but the actual "shifting moment" often came as a surprise. One participant, for example, says that "hope is the surprise of overcoming major destroyers of the culture as astounding facts happen that I never dreamed could happen in my entire lifetime." In accordance with Parse's third principle (1998), transforming is a deliberate shift in one's way of viewing the familiar. The meaning changes as the different perspectives shed new light on the situation. In this study the participants experienced a shift to new viewpoints and, in so doing, could not return to viewing the situation in the old way; rather, they shifted "in the new light" to other possibilities. One participant describes this shifting: "Hope is listening above the jungle with expansive sight for a beginning understanding of the meaning of life while letting go of stupid worries in order to be truly free." Another participant speaks of hope as "shape shifting" where people can change themselves physically to an animal, bird, or tree—to whatever they want to change themselves into.

Authors such as Maslow (1971) speak of "small mystical experiences, moments of ecstasy" (p. 48) in which there are qualitative jumps in normal modes of perceiving . . . where one experiences an ultimate holism with the cosmos. A participant says, "Hope means surviving . . . and being embodied in the cosmology. The cosmology is 'stars with earth sites' that show us all the sacred sites and ceremonies associated with those sites. There is a connectedness, a continuum, the past, present, and the future, not only in land but in experience and practices." Another participant, speaking of hope, said it "gives you awesome power" so that you bring forth "a resiliency of repeated tragedy and come out of it to fly and soar like the eagle and know anew who [you] really [are]."

Engaging Affiliations

In this study, *engaging affiliations* is the coming together and moving apart in *connecting-separating.* (See Table 2.) The paradoxical rhythm of connecting-separating is being with and apart from others, ideas, objects, and situations all-at-once (Parse, 1998). The rhythms of engaging affiliations, according to the participants, require handling what comes, and these are often arduous and feel like crosses to bear. Yet helpers of many directions also come in colors and inspire "dreaming forward and backward." The engagements described by the participants involved actions not unlike what Arrien (1993) has described as the paths of the warrior, teacher, healer, and visionary. Such paths involve universal essentials such as the following: showing up, or choosing to be present; paying attention to what has heart and meaning; telling the truth without blame or judgment; and being open rather than attached to outcome. Not claiming these essentials brings forth what Arrien (1993) describes as the shadow. The shadow is what a person does not yet know, which is partly personal and partly collective and which brings concomitant difficult struggles, tiring failures, and inanity or emptiness. The possibilities in claiming the essentials in engaging affiliations is like learning the essentials of brushwork to become a painter:

> A youth who likes to study will in the end succeed. To begin with he should know that there are Six Essentials in painting. The first is called spirit; the second, rhythm; the third, thought; the fourth, scenery; the fifth, the brush; and the last is the ink. (Ching Hao, fl. 925)

Among these essentials is the essential of rhythm. Amid the rhythm of engaging affiliations, however, "life has its tricksters," not unlike those described by Sneve (1997) who weave webs of trickery and deceit that confound the journey. Life also has its bullies, who condition whole enclaves of other human beings to commit large-scale cruelty (Bly, 1996). Persons may also for a time be "paralyzed" by sloth, a sort of living death, where even with great pain they cannot say, "That is enough" and redirect life accordingly (Bettelheim, 1960). In life there are also persons with great desire, *wachea*, and fortitude, *wachta*, for connective knowing (Brokenleg, 1997). Likewise, as Woodman and Dickson (1996) say, life includes those who "marry reason and order to creativity, and embrace the chaos that can ultimately lead to wisdom and transformation."

According to Parse (1981), connecting-separating involves a rhythmical pattern of relating where a person is connecting with one phenomenon and simultaneously separating from others. In separating from one affiliation and dwelling with another, a person integrates thought, becomes more diverse, and seeks new unions. In this study, the participants had a great desire for engaging affiliations the right way, for not feeling a failure when failing to make right affiliations, and for learning through intergenerational connecting.

Encircling the Legendary with Fortification

In this study, *encircling the legendary with fortification* is *mythologems unfolding unequivocal potency* in *languaging powering*. (See Table 3.) Native Americans perceive and live life in a circular way, as opposed to a linear way. The circle is no formula for living per se, but it keeps them close to "divine" power. According to Deloria (1974), "Life's sequences relate to the integrity of the circle, not the directional determination of the line. It encompasses, it does not point" (p. 12). The circle fortifies that which is treasured, but it does not require it. Native Americans have the freedom to conceptualize religion in individual ways and do so (Atwood, 1991). Thereby, religious and cultural mythologems unfold unequivocal potency. An example of a mythologem among Native Americans is that the spirit entities take on specific heritages for teaching purposes. Such legendary mythologems and ceremonies are languaged through ritual, song, dance, and art to encompass and fortify that which is most valued and treasured. These entities were further described by participants in this study when they spoke of "familial bonds," being "pulled forward by repeating ways" and "looking forward and returning to the culture."

According to Parse (1998), people in close association who have common ties and interests cocreate and perpetuate language and living patterns; thus, although unique realities are structured by each individual, these are cocreated through mutual process with others. Languaging is reflective of the interconnectedness of humans from generation to generation (Gadamer, 1993; Hall, 1976). Speaking–being-silent and moving–being-still are two paradoxical processes of languaging (Parse, 1992) and are signs or symbols expressing meaning (Sapir, 1966). Powering, according to Parse (1998), is a continuous rhythmical process incarnating intentions and actions in moving with possibilities. Pushing-resisting is an essential rhythm of powering all-at-once "in every moment of life in all relations of all beings" (Tillich, 1954, p. 42). Since human orientation is toward the future, powering is fundamental to being (Tillich, 1954). Languaging powering is the abstract construct that best describes encircling the legendary with fortification. It is speaking–being-silent and moving–being-still arising with the all-at-once pressing on as the legendary incarnates the will-be.

The traditions of the Native Americans in this study, whether in the form of sacred ceremonies or in cultural teachings, represent valued intentions and actions that inspire creatively moving with the future. The traditions have their own pushing-resisting patterns where "waiting" is almost like hope itself, as is honoring the "finality of decisions" in letting whatever happens happen.

For Native American participants, the human condition is a search for the "good way." The stories and findings of this study on the meaning of hope express an invisible mystery at the center of every life, much like Hillman's (1996) fundamental question, "What is it, in my heart, that I must do, be, and have? And why?" Jung as quoted in Hillman (1996) says, "In the final analysis, we count for something only because of the essential we embody, and if we do not embody that, life is wasted" (p. x). The essential emerges in the copresence of the today, yesterday, and tomorrow with a timelessness that surfaces "backward as well as forward" meanings in life stories (Hillman, 1996). Native Americans in this study see hope as something more than the illusion of the individual living a plot written by a genetic code, ancestral heredity, traumatic occasions, parental unconsciousness, or societal accidents.

The meaning of hope is lived, as participants have put it, "in dreaming forward and backward, in experiencing guidance from the spirits of many directions, and in living out the unique gifts of personhood, not for personal gain but for those who follow and to see how that fits in with those that have gone before." Their knowing comes not by knowledge alone but by wisdom. The expression of the wisdom in regard to hope lifts them and the reader to a higher plane of existence.

The meaning of hope for Native Americans is likely to overlap with descriptions of other groups of participants. The researcher was somewhat surprised by the participants' language being at such a high level of discourse from the start. Perhaps the high level of abstraction is related to the fact that the ideals that pervade the thought and life of the people of the Sioux Nation uplift universal connectedness.

Research and practice implications drawn from the findings, along with the findings from the other studies reported here, will be discussed in the final chapter of this book.

References

Arendt, H. (1958). *The human condition.* Chicago: The University of Chicago Press.

Arrien, A. (1993). *The four-fold way: Walking the paths of the warrior, teacher, healer and visionary.* New York: HarperCollins.

Atwood, M. D. (1991). *Spirit healing: Native American magic and medicine.* New York: Sterling.

Bettelheim, B. (1960). *The informed heart.* Glencoe, IL: Free Press.

Bly, C. (1996). *Changing the bully who rules the world: Reading and thinking about ethics.* Minneapolis, MN: Milkweed Editions.

Bray, B. (1997). In A. Garrod & C. Larimore (Eds.), *First person, first peoples: Native American college graduates tell their stories.* Ithaca, NY: Cornell University Press.

Brokenleg, M. (April 30, 1997). *Response—Hope: Native American Study,* Bush Faculty Luncheon Presentation, Augustana College, Sioux Falls, SD.

Deloria, V. (1974). Foreword. In R. K. Dodge & J. B. McCullough, *Voices from WaH'Kon-taH: Contemporary poetry of Native Americans.* New York: International Publishers.

Doll, D. (1994). *Vision quest: Men, women and sacred sites of the Sioux nation.* New York: Crown Publishers.

Gadamer, H.-G. (1993). *Truth and method* (2nd rev. ed.) (Translation revised by J. Weinsheimer & D. G. Marshall). New York: Continuum.

Gustafson, F. R. (1997). *Dancing between two worlds: Jung and the Native American soul.* Mahwah, NJ: Paulist Press.

Hall, E. T. (1976). *Beyond culture.* Garden City, NY: Doubleday/Anchor.

Hao, C. (fl. 925). Notes on brushwork. From *The spirit of the brush* (Shio Sakanishi, Trans.). [Wisdom of the East Series, 1957].

Hillman, J. (1996). *The soul's code: In search of character and calling.* New York: Random House.

Maslow, A. H. (1971). *The farther reaches of human nature* (2nd ed.). New York: Viking.

Parse, R. R. (1981). *Man-living-health: A theory of nursing.* New York: Wiley.

Parse, R. R. (1992). Human becoming: Parse's theory of nursing. *Nursing Science Quarterly, 5,* 35–42.

Parse, R. R. (1998). *The human becoming school of thought.* Thousand Oaks, CA: Sage.

Sapir, E. (1966). *Culture, language, and personality.* Berkeley: University of California Press.

Sneve, V. D. H. (1989). I watched an eagle soar. In V. D. H. Sneve & S. Gammell, *Dancing teepees: Poems of American Indian youth.* New York: Holiday House.

Sneve, V. D. H. (1997). *The trickster and the troll.* Lincoln, NE: University of Nebraska Press.

Tillich, P. (1954). *Love, power, and justice.* New York: Oxford University Press.

Woodman, M., & Dickson, E. (1996). *Dancing in the flames.* Boston: Shambhala.

Chapter 15

Hope for American Women with Children

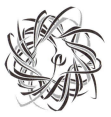

LYNN ALLCHIN-PETARDI

P A R T I C I P A N T S

Women with children were chosen as a participant group for this research because of the personal interest of the researcher. The women had some things in common: Each was a mother, was 30 years old or older, lived in the United States, knew the researcher, and was eager to participate and talk about hope in her life. Each woman's situation was also unique. Some women were married, some divorced. Several had four children; at least half had only two. One woman's children were adopted. Several participants lived in the South, several in the Midwest, and two in the East. They were similar but unique and each told a story of hope in her life.

D I A L O G I C A L   E N G A G E M E N T

The dialogical engagements took place in quiet places convenient to both the participant and the researcher. The dialogues were audiorecorded. A few times the taping was stopped while the participant shed tears and then was restarted when she was ready to continue. What surfaced in each dialogue was a personal expression of each participant's experience of hope. The name of each participant has been changed to protect her privacy.

E X T R A C T I O N - S Y N T H E S I S

Abby's Story

Abby is a mother of four who voluntarily left her job after her first child was born. She has continued to work as a freelance writer and has dedicated time and energy to a national women's organization. She helped start the local chapter of this organization in her hometown. Abby lives in a large midwestern city with her husband and four children under the age of 10. Hope for Abby is like a wish or a prayer; it is something she does when she feels she has no control over the situation, when she can't change something. She has a friend with ovarian cancer, and Abby hopes for this friend's well-being but realizes she really has "no control over that." Abby doesn't say "hope" a lot; she prefers to take action. "To take care of something, like I'm not just going to hope things turn out well. I'm going to work on that. . . . It seems like an inactive thing, to hope." Hope is like prayer too, but Abby thinks only very important things should be prayed for. "Sometimes I think: well, don't rely on God. Take care of that yourself. Go to Him for the big stuff." According to Abby, people with hope are more positive than people with no hope. People with hope "think things will work out." She also thinks hope is always present, even if you don't recognize it; people are always hoping things are going to work out.

Essences: Participant's Language

1. Hope is like a wish or a prayer, something the participant does when she has no control over something, when she can't change something. Hoping

is what you do when there is nothing else you can do. It is inactive; alone hope doesn't change much.
2. People with hope are more positive than people with no hope. If one has no hope that things will work out, then one is depressed.
3. Hope is always present and it may be unconscious and subtle, but it is always there.

Essences: Researcher's Language

1. A longing arises amid formidable ambiguous futility.
2. Optimistic expectancy emerges with the despair of inexpectancy.
3. Persistent envisaging surfaces at many realms.

Proposition. Hope is a longing arising amid formidable ambiguous futility, as optimistic expectancy emerges with the despair of inexpectancy, as persistent envisaging surfaces at many realms.

Bonnie's Story

Bonnie is a very busy mother of two elementary school–aged children. She is employed full-time and attends graduate school on a part-time basis. She lives with her husband and children near a large midwestern city. Hope is always present for Bonnie. Because in daily life there are many unknowns, Bonnie is always, on every level, hoping for her family's happiness, health, and productivity. These are the important parts of her life and what she hopes for most. Bonnie also has "concerns for the profession that I have taken such sacrifices for." She is hopeful that as more nurses are educated at an advanced level the profession will be enhanced. Hoped-for outcomes are worth working toward. Whether the outcome is to have children who are "good productive citizens" or a profession that is "person-centered," Bonnie strives each day to make these things happen.

Essences: Participant's Language

1. Hope is being with family and others in a way that models goodness and caring.
2. Hope is ever-present and pervasive in the participant's life. In an era of uncertainty and many unsavory influences, it is a wishing for happiness, health, and productivity.

Essences: Researcher's Language

1. Inspiration arises with benevolent connections.
2. Persistent envisaging of contented accomplishments emerges amid repugnant ambiguity.

Proposition. Hope is an inspiration arising with benevolent connections, as persistent envisaging of contented accomplishments emerges amid repugnant ambiguity.

Claire's Story

Claire is the mother of two children and has recently returned to work full time. She and her husband have lived apart for several years and she has started divorce proceedings. Claire is actively involved with her community and church and helped start a local chapter of a national women's organization. She lives with her two young children in a large midwestern city. Hope for Claire comes from inside herself. "I try not to put too much hope in other people; I try to keep it more on what I can do." She prefers to work on her own to get things done. Claire is a strong, self-sufficient woman who does not like to depend on others because of past incidences when others have let her down or not followed through on something she had wanted to happen. "If you lose hope you can find hope again, and if you're hopeful, you can lose it somewhere down the line and be disappointed." She thinks she must be realistic about what can and cannot be done in any given situation. People who "have no hope, have nothing," according to Claire, and she is unsure whether she has ever had hope in her life.

Essences: Participant's Language

1. Hope comes from inside the participant and rests with her, as others don't give her hope. She consistently relies on herself, and being realistic about what can and cannot be done helps alleviate disappointment.
2. If one has hope, it can be lost; if one loses hope, it can be found again.
3. If you have no hope, you have nothing, yet the participant is unsure whether or not she has ever had hope in her life.

Essences: Researcher's Language

1. Personal affirmation emerges with easing discontentedness.
2. Expectancy arises as an all-at-once surfacing and dissipating.
3. Envisaging surfaces with shadows of vacuous ambiguity.

Proposition. Hope is a personal affirmation emerging with easing discontentedness as an all-at-once surfacing and dissipating expectancy arises with envisaging amid shadows of vacuous ambiguity.

Donna's Story

Donna is the divorced mother of two high school–aged children. She works full time and attends graduate school on a part-time basis. She lives with her children in a suburban area of a large midwestern city. Hope doesn't appear in Donna's life "unless there is something negative I want to hope to change." Hope means something bad has happened to cause Donna to want to change that for the better. For Donna, hope can be associated with the terribly bad things in life like finding a loved one not breathing. Hope can also be associated with the really insignificant incidents in life, such as buying hosiery that won't run. Donna cannot just hope for something to occur or change, however. Once the situation presents itself and she figures out what she wants, Donna will hope for that outcome and work to make it happen. She feels "like I kind of have to make that outcome happen to the degree that I can." She sees hope tied to dreams and wishes, and one must do some planning to make them come true. Things won't "happen by just sitting there and wishing it would happen. . . . You try to find out ways to help that hope, that dream, to come true or that vision to come true." Donna feels she must act and work toward what she hopes will happen.

Essences: Participant's Language

1. The impetus for hope is uncertainty when something negative and frightening happens that the participant wants to change to a positive direction.
2. Hope is an action thing that the participant sees as tied to dreams and wishes, in degrees or steps. First, she figures out what she wants, then she hopes for it, and, finally, she helps that hope to come true. She just can't hope and not act.
3. Hope is associated with really big things, like life and death, or really little things, something that is not important. Hope can be used to deny the reality of things.

Essences: Researcher's Language

1. Ambiguous possibles emerge with disconcerting alarm.
2. Contemplating with a vision arises with the resolute.
3. Persistent expectancy surfaces with varied perspectives.

Proposition. Hope is a persistent expectancy surfacing with varied perspectives, as contemplating with vision arises with the resolute, while ambiguous possibilities emerge with disconcerting alarm.

Emma's Story

Emma is a divorced mother of three children. She works full time in the healthcare field. She lives in a suburban area of a large midwestern city. Emma equates "hope with something that happens when you are faced with a negative outcome or an adverse circumstance, and hope is the thing that sees you through that negative time." She says people use hope to see "some improvement in the future from . . . the present circumstances." Emma's life has been blessed with minimal adversity, plus she has had the confidence that things will work themselves out and be all right. She believes "you make what happens for you. You create your future and hoping seems more passive to me." She thinks people use hope when they don't have the strength or ability to do something about their circumstances.

Essences: Participant's Language

1. Hope happens when the participant is faced with adverse circumstances, and it sees her through negative times as she is able to see some improvement in the future.

2. Hope is passive, yet the participant has confidence that things will be all right for her as she makes things happen for herself.

Essences: Researcher's Language

1. Expectancy emerges with formidable ambiguity amid possible amelioration.
2. Certitude surfaces with resolute perseverance.

Proposition. Hope is an expectancy emerging with formidable ambiguity amid possible amelioration, as certitude surfaces with resolute perseverance.

Fran's Story

Fran lives in a small city in the South with her husband and their four young children. She stopped working after the birth of her first child and currently works part time. She is active in her children's school and the community where she lives. Fran relates hope to major events in her life: marriage, graduate school, children, and crises. She hoped she could complete graduate school. She hoped her marriage was the right decision, that she would be happy. Fran has hoped for each of her children as they were born, hoped for their health and well-being. Hope for Fran is more than just an everyday wish for things to occur. She thinks of hope "as more of a deeper, more yearning desire for things than just an everyday wish for things to occur." Fran uses hope when she has no way of controlling an event or crisis. When faced with a situation that she says "is attainable through my own actions, I pretty much am thinking I can figure out how to do that, and I take steps to reach those goals I hope for." If she thinks she cannot work toward what is hoped for, she frequently will ask God for help in obtaining it.

Essences: Participant's Language

1. Hope is related to major events in life like graduate school, marriage, children, and crises; it is a deep yearning desire and not just an everyday wish for things to occur.
2. Hope is used when there is uncertainty and no way for the participant to actually control things. On the other hand, if she thinks something is attainable through her own actions, she tries to do that.

Essences: Researcher's Language

1. Expectancy arises with the notable as heartfelt longings.
2. Diligent perseverance surfaces amid formidable ambiguity.

Proposition. Hope is an expectancy arising with the notable in heartfelt longings as diligent perseverance surfaces amid formidable ambiguity.

Gayle's Story

Gayle is the mother of two young children. She and her husband live in a suburban area in the East. Gayle does not work outside the home but is very active in her church and community. Hope for Gayle occurs when she has no control over a situation. She likes to plan, to take control, but on occasion, this is not possible. There have been times when Gayle could not have control over a situation, when she felt she could not make things better. At these uncertain times she turns to hope. Gayle feels a certainty in her hope since her hope comes from God. "Because of that, my hope is not something I'm hoping is going to happen, but I'm certain is going to happen." Life events have led Gayle to turn her fears and desires over to God and to trust that He will provide. Things have worked out for Gayle in ways she "never could have envisioned" because she trusts God to fulfill her hopes.

Essences: Participant's Language

1. When troubled times occur for the participant, hope is not a wishful anticipation but a comforting certainty, because she has accepted the promises of Christ and the Scriptures into her life.
2. Knowing what she is going to do and being in control is important for the participant. When she has been out of control and has known there was no way for her to gain control, she has given her unsureness of things over to hope.

Essences: Researcher's Language

1. Solace emerges with steadfast envisaging of the divine.
2. Expectancy arises with the ebb and flow of changing possibles amid ambiguity.

Proposition. Hope is an expectancy arising with the ebb and flow of changing possibles amid ambiguity, while solace emerges with steadfast envisaging of the divine.

Hilda's Story

Hilda is married and has two elementary school–aged children. They live in a semi-rural area outside a large southern city. Hilda is in the process of starting a business from her home. She is active in her children's schools and her community. Hope for Hilda is looking to desired ideals in her life that she wants "to be closer to in terms of being happier, more satisfied," and being able to work toward those ideals. She talks about a time in her life when she was very dissatisfied with herself. At that point she decided to take steps to ensure that she obtained what she hoped for herself. She knew what she wanted and worked to change herself. She worked to change her life to reach her ideal, her hoped-for goals. The active participation of working toward a hoped-for ideal gives Hilda a sense of control over her life. She sees what she has, sees what she wants, what she hopes for, and then takes steps to reach that hoped-for goal. She sees this as "hopefulness in the sense I can take action to change things. I have a sense of control over my life and something to strive for." The hope helps Hilda to "keep going and keep working toward" her ideal.

Essences: Participant's Language

1. When the participant's life held uncertainties, she looked at ideals and took actions to change her life in the way she wanted it to go. For her, hope is traveling toward her ideals, and changing her life for the better, and this gives her a sense of control over her life.
2. Hope is reaching a strived-for goal.

Essences: Researcher's Language

1. Expectancy arises with the resolute perseverance of clarifying ambiguity.
2. Inspiration surfaces with attainment of the envisaged.

Proposition. Hope is an inspiration surfacing with attainment of the envisaged, as expectancy arises with the resolute perseverance of clarifying ambiguity.

Irma's Story

Irma is a divorced mother of two grown children. She has been working as a professional and lives in a large urban area in the South. Irma views hope as a paradox in that "it does conjure up a lot of sadness because it has been very difficult; it's a struggle and yet with that sadness there's also a real joy and a balance between those two. But there is definite sadness, so hope, it conjures up a lot of sadness." This sadness is pervasive, but it is balanced with "contentment and satisfaction." For Irma, it is hope that drives her forward. She grew up in a family that expected her to carry on a very traditional female role: wife and mother. Irma always wanted more than this. Hoping for a different future helped move her forward into a future that she views as more satisfying. Hope is also seen as faith by Irma. She thinks God will help her see opportunities and be open to them.

Essences: Participant's Language

1. Hope is a paradox; it has both a negative and positive connotation. It brings up a pervasive sadness but also brings joy.
2. Hope is a process of reaching beyond; it has been a driving force of moving the participant forward into a future that at times she could not define.
3. Hope leads to a faith that the participant can become whatever she was meant to be, a faith that God will help her see and be open to opportunities and learning.

Essences: Researcher's Language

1. Expectancy emerges with the elated and sorrowful all-at-once.
2. Propelling with the possibles surfaces amid formidable ambiguity.
3. Aspirations arise with divine certitude.

Proposition. Hope is an expectancy emerging with the elated and sorrowful all-at-once, as propelling with the possibles surfaces amid formidable ambiguity, while aspirations arise with divine certitude.

Jenna's Story

Jenna is a married mother of two, living with her family in a suburban area in the East. Jenna has always worked full time in her profession, taking time off only after the birth of each child. Hope for Jenna "is woven into my daily existence" and is "the belief that there will be another chance, another opportunity, something might improve." During crises, Jenna tries to "reframe" the obstacle, thinking "tomorrow is another day or maybe I can try doing it another way." She is hoping that things will work out the way she wants them to. Hope has enabled Jenna to face her crises and look toward the next day even in her most difficult times. At times Jenna has had no hope and this has been horrible. "It is like falling into a black grease pit which is incredibly hard to climb out of." Usually, though, she is able to have hope for a better situation. Jenna says she feels lucky in that "somehow I am able to have hope at my most difficult times." The hope may be "slow in kicking in; so far it has never failed me."

Essences: Participant's Language

1. Hope is woven into the participant's daily existence; she believes there will always be another chance, another opportunity for improvement, or that things will work out the way she wants them to.
2. Hope enables the participant to face crises and look forward to the next day, and it helps her keep going even in the most difficult times.
3. When the participant has hope, she is able to work toward what she wants, but when she has no hope, it's like falling into a black grease pit.

Essences: Researcher's Language

1. Integral promise arises with the certitude of amelioration of the ambiguous.
2. Expectancy amid the arduous surfaces with perseverance.
3. Envisaging coveted achievements emerges amid vacuous despair.

Proposition. Hope is an expectancy amid the arduous surfacing with perseverance, as an integral promise arises with the certitude of amelioration of ambiguity, while envisaging coveted achievements emerges amid vacuous despair.

FINDINGS AND RELATED LITERATURE

Three core concepts are evident in the ten propositions: *envisaging possibles, resolute perseverance,* and *formidable ambiguity.* Table 1 shows the core concepts, the structure, and heuristic interpretation in progressive levels of abstraction.

The core concept of *envisaging possibles* was apparent in each participant dialogue, story, and proposition. In her own unique way each participant expressed her view of the possibles considering the was, is, and will-be all-at-once. Envisaging possibles at the theoretical level is imaging (Parse, 1981, 1992, 1995).

TABLE 1.
Progressive Abstraction of Core Concepts with Heuristic Interpretation

Core Concepts	Structural Transposition	Conceptual Integration
Envisaging possibles	Contemplating potentials	Imaging
Resolute perseverance	Tenacious abiding	Powering
Formidable ambiguity	Arduous diversity	Enabling-limiting originating

Structure

The lived experience of hope is envisaging possibles with resolute perseverance amid formidable ambiguity.

Structural Transposition

Hope is contemplating potentials with tenacious abiding amid arduous diversity.

Conceptual Integration

Hope is imaging the powering of enabling-limiting originating.

Participants described their lives in light of looking for desired ideals, hoping for different futures, and looking forward even in difficult times. They gave unique meaning to the now as it related to the was and will-be. Envisaging possibilities was uniquely evident in each participant proposition as follows:

1. optimistic expectancy emerges . . . as . . . envisaging surfaces
2. envisaging of contented accomplishments emerges
3. expectancy arises with envisaging
4. contemplating with a vision arises
5. expectancy emerging
6. expectancy arising
7. expectancy arising with envisaging
8. attainment of the envisaged as expectancy arises
9. expectancy emerging
10. envisaging coveted achievements emerges

Envisaging possibilities, integrated as *imaging*, is coming to know the explicit-tacit all-at-once. It is a coming to know the will-be as what is known and what is unknown surface simultaneously. In her study of the lived experience of hope, Parse (1990) conceptualized anticipating possibilities through envisioning the not-yet as imaging. Her participants "persistently pictured alternative ways of becoming" (p. 15), just as the participants in this study did. Both groups of participants spoke of various possibles in the not-yet. Imaging is viewing the will-be in light of the present, as each participant uniquely comes to understand his/her situation and what is hoped for. Bunkers's (1998) study about considering tomorrow for women who are homeless conceptualized the core concept contemplating desired endeavors as imaging. Bunkers states, "Contemplating desired endeavors is creating actuality out of possibility in living the now with hopes and dreams of the not-yet" (p. 59). Participants in both studies shared their thoughts and hopes about the not-yet and how they looked at new ways of being in the not-yet.

The core concept of *resolute perseverance* was also apparent in all ten participant dialogues, stories, and propositions. Each participant spoke about working toward her hoped-for goal. At times the notion of perseverance is very clearly stated by participants and at other times it is stated more subtly. Perseverance can be thought of as a pushing onward, striving, or propelling with what is hoped for. Resolute perseverance at the theoretical level is *powering* (Parse, 1981, 1992, 1995). Powering is a forging onward and a continuous unfolding (Parse, 1981) as one moves beyond the now and contemplates and ventures with the will-be. Resolute perseverance was stated uniquely for each participant as follows:

1. persistent
2. persistent
3. personal affirmation
4. persistent
5. resolute perseverance
6. diligent perseverance
7. emerges with steadfast
8. resolute perseverance
9. propelling with the possibles
10. surfacing with perseverance

Resolute perseverance as powering is inherent to being. Powering is the way individuals move from the now with the not-yet. As these women hoped for certain things within a situation, they looked at what was and what could be, as they saw it, and moved in unique directions to reach what was desired. Powering is seen in the core concept of directing intentions to nurture in Mitchell and Heidt's (1994) study about the lived experience of wanting to help another. Mitchell and Heidt indicated that powering was related to how the participants decided to live with others. Powering is described as "turning toward the not-yet in light of possibilities, intentions, fears, and hopes" (p. 124). Participants in both research studies viewed the present, as it was known to them, and looked to the not-yet. In this study, participants viewed a variety of ways that their own situations could turn, but each looked to the not-yet and what was desired.

The last core concept, *formidable ambiguity*, was also present in each participant dialogue, story, and proposition. This concept can be viewed as the participants' ability to view their difficult situations in more than one way. The particular situation was unique for each participant, but all situations were identified as personally insurmountable and all-at-once surmountable as each participant knew there was more than one path to move beyond the ambiguity. As participants dwelled with their circumstance, each sorted through the ambiguity. Among the varied ways each situation could flow were opportunities and restrictions for each participant. The opportunities were not always clearly evident to the participant, nor were the inherent restrictions that occur when opportunities arise. In deciding which opportunity to pursue, and which restriction to live with, participants lived with the certainty of what they hoped for and the uncertainty of what their choices would entail in the will-be. As choices were made to create anew, participants were both enabled and limited by their decisions to be one way or another with their situation. Participants chose the direction they wanted to move, thereby limiting movement in another direction. Formidable ambiguity at the theoretical level is *enabling-limiting originating* (Parse, 1981, 1992, 1995). Enabling-limiting is a rhythmical pattern where each participant chooses a direction in which to move and, simultaneously, chooses to limit movement in another direction. Originating is the process of unfolding, that is, creating new ways of living. Of the two paradoxes coexisting within originating, certainty-uncertainty surfaced in this research.

In certainty-uncertainty, participants made clear their intention in the situations while simultaneously living the ambiguity of unknown outcomes. Enabling-limiting originating, then, is the process of living the opportunities and all-at-once restrictions with the certainty-uncertainty in creating anew. As participants experienced events in their lives, they lived their valued choices, often certain of their values but uncertain of what their valued choices would entail in the will-be. Formidable ambiguity was stated uniquely for each participant as follows:

1. formidable ambiguous futility
2. repugnant ambiguity
3. vacuous ambiguity
4. ambiguous possibles
5. formidable ambiguity amid possible amelioration
6. heartfelt longings . . . surface amid formidable ambiguity
7. ebb and flow of changing possibles amid ambiguity
8. clarifying ambiguity
9. formidable ambiguity
10. certitude of the amelioration of the ambiguous

Formidable ambiguity, integrated as enabling-limiting originating, is the process of humans moving in a chosen direction as they create anew. Here, participants chose a hoped-for direction, while simultaneously restricting themselves in other directions, as they worked to make a new way for themselves and others. Mitchell (1990), in her study of the lived experience of taking life day by day in later life, describes glimpsing a diminishing now amidst expanding possibles as enabling-limiting. Mitchell identifies enabling-limiting as her "participants contemplated options and possible consequences of decisions faced in everyday relating with others" (p. 34). Participants in both studies contemplated their unique options and possible consequences as they alone saw them. As participants viewed options and made choices, they were simultaneously enabled to move in one direction and limited to move in other directions in creating new ways of becoming. Participants in this study gracefully acknowledged the fact that as they hoped for specific ways, other ways were, sometimes gladly, closed or lost to them.

In Bunkers's (1998) study of considering tomorrow, participants described resilient endurance amid disturbing unsureness as originating. She stated that resilient endurance amid disturbing unsureness "involves knowing and not-knowing one's possibilities and moving with the not-yet in confidence while pausing with the realization of unpredictability" (p. 61). Originating is a continuous process of inventing different ways of being, and, in this regard, both groups of participants describe choosing new ways from what is known and unknown all-at-once.

Implications for research and practice are discussed in the final chapter of this book.

REFERENCES

Bunkers, S. S. (1998). Considering tomorrow: Parse's theory-guided research. *Nursing Science Quarterly, 11,* 56–63.

Mitchell, G. J. (1990). The lived experience of taking life day-by-day in later life: Research guided by Parse's emergent method. *Nursing Science Quarterly, 3,* 29–36.

Mitchell, G. J., & Heidt, P. (1994). The lived experience of wanting to help another: Research with Parse's method. *Nursing Science Quarterly, 7,* 119–127.

Parse, R. R. (1981). *Man-living-health: A theory of nursing.* New York: Wiley.

Parse, R. R. (1990). Parse's research methodology with an illustration of the lived experience of hope. *Nursing Science Quarterly, 3,* 9–17.

Parse, R. R. (1992). Human becoming: Parse's theory of nursing. *Nursing Science Quarterly, 5,* 35–42.

Parse, R. R. (Ed.). (1995). *Illuminations: The human becoming theory in practice and research.* New York: National League for Nursing Press.

Chapter 16

The Findings and Beyond

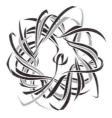

ROSEMARIE RIZZO PARSE

The nine-country, 130-participant, translinguistic research study on the lived experience of hope using the Parse research method yielded fascinating findings. In this chapter, the author synthesizes the findings, relates them to the human becoming principles of meaning, rhythmicity, and transcendence, draws implications for further research, and discusses challenges with conducting translinguistic nursing research.

Table 1 shows the findings, the structures formulated from the participants' descriptions in each of the thirteen studies. It is clear from a careful study of these findings and the stories that led to them that the lived experience of hope is a universal phenomenon arising in personal uniquenesses and understood similarly by people of different heritages. Participants from various countries describe hope in unique ways, yet with similar meanings. Participants from nine countries and several cities in the United States, as diverse as women with children in the United States and persons living in a leprosarium in Taiwan, described hope in light of the potential of no-hope. They all shared their stories of hardships and the personal difficulties that are present with inspiring possibilities. The descriptions of hope show that opportunities and restrictions arise mutually with turmoil and contentment in creating anew, and that intimate engagements are important in fortifying the persistence of expectancy in day-to-day living. The participants speak of experiences that are arduous, restrictive, adverse, disheartening, anguishing, ambiguous, tumultuous, and despairing, but they add that simultaneously present are experiences of contentment, vitality, liberation, nurturance, and inspiration. All participants have expectations that their lives will be different, which reflects an awareness of change as ongoing. They also indicate belief in the not-yet with wished-for options but with no guarantees.

The participants' stories enhance understanding of lived experiences of hope, thus, of health and quality of life. All human experiences, like hope, incarnate health, and, from a human becoming perspective, health and quality of life can be described only by the individual living the life (Parse, 1981, 1994, 1998). Health is the living experience of ongoing human-universe change. Hope is a living experience of health inextricably connected to quality of life (Parse, 1990a). Evidence from the participants' stories shows hope as an ever-present expectancy enduring all-at-once with the arduous, reflecting paradoxical changing health patterns cocreated as individuals live the meanings of their situations in moving beyond the moment. The meanings of hope described by participants are their structured realities arising in confirming–not-confirming cherished beliefs with speaking–being-silent and moving–being-still. Unique rhythmical patterns of relating as described by participants are paradoxical, incarnating being with and away from close others, while living all-at-once the opportunities and restrictions of pushing onward with the expanding horizons that unfold with new endeavors. Each participant's story weaves a personal understanding of hope, as each person shares meanings, cocreates rhythms, and cotranscends with possibles. Understandings of how human experiences are lived fortify knowledge of the meaning of human becoming (Parse, 1981, 1992, 1995b, 1998).

TABLE 1.
Structures of Hope

Australia	Hope is anticipating possibilities amid anguish, while enduring with vitality in intimate affiliations.
Canada	Hope is persistently anticipating possibilities amid adversity, as intimate engagements emerge with expanding horizons.
Finland	Hope is persistent anticipation of contentment arising with the promise of nurturing affiliations, while inspiration emerges amid easing the arduous.
Italy	Hope is expectancy amid the arduous, as quiescent vitality arises with expanding horizons.
Japan	Hope is anticipation of expanding possibilities, while liberation amid arduous restriction arises with the contentment of desired accomplishments.
Sweden	Hope is envisioning possibilities amid adversity, as persistent expectancy arises with nurturing affiliations.
Taiwan	Hope is anticipating an unburdening serenity amid despair, as nurturing engagements emerge in creating anew with cherished priorities.
United Kingdom	Hope is anticipating cherished possibilities while persevering amid adversity with benevolent affiliations.
United States	
New York	Hope is the envisioning of nurturing engagements while inventing possibilities.
North Carolina	Hope is picturing attainment in persisting amid the arduous, while trusting in potentiality.
South Dakota and Illinois	Hope is envisioning possibilities amid disheartenment, as close alliances with isolating turmoil surface in inventive endeavoring.
South Dakota (Sioux Indian Nation)	Hope is transfiguring enlightenment arising with engaging affiliations, as encircling the legendary surfaces with fortification.
Various states	Hope is envisaging possibles with resolute perseverance amid formidable ambiguity.

The understandings gleaned from this nine-country study offer insight into the meaning of hope as structured by people living with a variety of situations. The findings expand the extant knowledge about hope (as evident in Chapter 2 of this book, where there is an extensive review of literature) and shed light on human experiences in general in the following ways:

1. Envisioning a different way of becoming accompanies discomfort and adversity.
2. People experience and describe an awareness of change as ongoing.
3. Expectancy is persistent and ever-present.
4. Engagements with others and ideas fortify moving on.
5. Opportunities and restrictions prevail with wishes for something yet-to-be.

Interpretation of the findings of this study took place within the context of the human becoming school of thought as the horizon for interpretation. While the findings add to the general knowledge base on hope, the interpretation in relation to the human becoming school of thought enriches the theory base of nursing science. These understandings provide a more fully developed knowledge repertoire of the lived experience of hope from which nurses and others can draw in living the art of human becoming. In bearing witness with the changing health patterns of others, nurses and other healthcare professionals with a human becoming perspective live the dimensions of the practice methodology (illuminating meaning, synchronizing rhythms, and mobilizing transcendence) through true presence. (For details, see Parse, 1981, 1990a, 1992, 1997, 1998.)

R E C O M M E N D A T I O N S
F O R   F U R T H E R   R E S E A R C H

There are many implications for further research from the findings of these thirteen studies on hope. All of the core concepts lend themselves to further inquiry using the Parse method; for example, anticipating possibilities amid anguish might be studied as the lived experience of leaving a familiar situation, and nurturing affiliations might be studied as the lived experience of caring about another.

Table 2 shows core concepts gleaned from the thirteen studies, along with possible research phenomena related to health and quality of life.

Research on these phenomena all add to the knowledge about universal lived experiences. Studies on lived experiences broaden understandings of health as a process of human becoming. Continuing to extend understanding is a way to build knowledge with qualitative research (Parse, 1995a, 1996).

TABLE 2.
Core Concepts with Possible Research Phenomena

Core Concepts	Possible Research Phenomena
expectancy amid the arduous	living with changing expectations
persistent expectancy	leaving a familiar situation
persistent anticipation of contentment	dreaming about tomorrow
	wishing for something to happen
persistently anticipating possibilities amid adversity	feeling optimistic despite difficulties
	feeling confident
anticipating possibilities amid anguish	
anticipating cherished possibilities	
anticipating an unburdening serenity amid despair	
anticipation of expanding possibilities	
envisioning	
envisioning possibilities amid adversity	
envisioning possibilities amid disheartenment	
envisaging possibles	
picturing attainment	
inspiration amid easing the arduous	
expanding horizons	
enduring with vitality	feeling alive
quiescent vitality	feeling exuberant
encircling the legendary with fortification	feeling strong
	feeling tired
	feeling rested
benevolent affiliations	caring about another
intimate affiliations	feeling cared for
promise of nurturing affiliations	being attentively present to another
nurturing engagements	loving someone
nurturing affiliations	feeling loved
engaging affiliations	feeling close to another
close alliances with isolating turmoil	grieving the loss of someone close

TABLE 2. *(CONTINUED)*
Core Concepts with Possible Research Phenomena

inventive endeavoring inventing possibilities creating anew with cherished 　priorities	creating something new achieving a goal
transfiguring enlightenment	seeing something different in a 　familiar situation changing a view in light of a new 　insight
liberation amid arduous restriction	feeling peaceful feeling unburdened feeling relieved feeling uplifted feeling calm feeling confined feeling free
contentment of desired 　accomplishments	feeling satisfied feeling contented
resolute perseverance persevering amid adversity persisting amid the arduous	persisting with what is holding to a conviction no matter 　what
formidable ambiguity	taking a chance having courage living on the edge
trusting in potentiality	feeling trusted trusting another believing in yourself having faith

CHALLENGES WITH TRANSLINGUISTIC NURSING RESEARCH

There are many challenges when conducting translinguistic qualitative nursing research with multiple coinvestigators. Linguistic and procedural differences arise in the conceptual, ethical, methodological, and interpretive phases of research. The first challenge is conceptual, to ascertain whether the phenomenon has a similar meaning in the languages of the researchers. In the hope study, the challenge was to ascertain whether hope meant the same in the five non-English-speaking countries. In Sweden, the word is *hopp*; in Italy, *speranza*; in Taiwan, the symbols for hope also mean "mending a torn fishnet," and so on. Conceptualizations in different languages are different, so it is vitally important for all coinvestigators to understand the meaning of the phenomenon before undertaking a translinguistic research project. Hope is a concept that all bilingual coinvestigators in this study understood as essentially the same lived experience in any language.

Ethical procedures related to protection of participants vary widely around the world. In most countries no ethics panel reviews the research protocol for protection of participants. Standard ethical procedures were implemented in this hope study. It was agreed on by a university review board that there were no activities in the research protocol that would bring harm to the participants and that the consent that each participant either signed or agreed to orally would offer sufficient information regarding risks and benefits, purpose and length of the study, the right to withdraw at any time, and assurances of confidentiality and anonymity.

The methodological and interpretive phases of research are perhaps the most tedious and yet offer the most rewarding challenges. These phases include data gathering, data analysis-synthesis, and interpretation of findings. For good sciencing to be achieved there must be assurances that the conduct of the processes of the method is appropriate and that there is accurate translation and interpretation of findings.

For the hope study, the principal investigator discussed the Parse method (1987, 1990b, 1995a, 1995b, 1997, 1998) (the qualitative phenomenological-hermeneutic method used in the study) with each coinvestigator, since its data gathering and data analysis-synthesis are unique processes. Dialogical engagement, the data gathering process, requires explanation and practice in that it is not an interview but a special way of being truly present as participants describe lived experiences. It is a challenge for all scholars who conduct research with this method. The extraction-synthesis and heuristic interpretation processes of this method are difficult and time-consuming and require guidance. The coinvestigators were responsible for accurate translations—some did their own and most had others familiar with English check their translations. The coinvestigators gave their translations of the dialogues or a summary of them to the principal investigator with a beginning attempt at the extraction-synthesis, which is a process of culling the essences of the dialogue, stating them in the language of the participants, and then raising them to a higher level of discourse. The principal investigator then collaborated in revising these to the specifications of the method. These were returned to the coinvestigators to ensure consistency with the meaning participants gave to the experience of hope. There was much discussion and many revisions to achieve this consistency.

Synthesis of multiple studies of one phenomenon using the Parse method is a new endeavor. It was important to achieve some conclusions without over-blending the distinct ideas in the different segments of the study. The interpretation of findings required intense communication. Communication throughout the project took place through mail, e-mail, facsimile, telephone, and face-to-face meetings. There was one face-to-face meeting of the principal investigator and coinvestigators each year. The hope project took four years of rather intense concentration for the principal investigator and periods of intense concentration for the coinvestigators. Trust between the principal investigator and the coinvestigators was evident throughout the project. Each person's work was honored and respected.

The challenges in the conceptual, ethical, methodological, and interpretative phases of translinguistic research require attention in order to avoid overwhelming confusion. Know that an undertaking such as this is not for the faint-hearted—it is rigorous and tedious—but there are many moments of joy in the process. It is exciting to uncover the meaning of a phenomenon from persons living on four continents of the world. Translinguistic research is on the forefront of investigative possibilities, because global connections continue to exceed expectations as the twenty-first century approaches.

REFERENCES

Parse, R. R. (1981). *Man-living-health: A theory of nursing.* New York: Wiley.

Parse, R. R. (1987). *Nursing science: Major paradigms, theories, and critiques.* Philadelphia: Saunders.

Parse, R. R. (1990a). Health: A personal commitment. *Nursing Science Quarterly, 3,* 136–140.

Parse, R. R. (1990b). Parse's research methodology with an illustration of the lived experience of hope. *Nursing Science Quarterly, 3,* 9–17.

Parse, R. R. (1992). Human becoming: Parse's theory of nursing. *Nursing Science Quarterly, 5,* 35–42.

Parse, R. R. (1994). Quality of life: Sciencing and living the art of human becoming. *Nursing Science Quarterly, 7,* 16–21.

Parse, R. R.(1995a). Building the realm of nursing knowledge. *Nursing Science Quarterly, 8,* 51.

Parse, R. R. (Ed.). (1995b). *Illuminations: The human becoming theory in practice and research.* New York: National League for Nursing Press.

Parse, R. R. (1996). Building knowledge through qualitative research: The road less traveled. *Nursing Science Quarterly, 9,* 10–16.

Parse, R. R. (1997). The human becoming theory: The was, is, and will be. *Nursing Science Quarterly, 10,* 32–38.

Parse, R. R. (1998). *The human becoming school of thought.* Thousand Oaks, CA: Sage.

Index

About the Author

Rosemarie Rizzo Parse, RN, PhD, FAAN, is professor and Niehoff Chair at Loyola University Chicago. She is founder and editor of *Nursing Science Quarterly*, president of Discovery International, Inc., which sponsors international nursing theory conferences, and founder of the Institute of Human Becoming, where she teaches the ontological, epistemological, and methodological aspects of the human becoming school of thought. Previous works include *Nursing Fundamentals, Man-Living-Health: A Theory of Nursing; Nursing Science: Major Paradigms, Theories, and Critiques; Nursing Research: Qualitative Methods* (coauthored); *Illuminations: The Human Becoming Theory in Practice and Research; The Human Becoming School of Thought: A Perspective for Nurses and Other Health Professionals.* Her theory is a guide for practice in healthcare settings in Canada, Finland, Sweden, and the United States; her research methodology is utilized as a method of inquiry by nurse scholars in Australia, Canada, Denmark, Finland, Greece, Italy, Japan, South Korea, Sweden, the United Kingdom, and the United States.

Dr. Parse is a graduate of Duquesne University in Pittsburgh and received her master's and doctorate from the University of Pittsburgh. She was a member of the faculty of the University of Pittsburgh, was dean of the Nursing School at Duquesne University, and, from 1983 to 1993, was professor and coordinator of the Center for Nursing Research at Hunter College of the City University of New York. She has consulted throughout the world with doctoral programs in nursing and with healthcare settings that are utilizing her theory as a guide to practice and research.